# Praise for *Keto for Cancer*

"*Keto for Cancer* is an incredible guide for cancer patients and anyone attempting the ketogenic diet for the metabolic management of disease or just overall health benefits. This book addresses at least 95 percent of the questions I get on a daily basis. A must-read resource for anyone interested in ketogenic diets, cancer, exogenous ketones, and personalizing their nutritional ketosis strategy."

—**DOMINIC D'AGOSTINO**, PhD, leading scientist
on ketogenic metabolic therapies

"In an era when interest in ketogenic diets has erupted and misinformation abounds, Miriam Kalamian has brilliantly cut to the facts for cancer patients and their caregivers. *Keto for Cancer* is a clear, concise, and invaluable resource that describes both the science and implementation of these metabolic therapies. Underlying it all is the heart of a mom who has experienced the ultimate tragedy and has chosen to give additional meaning to her son, Raffi's, life."

—**JIM ABRAHAMS**, The Charlie Foundation for Ketogenic Therapies

"*Keto for Cancer* reveals how a ketogenic diet powerfully targets cancer at its metabolic core. . . . Miriam Kalamian's exemplary achievement brings clarity to this emerging science and makes implementation of this information straightforward and uncomplicated."

—**DAVID PERLMUTTER**, MD, FACN, author of #1 *New York Times* bestseller
*Grain Brain* and *The Grain Brain Whole Life Plan*

"*Keto for Cancer* is comprehensive and has appropriate cautions about the limits of the approach. . . . It's a complete how-to book for others in this terrible position and is imprinted with her love for her son."

—**EUGENE J. FINE**, MD, professor of clinical radiology,
Albert Einstein College of Medicine

"*Keto for Cancer* offers hope for healing to cancer patients by offering them a personal plan for success that implements the powerful symbiosis of natural strategies such as the ketogenic diet, fasting, and supplementation."

—**JIMMY MOORE**, health podcaster;
international bestselling author of *Keto Clarity*

"I'm confident that [this book] will become the go-to resource for the practical application of the ketogenic approach. *Keto for Cancer* will undoubtedly pave the way for improved health in many chronically ill patients."

—**PATRICIA DALY**, coauthor of *The Ketogenic Kitchen*

"A well-researched yet easy-to-understand approach to the science underpinning the metabolic foundations of cancer. A must-read, not only as stepwise guide for patients but for all physicians, particularly those skeptical of the therapeutic benefits of the ketogenic diet."

—**JOSEPH C. MAROON**, MD, clinical professor of neurosurgery, University of Pittsburgh Medical Center

"Miriam Kalamian has written an excellent and complete guide to ketogenic therapy in cancer treatment. . . . I especially recommend this book to patients and their relatives, but it has also become a valuable reference for my own clinical work with patients."

—**DR. RAINER J. KLEMENT**, PhD, Department of Radiation Oncology, Leopoldina Hospital Schweinfurt, Germany

"Miriam Kalamian's *Keto for Cancer* provides the most comprehensive and organized step-by-step information to easily understand and efficiently implement a lifesaving ketogenic diet. The book is an academic, scientific primer for clinicians (who will greatly benefit from the lucid, crisp explanations), as well as a detailed, easy-to-follow manual for patients and their families to carry out their daily anticancer ketogenic diets. This diligent, gifted work gives real life and authentic hope to its readers in a unique tour de force which will remain a landmark for generations."

—**J. WILLIAM (WILL) LaVALLEY**, MD, Molecular Integrative Oncology

"Cancer nutrition expert Miriam Kalamian has poured every ounce of her hard-earned wisdom, deep scientific knowledge, and compassion into *Keto for Cancer*. Within this masterful guide, she explains how ketogenic diets limit tumor cell access to key nutrients while nourishing healthy cells, quieting inflammation, and improving quality of life. Let Kalamian empower you to take aim at cancer's soft underbelly and begin reclaiming your health."

—**GEORGIA EDE**, MD, Psychiatrist and Nutrition Specialist

"I had the pleasure of first meeting Miriam at a conference in Berkeley a few years back, she was speaking on a panel about the ketogenic diet and cancer. Her story touched me deeply as did her articulate way of expressing how to implement a ketogenic diet. Since then, I have watched Miriam reach superstardom with her brilliant mind and compassionate heart. This book is a culmination of what she has learned, shared, gleaned from others, and inspired in the world of both bench (her collaborations with world renowned researchers) and bedside (real-life application by respected clinicians) medicine. This is the most thorough discussion on ketogenic diet and cancer in the industry and I expect it to continue to inspire change in how we approach cancer today."

—**NASHA WINTERS**, ND, coauthor of *The Metabolic Approach to Cancer*

# KETO for CANCER

## Ketogenic Metabolic Therapy as a Targeted Nutritional Strategy

**Miriam Kalamian**, EdM, MS, CNS

FOREWORD BY

**Thomas N. Seyfried, PhD**

Chelsea Green Publishing
White River Junction, Vermont

Copyright © 2017 by Miriam Kalamian.
All rights reserved.

No part of this book may be transmitted or reproduced in any form by any means without permission
in writing from the publisher.

Photograph on page v by Miriam Kalamian.

Project Manager: Patricia Stone
Developmental Editor: Makenna Goodman
Copy Editor: Jennifer Lipfert
Proofreader: Nanette Bendyna
Indexer: Shana Milkie
Designer: Melissa Jacobson

Printed in Canada.
First printing September 2017.
10 9 8 7 6          23 24 25

**Our Commitment to Green Publishing**

Chelsea Green sees publishing as a tool for cultural change and ecological stewardship. We strive to align our
book manufacturing practices with our editorial mission and to reduce the impact of our business enterprise
in the environment. We print our books and catalogs on chlorine-free recycled paper, using vegetable-based
inks whenever possible. This book may cost slightly more because it was printed on paper that contains
recycled fiber, and we hope you'll agree that it's worth it. *Keto for Cancer* was printed on paper supplied by
Marquis.

**Library of Congress Cataloging-in-Publication Data**
Names: Kalamian, Miriam, author.
Title: Keto for cancer : ketogenic metabolic therapy as a targeted nutritional strategy /
   Miriam Kalamian, EdM, MS, CNS ; foreword by Thomas N. Seyfried, PhD.
Description: White River Junction, Vermont : Chelsea Green Publishing, [2017]
Identifiers: LCCN 2017023265 | ISBN 9781603587013 (paperback) | ISBN 9781603587020 (ebook)
Subjects: LCSH: Cancer—Diet therapy. | Ketogenic diet. | Integrative medicine. |
   BISAC: HEALTH & FITNESS / Diseases / Cancer. | COOKING / Health & Healing /
   Cancer. | HEALTH & FITNESS / Nutrition.
Classification: LCC RC271.D52 K35 2017 | DDC 616.99/40654—dc23
LC record available at https://lccn.loc.gov/2017023265

Chelsea Green Publishing
85 North Main Street, Suite 120
White River Junction, VT 05001
(802) 295-6300
www.chelseagreen.com

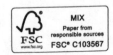

MIX
Paper from
responsible sources
FSC® C103567

This book is dedicated to my son, Raffi.

RAFFI KALAMIAN WALSH
BORN FEBRUARY 18, 2000
DIED APRIL 17, 2013

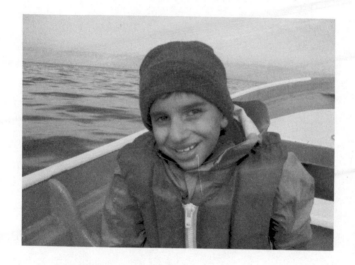

Raffi, the sunsets we shared could be
enjoyed only in the moment, but the light
you brought to this Earth shines on.
You will always be my hero!
I'm grateful to have been your mom.

# Contents

# Foreword

I t is an honor for me to write the foreword to Miriam Kalamian's deeply important book, *Keto For Cancer*. Miriam has produced a masterpiece that translates decades of research on the anticancer therapeutic benefits of ketogenic diets and calorie restriction in preclinical models to a practical guide for people with cancer and practitioners who are increasingly drawn to the science behind this metabolic approach. The information in her book moves far beyond the limits of conventional anticancer nutrition to include the use of food as medicine, a concept first elucidated by Hippocrates, the father of modern medicine.

Miriam's book comes at a critical time in our quest to manage cancer, as the cancer field is now stagnating under the weight of traditional therapies (radiation and chemotherapy) that result in unacceptable toxicity and impairment in quality of life, often with little improvement in survival. Even the new immunotherapy drugs are proving to be unacceptably toxic, marginally effective, and inordinately expensive. The rate of increase in deaths from cancer over the last five years (3.4 percent) is now twice the rate of increase in new cases (1.7 percent). According to data from the American Cancer Society, cancer deaths have reached epidemic proportions, with over 1,600 people dying each day in the United States alone. Too often, five-year survival statistics masquerade as a cure, allowing the conventional community to dodge any discussion of long-term survivorship, especially in those people with aggressive or metastatic disease.

How could this situation exist even with the enormous investment in resources and the decades of research directed at cancer therapies supported by the NIH, the pharmaceutical industry, and the many private cancer research groups, many of which are founded by people who have lost loved ones to this disease? This unacceptable state of affairs is due largely to the prevailing but flawed dogma that cancer is a genetic disease. Massive evidence shows the large impact that environmental influences have on the initiation and progression of this disease. Cancer treatment centers use buzzwords like personalized medicine, targeted therapies, and cancer mutation screening to imply that cancer is under their control. These are hollow words linked to a fundamental misunderstanding of the origin of cancer. Emerging evidence indicates that cancer is primarily a metabolic disease arising from a disruption in the ability of the cell to obtain the energy it needs to survive and proliferate from normal cellular respiration. Although the cancer research community acknowledges this aberration, it fails to connect the dots leading back to the origin of most cancers. That is, most cancer cells obtain their energy from the process of fermentation, which was the way primitive living organisms survived before oxygen became abundant in Earth's atmosphere some 2.5 billion years ago. It is cancer's protracted reliance on fermentation energy that leads to the many genetic mutations seen in cancer cells. In other words, the mutations are not the *cause* of cancer but instead are the *downstream effect* of the disturbed respiration that drives compensatory fermentation and even evasion from immune system surveillance.

Cancer mutations are "red herrings" that divert attention away from the real problem, which is a reliance on fermentation for growth and survival. It is no wonder that cancer therapies based on the gene theory have had so little success in managing the disease. Damage to cellular respiration, thus causing a reliance on fermentation, can arise from any number of provocative agents, including carcinogens, radiation, tissue inflammation, viral infections, focal hypoxia, rare inherited mutations, or simply age. Fermentation metabolism also makes tumor cells resistant to radiation and chemotherapies by strengthening their inherent antioxidant defenses. Miriam's book provides a nutritional strategy to manage cancer based on the metabolic origins underlying most tumor cells. Cancer is not many diseases, as some would suggest, but it is a singular disease of abnormal energy metabolism regardless of the cell or tissue of origin.

It is now recognized that both glucose and glutamine, an amino acid, are the prime fuels that drive fermentation metabolism in most tumor cells. In addition to generating energy, these fuels are also the precursors for the synthesis of lipids, proteins, and nucleic acids, which pave the way for rapid tumor cell proliferation. It follows that the most logical therapeutic strategy for managing cancer centers on restricting glucose and glutamine. The low-carbohydrate, high-fat ketogenic diet is an alternative, nontoxic metabolic strategy for targeting those tumor cells that depend on fermentable fuels for their growth and survival. Therapeutic ketosis starves tumor cells of glucose while elevating blood levels of ketones, a metabolic fuel that enhances the health of normal cells. Tumor cells, however, cannot use ketones for energy because of defects in oxygen respiration. Ketogenic diets also enhance the therapeutic action of glutamine-targeting drugs, and there is evidence that ketogenic metabolic therapy sensitizes tumor cells, in effect targeting them for destruction without producing collateral toxic damage to normal cells. Recent studies from an oncology clinic in Istanbul, Turkey, showed that a ketogenic diet used together with a cocktail of glucose-targeting drugs and procedures that increase oxidative stress in tumor tissue could successfully manage a broad range of advanced stage IV metastatic cancers, including breast, colon, ovary, lung, and pancreas. The ketogenic diet has also been shown to enhance the therapeutic efficacy of low-dose chemotherapy while simultaneously reducing toxicity to normal cells, tissues, and organs. It therefore becomes essential for cancer patients and their caregivers to recognize and understand how therapeutic ketosis using ketogenic diets can be used for managing cancer while also improving quality of life.

Miriam Kalamian is exceptionally well qualified to instruct cancer patients, their family members, and their oncology teams in using therapeutic ketosis as either an adjunctive or alternative approach for managing cancer. Miriam experienced firsthand the therapeutic effects of the ketogenic diet over a decade ago when she initiated the diet as a nutritional strategy for her own son. Indeed, her book is dedicated to Raffi, and the passion she has for sharing this experience is palpable. Managing Raffi's brain tumor with a ketogenic diet put her on the path to learning the science behind the therapy and helped her to face the many challenges she encountered as an advocate for her son. I consider Miriam Kalamian a foremost authority in the emerging field of metabolic therapies for cancer. Her book addresses every question or concern that cancer patients might have in using a ketogenic metabolic strategy for managing their cancer. Being part of the team takes on new meaning as the person with cancer now plays an active role in the management of the disease. Miriam has provided cancer patients with a playbook that lays out the moves and strategies necessary for the nontoxic management of their disease. It is my view that therapeutic ketosis that revolves around ketogenic diets should be incorporated into the standards of care in oncology. Miriam Kalamian's book is an essential resource for any cancer patient, caregiver, or oncologist with an interest in metabolic therapy.

THOMAS N. SEYFRIED, PhD
Professor
Boston College
Chestnut Hill, MA

# Preface

I t was Christmas Eve in 2004. We were far from home and still reeling from the news that our young son had a brain tumor. Chemotherapy would begin right after the holiday, and my husband and I were sent off with strict instructions to "stay off the internet." On Christmas Day, with Raffi occupied by his new toys, I stole away and took my first forbidden peek with the hope that I would learn something—anything—that would ease the terror building up inside me. Instead I was devastated by what I found: That one little life, more precious to me than my own, was doomed to slip away.

A few days later we returned to the hospital, where Raffi was started on 14 months of weekly chemotherapy. When that protocol failed we moved on to another . . . but to no avail. We put him through multiple risky surgeries, but the tumor was relentless. I can't even begin to describe how devastating it was to watch our young child be taken apart, piece by precious piece.

Unfortunately, our experience is far from unique. In fact, it's all too common.

In January of 2007 Raffi started yet another treatment—this time, as part of a clinical trial testing a potent cocktail of anticancer drugs. Within a few weeks my normally cheerful little guy had several distressing new symptoms: He was nauseous, fatigued, and unable to focus. He spent most of the day sleeping. Six weeks into the protocol I tried to wake him from a long nap to ask if he needed to use the bathroom. His knees buckled when he tried to stand up, and when he opened his mouth to speak, all that came out was gibberish. These were both signs of increasing hydrocephalus (excessive buildup of fluid in the brain), a life-threatening condition often associated with tumor growth. We rushed him to the hospital, where he underwent an emergency surgery to place a shunt to relieve the pressure. An MRI prior to the surgery confirmed what my gut had already told me: Raffi's tumor was still growing and had invaded new areas.

While Raffi was in the hospital, I learned from a nurse that one of the drugs in the trial cocktail was especially toxic to the kidneys. In fact I had to wear gloves when changing him, and his wet diapers were disposed of in a special container designed for toxic waste.

A few days after the surgery, Raffi was released. We returned to my mother's home, where we had been living for the previous four months to be closer to the hospital where Raffi was receiving his care. Once he was settled in, I went online to learn more about that toxic drug. In answer to my request for more information, another mom who was active on one of the sites I visited sent me the link to a press release about the drug. I tried to print the article out, but my mother's ancient printer wouldn't cooperate. A few days later when I returned to the site to look again at the release, in its place I discovered a *new* article that hit me like a freight train. Purely by chance I had stumbled upon a paper from Dr. Thomas Seyfried's lab at Boston College. It reported that mice fed a calorie-restricted ketogenic diet over an eight-week period showed a significant slowing in the progression of a deadly type of brain tumor known as *glioblastoma multiforme*.

I was well aware of the drawbacks of this type of research: These were mice, not people, and the study lasted only eight weeks. But reading the brief summary lifted my heart, allowing a ray of sunshine into that place of dark despair. I tried not to get too excited. "Another dead end," I told myself, at the same time finding it impossible not to follow up on this unexpected lead.

Tentatively I emailed the author of the paper, fully expecting him to crush my seed of hope. Instead, almost immediately I received a response from the lab's director—Dr. Thomas Seyfried himself. (Dr. Seyfried and I have become good friends over the years. He even wrote the foreword to this book.) The passion that Dr. Seyfried has for his work sprang from the page: He was *certain* that the ketogenic diet had enormous potential as a cancer therapy. He shared with me the research that had led to this most recent study and connected me with resources from The Charlie Foundation, a nonprofit organization devoted to the use of the ketogenic diet for epilepsy. I wasn't aware of it at the time, but that day turned out to be a crucial turning point in my quest for a better life for my son.

In the following weeks and months, I came to understand that I (like the overwhelming majority of people) had accepted the widely held belief that cancer was a genetic disease of mutated cells. Dr. Seyfried held a different view: According to himself and a tiny cadre of other researchers, cancer was a metabolic disease that arose from defects in mitochondria, the tiny power-houses in cells responsible not only for producing energy but also for directing signals that tip the fate of a cell toward either health or disease. Dr. Seyfried had reinvigorated the work of German physiologist Otto Warburg, one of the earliest cancer researchers, who long ago had observed that cancer cells utilize glucose differently from normal cells. Instead of taking advantage of the highly evolved and efficient energy-generating process known as the Krebs cycle, cancer cells thrive by running huge amounts of glucose through an important but primitive energy pathway known as *glycolysis*. (Read more about this in chapter 3.) In honor of the early researcher, his indisputable observation is still known as the Warburg effect.

It took me several weeks to gather enough information—and courage—to start Raffi on the ketogenic diet. At that time, I couldn't rally any support from the professionals who had the most experience in the use of the diet in the treatment of epilepsy. Even though they supported us in theory, the reality was that the liability was too high for them to engage with me. In the cancer clinic the situation was even worse, and I came up against a formidable wall of resistance and intimidation. Raffi's prominent specialist shook his head: "It won't work." He handed me off to one of his colleagues who declared, "That diet's for fat people. Stick to the plan" (even though he had not presented an acceptable plan). "Let him go," another oncologist bluntly stated.

Thankfully, Raffi's local team held a much more sympathetic view. With so much at stake and so few options, what did we have to lose? Twenty-seven months after his diagnosis, Raffi began the ketogenic diet under the watchful eye of his amazing pediatrician and supportive local oncologist. Here's what happened: *In only three months*, an MRI showed that Raffi's tumor had shrunk for the first time since the beginning of his ordeal. We were stunned. How could something as simple as a different mix of familiar foods succeed when everything else had failed? Raffi's success spurred me on to learn as much as I could, and by the end of the summer I was enrolled in a graduate nutrition program at Eastern Michigan University. I threw myself into studying the nuts and bolts of nutrition science: biology, biochemistry, and nutrition practice. But unlike my peers who would go on to become registered dietitians in hospital, clinic, or community settings, I was laser-focused on learning all I could specifically related to the science of macronutrient metabolism. There was precious little in the textbooks about ketosis, and most of that was portrayed negatively as the downstream effect of starvation or poorly controlled diabetes. Now, as a "keto-for-cancer" specialist ("keto" is short for ketogenic [key-ta-*gen*-ic; or kētə'jenik]), I can look back on how following my passion contributed to a longer and healthier life for my own son and ultimately for the hundreds of other people with whom I've worked over the past decade.

My experience in implementing the diet for my son also opened my eyes to a huge flaw in the current medical model: Conventional care treats the herd, not the individual, and the succession of only partially effective therapies falls far short of the implied promise of a cure. "Personalized medicine" and "targeted therapies" are great buzzwords in the conventional cancer community, and they may even lead you to believe that your treatment is on the cutting edge, but once you commit, you may discover that most of this talk is aimed at drumming up funding and support for clinical trials of new pharmaceuticals. Yet a cancer cure in pill form is far from a reality for most. If these new drugs don't repair the ongoing genetic damage or improve your immune system's efficiency at wiping out diseased cells, then you've only kicked the can down the road.

I would have given anything to have known about the ketogenic diet at the time of my son's diagnosis, but in 2004 the use of the diet as cancer therapy had barely crossed the "speculation" threshold. Compare that to what you can find today by conducting even the simplest of internet searches! Certainly, the ketogenic diet is more visible to a much wider audience now than it was a decade ago, but it's still necessary to ask: Is it the right plan for *you*? Before you begin the diet, take the time to read through the list of limiting conditions (outlined in chapter 4, "Considering Contraindications," page 39) and tell your medical team that you are considering this change to your diet. This is an important step to take even though the mere *thought* of broaching this subject with your team might make you uncomfortable. Yes, you run the risk that you'll run into the same negativity that I experienced, but at least you'll learn if they have any valid concerns. In chapter 6 I'll give you some tips on how to approach this discussion.

In this book I answer the most common questions: Where do I start? How can I do this safely? How do I get up to speed quickly? How long before I know if it's working? This comprehensive guide breaks the steps down into bite-sized pieces: a list of keto-friendly foods, an action plan, resources, tools to develop a personal diet prescription, and a system for tracking and monitoring your progress. I include tips on how to ease the transition into this new way of life while navigating the hazards of the "non-keto" world. I'll also begin the discussion of how to improve mental and physical health by incorporating other healthy habits into a total anticancer, pro-health lifestyle. That leaves one crucial element that you'll need to bring to the table: your strong commitment to the plan.

As you'll learn, the science behind the diet is sound. In the scientific community, conferences now feature presentations highlighting the results of this new research. We owe a lot to the people who are moving the research forward. The growing list includes talented and passionate researchers, out-of-the-box thinkers and visionaries—many of whom you'll meet later in this book. The fact that *any* research moves forward is a testament to the dedication of these individuals given that diet studies receive very little funding from the public sector and virtually *no* funding from the pharmaceutical industry.

Researchers are thus forced to spend countless hours of their time writing grants and giving presentations to groups of potential funders. It's a hard sell. After all, there's no profit in proving that a simple diet can have as powerful an effect on outcomes as an expensive drug. And don't hold your breath waiting for the day that prime-time advertisers direct you to "talk to your doctor" about the ketogenic diet!

In health,
**MIRIAM KALAMIAN**,
EdM, MS, CNS

# Acknowledgments

I wish to acknowledge the many contributors who brought this book to life.

Peter Walsh, for his many roles: content researcher, editor, family chef—as well as husband and fellow traveler in our son Raffi's journey. Thank you, Peter, for your encouragement and support in bringing what we've learned to others in need.

Thomas Seyfried, PhD, for his groundbreaking research presenting evidence that cancer is primarily a disease of mitochondrial metabolism. Dr. Seyfried's knowledge, and his willingness to share what he knew with a mom, gave us extra time with our son. Thank you, Tom, for your tireless efforts in testing metabolic therapies that push back against this devastating disease.

Dominic D'Agostino, PhD, and Angela Poff, PhD, for their boundless enthusiasm and dedication to furthering our understanding of ketogenic metabolic therapies. Thank you, Dom and Angela, for all your efforts directed at advancing and promoting this important body of work.

Blaise Favara, MD, Raffi's beloved pediatrician. Thank you, Blaise, for your incredible support, genuine warmth, and great sense of humor. You helped us through some very tough times.

William LaValley, MD, for his very thorough and exacting review of this book. Will, your understanding of integrative oncology runs very deep and your support of the ketogenic diet means a great deal to me. I'm grateful that our paths finally crossed.

Kara Fitzgerald, ND, and Romilly Hodges, MS, for their thoughtful review and many valuable suggestions. Thank you both for your willingness to share valuable insights gained from your clinical experience with the ketogenic diet. Your critical thinking will help build better practice guidelines for the use of this diet for cancer and other metabolic diseases.

The Abrahams family for establishing The Charlie Foundation. Charlie's story continues to be a source of inspiration and support to families of children with epilepsy. Thank you, Jim and Nancy, for extending that support to the growing number of people using ketogenic metabolic therapy for a wide range of other devastating diseases.

Beth Zupec-Kania, RDN, for her mentoring and willingness to step out of the box to work with me soon after the start of our own journey. Thank you, Beth, for answering my many questions and setting us on the right track.

Ellen Davis, MS, for her feedback, encouragement, and support. Thank you, Ellen, for all you do in bringing vetted keto information to the public.

Becky Lellek, my friend and colleague, for gently shaping the language I use to coach, encourage, and motivate my clients. Thank you, Becky, for warming my heart with your genuine smile, even on grayest of days!

John Freeman, MD, for keeping the ketogenic diet alive during challenging times. Dr. Freeman was a strong advocate for the ketogenic diet even when it was unfairly disparaged by most of his peers. (Dr. Freeman was named Professor Emeritus by Johns Hopkins University in 2007. He died on January 3, 2014.) Thank you, Dr. Freeman, for your lifetime of work and also for reminding us all that "First they ignore you, then they laugh at you, then they fight you, then you win."

The team at Chelsea Green Publishing: Makenna Goodman (developmental editor), Jennifer Lipfert (copy editor), Nanette Bendyna (proofreader), Shana Milkie (indexer), Melissa Jacobson (designer), and Patricia Stone (project manager). Thank you for your many contributions. Without a doubt, your input shaped my manuscript into a more coherent and powerful book!

# Introduction

We were sitting in a therapist's office with our four-year-old son. Something was up with Raffi, and we needed to get a handle on it. Over the previous few months, he'd become increasingly withdrawn and unable to focus. He could no longer tolerate even a few minutes away from my side. To us and to the professionals who evaluated him, it looked like a classic case of attachment disorder. We'd adopted Raffi as a toddler, and the diagnosis seemed to fit. We were hopeful that with the therapist's help we'd get through this latest wrinkle.

Then I got the call. I'd forgotten to turn off my cell phone when our therapy session began. I glanced at the caller ID and saw that it was Raffi's pediatrician. Raffi's recent eye exam had uncovered a condition known as optic nerve pallor. The most likely cause was poor nutrition; this made sense given that Raffi was malnourished and suffering from rickets when we adopted him. But quick on the heels of this discovery, Raffi had experienced a trio of brief but disabling headaches. Erring on the side of caution, the pediatrician had ordered an MRI to rule out any brain abnormalities. The plan: If there was a problem, the radiologist would alert the pediatrician right away, but if the scan was normal, we'd get the report the following day. It had now been more than 24 hours since Raffi's scan, so of course I expected to hear "all clear." Instead, our world was hit with an atomic blast as we listened to the news: "I'm so sorry to tell you this. Raffi has a brain tumor. I can't believe the radiologist didn't call me right away. But listen carefully: This tumor is very large, and you need to get him to the children's hospital—right now. I called ahead. They're waiting for you." That ended our therapy session and the world as we knew it. Before we even had time to process what we'd heard, we were on the road, driving 16 hours through a blizzard. By the next afternoon our son was in the hospital undergoing a biopsy. We were handed the pathology report on Christmas Eve and sent home for the holiday.

## Of Course We Asked, "Why Raffi? Why *Our* Child?"

Sometimes there's an obvious answer to this agonizing question. Did you work with asbestos? Then mesothelioma should come as no surprise. Lifelong smoker? Of course that raises the risk of respiratory disease, including cancer. But what if you've never smoked a cigarette in your life and you learn you have stage IV lung cancer? Whatever brought you to this point, your life now depends on how you move forward.

In truth, your current situation is most likely linked to the convergence of many events: a perfect storm that reflects a life spent in a complex and challenging environment. Your past exposure to toxins and your choice of nutrients have initiated changes in your body as well as changes in downstream cellular activities (such as signaling pathways) that impact your overall health. Yet there is a huge and as-yet-unpredictable variation in any individual's response to the sum total of their experience. Yes, genetic risk factors can be passed down from parent to child, but savvy researchers are just beginning to wake up to what integrative health care practitioners already know: Your health is inextricably tied to whether the interaction of genes with the environment helps maintain balance or, instead, tips the scale toward disease. Integrative practitioners also believe that you can commit to meaningful changes in diet and lifestyle well beyond the mainstream mantras "eat a balanced diet" and "move more."

## Epigenetics

Epigenetics, a subspecialty within the field of genetics, is the study of how our environment, including the foods that we choose to take into our bodies, can change the expression of our genes. Cancer researchers have discovered a myriad of cellular proteins that behave badly when stressors, such as reactive oxygen species (called ROS), are produced in amounts that damage cellular signaling, either by increasing activity in pathways associated with cancer progression or by inhibiting pathways associated with gene repair and cellular health. Pharmaceutical companies and the institutions they support are focused on developing profitable new drugs that inhibit discrete cancer progression pathways. The drawback: Altering signals in one pathway at a time without addressing the underlying problem is akin to trying to fix a wobbly table by sawing away at the legs instead of recognizing that the floor is uneven.

It's increasingly clear that diet plays a huge role in certain cancers. Researchers have known for years that excess weight raises the risk of certain cancers (including colon, breast, and prostate) and that the incidence of these cancers increases as we age. Why do these diseases pick up speed as we grow older? Most theories assume that the failure to clear or repair pre-cancerous cells is just another downstream effect of aging. But there's another theory—the metabolic theory of disease. Metabolic theory, the focus of this book, shines a light on the growing body of evidence pointing to the three "I's" (inflammation, insulin resistance, and immune system failure) as the underlying causes of the downward spiral that leads to what we generally accept as diseases of aging—cancer included.

## Get in the Game!

Cancer treatment needs a team. But what if you find that you're not even offered a spot on the bench? Instead, you, the patient, are expected to be a spectator: Sit in the bleachers and root for your team, but don't you dare step onto the field! Even the language used in conventional medicine reinforces the expectation that you'll receive treatment as a passive bystander. By all means, if you've broken a bone, stand back and let the pros do their work. But if you've been handed a cancer diagnosis, you have the *right* to be on that field.

Make no mistake. You're about to jump into a rough game without a referee to ensure that everyone plays by the rules. In fact, there are no rules. If you've spent any time researching cancer on the internet (and I'll bet you have), then you already know how quickly that playing field turns into a minefield of conflicting ideas, misguided advice, and outright quackery.

But you now hold in your hands a playbook that lays out the moves and strategies that will help you through the challenges ahead. As you'll soon see, ketogenic metabolic therapy is one of the most powerful strategies you can launch in your quest to manage your cancer. (Note that I say "manage," not "cure": Most cancers—even those with decent survival rates—reemerge at some point in the future driven by a small population of cells that evade treatment and capitalize on mutations that allow them to survive, thrive, and spread. Or you may find yourself with an entirely new but closely related cancer, often a side effect of treatments such as chemo and radiation that damage normal cells along with diseased ones. That's why you need a game plan that works for a lifetime!) Finding the ketogenic diet is the easy part. Acquiring the tools and knowledge to implement these changes, and others, requires commitment and effort. This book is a good first step.

## The Importance of Language

Language is powerful. In medicine, it shapes thoughts and actions. If you use the language of war for illness, as in "fighting" cancer, then expect significant casualties, with both sides contained in a single body—your body. Focus instead on "winning" the game. In doing so, you are more likely to choose actions that protect you, the most valuable player. That said, if it suits you to use the language of war, think in terms of developing the most effective maneuvers and strategies, those that protect your most valuable assets over a lifetime. In other words, focus your attention on bringing your body back into the best balance possible given the strengths and limitations of your current life situation.

Language also reflects beliefs: Patients (or should I say "patience"?) are expected to receive treatment passively: "Doctor knows best." You are seldom encouraged to ask questions or share what you're learning. Meditation guru and writer Jon Kabat-Zinn illustrates a perfect example of the wall that exists between doctors and patients in describing a program he developed to encourage medical students to deepen communication with the people they treat. He instructed the students to close their sessions with patients by asking, "Is there anything else you would like to tell me?" When he reviewed the videotapes of these sessions, Kabat-Zinn noted with amusement that the students said the words as they were told, but were visibly shaking their heads "no" at the same time. Nothing subtle there about their body language![1]

The language of medicine also places the utmost importance on doctors' *training*, not their *education*. Physicians hold fast to the tenets of this training even when the prognosis is poor or it's clear that the patient is not getting better. For a doctor's view of training versus education, read *Honest Medicine* by Julia Schopick (www.honestmedicine.com). In her book, Schopick includes a chapter written by Burt Berkson, MD, MS, PhD, who reveals the striking differences between his graduate school *education*, which encouraged critical thinking and participation in learning, and his medical school *training*, which enforced lockstep compliance with prevailing practice guidelines.[2] What will it take to remodel medicine's current disease management mindset, which relies almost entirely on drugs or procedures to treat each discrete symptom?

## The Current Standard of Care

There is *no question* that the current standard of care in cancer treatment falls far short of the goal of a cure and that many of the most commonly accepted treatment protocols seriously erode quality of life. So how can we improve this picture?

The pharmaceutical companies' approach is to spend billions of dollars in bringing new and very profitable drugs to market, often with the bar for success set very low. For example, in the treatment of extremely aggressive cancers, such as pancreatic or brain cancer, a new drug needs to improve overall survival by only a few months in order to be heralded (and marketed) as a "significant advance" over prior therapies, with little attention given to the huge sacrifices to quality of life that are often a part of this hellish bargain. You've seen those flashy ads—slick direct-to-consumer appeals that lead with an upbeat 10-second pitch for you to "talk to your doctor" about a new drug that offers the hope of living longer, while the remaining 20 seconds are devoted to a breathless reading of potential side effects, including death.

At the institutional level (i.e., cancer centers and university hospitals), oncology teams made up of surgeons and radiation and medical oncologists may use data from genetic testing of the tumor tissue, combined with such diagnostics as pathology reports and circulating cancer biomarker levels, to decide on a protocol that they feel is most likely to achieve a response. That sounds great on the surface, but let's look at what it really means to you personally. In a common scenario, the statistics may suggest that 30 percent of people with characteristics similar to yours will have a clinically significant response to a treatment. Of course, this is better than outright trial and error, but if you are among the 70 percent of people who are not "responders," you've just endured a treatment that weakened your system while leaving the stronger and more aggressive cancer cells free to grow and proliferate.

For a person with cancer, this shotgun approach may be dressed up as personalized medicine or a targeted therapy. In fact, these protocols are often simply your oncologist's educated guess as to what therapy will best address your disease and are based on medical algorithms that are still years away from accounting for the vast array of variations between one person and the next. Understand, too, that personal bias is also likely to influence your team's recommendations. For example, if the medical oncologist has a strong institutional presence and an established reputation, then his or her treatment recommendations may take precedence over those of less influential but equally knowledgeable members of the team.

The current Western medical paradigm pays lip service to the importance of shared decision-making, but many practitioners in mainstream medicine have yet to make significant headway toward providing truly patient-centered care. In fact, the chasm between doctors and patients threatens to grow even wider. Although some of this distancing is due to time and financial limitations beyond the providers' control, much of it can be attributed to increasing specialization and the challenges inherent in communicating ever more complex information. Yes, it's great to be under the care of the highest-rated doctors at the highest-rated centers specializing in your particular disease, but this may come at a high price if it squelches meaningful communication with the people who hold your life in their hands. Specialists lose, too, if they dismiss the notion that there is anything to learn from the people they serve.

Let me be clear: It is not my intent to disparage or denigrate the dedicated practitioners you will find in most conventional care settings. They most certainly want to provide you with the best care possible. The issue at hand is the lack of funding for research, including clinical trials, that will ultimately prove what effect the ketogenic diet and other metabolic therapies have on a disease that is unfortunately viewed by many as simply "bad luck."

## Alternative and Adjuvant Therapies

Given the failures and limitations in the standard of care, especially in late-stage or aggressive cancers, why don't low- or no-cost alternative and adjuvant (add-on) therapies come up in the conversations you have with your oncologist? And if you do bring them up, why are they so often dismissed out of hand as having "no evidence," despite what you might have read? You may believe that this is a conspiracy; that your oncologist is recommending a particular treatment due to personal gain, such as a kickback from a drug company. Unfortunately, while there may be those in the profession who are guilty of this, the vast majority of oncologists really are offering you what they believe to be the best care. The problem is that on Day One of their medical school training, they were handed a set of glasses with a filter that allows them to see only the particular style of "evidence-based medicine" approved by the people in charge of their studies. When these doctors then move into clinical practice, they are bound by convention to stick to these evidence-based guidelines in the treatment of cancer, almost as if one hand was tied behind their backs. Addressing the underlying issues that may heal the body is not their primary goal.

Given this scenario, "First, do no harm" may seem contradictory considering the collateral damage inflicted by most of the current conventional therapies. There would be *so much value* if the best of both worlds could be combined: your oncologist's expertise and institutional knowledge along with adjunctive and alternative therapies that offer immediate benefits, such as a healthier immune system and improved quality of life. Simply put, however, adjunct therapies don't yet have a cheerleading section in conventional care, even if they do show some grounding in science.

Consider the ketogenic diet. Despite the best efforts of its detractors, diet proponents (myself included) have been able to connect the dots between patient-based evidence, usually gathered from anecdotal information, and "preclinical data," the results of studies using animal models of disease. (In the development of pharmaceuticals, promising preclinical data are used to support moving to clinical trials with humans.) Fortunately, the ketogenic diet is available to all because, unlike conventional care, access isn't dependent on health insurance reimbursement or one's ability to shoulder huge out-of-pocket costs. We eat to live. The choice is in what we decide to eat.

The medical community doesn't see it this way. They want indisputable evidence from human clinical trials, choosing to ignore even the huge body of data supporting the ketogenic diet gleaned from the decades-long history of implementation in people with epilepsy. In fact, there is scientific evidence that, as used in epilepsy therapy, the diet is safe, feasible, and efficacious.[3,4,5] Can't we therefore speculate that the same safety and feasibility profile may also apply to other uses of this diet? There is already sound evidence that it does apply in cancer.[6,7] Nevertheless, you must first determine whether the diet is appropriate for you personally. I will walk you through a few exceptions to implementation of the diet in chapter 4 ("Considering Contraindications," page 39).

Impassioned researchers and clinicians have begun the process of running the ketogenic diet through the gauntlet of clinical trials that are needed to eventually move this therapy into evidence-based practice in cancer. Why, then, am I not content with waiting patiently for this to unfold?

*Because people with cancer don't have the luxury of time!*

## Disclaimer

I am a nutrition professional specializing in the implementation of the ketogenic diet for cancer. I am a nutritionist and educator, not a microbiologist, biochemist, or researcher. But I've combined aspects of all of these disciplines in what I offer in this book.

The information I present here (and on my websites and media recordings) should never be used to diagnose or treat disease and is not intended to take the place of medical advice. Seek advice and/or treatment if you have (or suspect you have) cancer or any other disease.

Although the ketogenic diet is an evidence-based dietary treatment for epilepsy, its use as a therapy for cancer and other diseases is strictly experimental. There is no guarantee that changing your diet will improve your condition or lengthen your life. In certain circumstances a ketogenic diet may not be a safe or appropriate choice. Before making changes to your diet, please seek the advice of your health care team.

I make no claim, express or implied, that the information I provide here is complete or free of errors. All material is also subject to misinterpretation. Neither I nor my heirs can be held responsible for your decision to adopt a ketogenic diet or other therapies using the information I provide either directly or indirectly in the text or in other resources cited throughout this book.

Please respect all copyright and trademark rules and regulations regarding the use of copyrighted material.

MIRIAM KALAMIAN, EdM, MS, CNS
Dietary Therapies LLC

# CHAPTER 1

# Cancer: Genetics or Metabolism?

I t sounded so great, at least in theory. The internationally organized Human Genome Project was a huge success, leapfrogging us forward in our understanding of our genetic roots. So in 2006 the United States went on to fund The Cancer Genome Atlas with the hope of zeroing in on a cure for cancer. Despite the initial anticipation and excitement that a cure was near, deconstructing this devastating disease has left the conventional oncology community still stuck "treating" cancer, not curing it. And treating it still comes at great expense— not only in terms of dollars spent but also, more importantly, in lives lost.

By 2015, after $375 million had been spent, the DNA (deoxyribonucleic acid, a cell's genetic instructions) of 10,000 tumors had been sequenced, and 10 million cancer-related mutations had been identified, science writer Heidi Ledford, in an important article in the journal *Nature*, concluded that, among other issues:

> Also a problem was the complexity of the data. Although a few "drivers" stood out as likely contributors to the development of

## The War on Cancer

Much like the Civil War, the "war on cancer" has dragged on far too long and at too great a human cost. How can we finally win it? Right now, conventional care is focused on narrow battles, but that's not how a war is won. When you're outsmarted on one front, do you keep pressing on? Or do you rethink your strategy?

cancer, most of the mutations formed a bewildering hodgepodge of genetic oddities, with little commonality between tumors. Tests of drugs that targeted the drivers soon revealed another problem: cancers are often quick to become resistant, typically by activating different genes to bypass whatever cellular process is blocked by the treatment.[1]

Here epigenetics is at work again, together with the random mutations that so commonly occur in the active sites of the targeted pathway. In combination, the two phenomena unfortunately tip the needle toward progression of the disease. Yet despite this dismal scenario, the international consortium that grew out of the project remains focused on developing new drugs, alone and in combination, that are somehow supposed to accommodate these 10 million cancer-related mutations (a number that may prove to be just the tip of the iceberg). Does it really make sense to continue to pursue a strategy to outwit cancer's ability to morph at will? And what proof do we have that cancer is actually a genetic disease? Of course, we know that genetic mutations drive cancer, but while searching for a cure related solely to mutations, might we have overlooked a much simpler possibility: that the answer may actually lie in cancer cell metabolism? In other words, is there an alternative explanation that can make sense of what we know to be the hallmarks of cancer?

## The Hallmarks of Cancer

In 2000 biologists Douglas Hanahan and Robert Weinberg published a paper identifying six traits common to most cancers and designating them as the "hallmarks of cancer."[2] These acquired traits include:

- Self-sufficiency in growth signals (Cancer cells control their own rate of proliferation.)
- Insensitivity to anti-growth signals (The cells do not respond to inhibitory signaling.)
- The ability to evade *apoptosis* (Cancer cells escape "cell suicide," a self-culling attribute of normal cells.)
- Limitless replicative potential (No explanation needed.)
- Sustained angiogenesis (Cells in a cancerous tumor stimulate the growth of new blood vessels needed to sustain them.)
- The ability to invade and *metastasize* (Cancerous tumor cells can spread and travel from the original site of tumor development.)

After another decade of investigation, the authors suggested the following additional characteristics of the cell and its environment that lead to cancer development and progression:[3]

- metabolic pathway dysregulation (cell signaling gone awry)
- immune system evasion (with help from mutations that disable surveillance)
- genomic instability (subject to mutations)
- inflammation (specifically, of the tumor microenvironment)

In 2005 biologist Dr. Thomas Seyfried and his colleague Dr. Purna Mukherjee were leaders in reexamining another characteristic of most cancer cells: That is, to produce energy, they preferentially ferment glucose in the cytoplasm even when there is sufficient oxygen to generate energy using the more efficient mitochondrial pathway. This particular characteristic of cancer is known as the "Warburg effect," named after German biochemist Otto Warburg. In a review paper published in the journal *Nutrition and Metabolism*, Drs. Seyfried and Mukherjee present a strong case in support of Warburg's central theory that cancer is a downstream effect of damage to mitochondria. They also describe the mechanism by which reactive oxygen species (ROS) from damaged respiration could produce mutations in the nucleus. Put simply, inefficiencies in cellular energy metabolism are compensated for by an increase in glucose fermentation, and this change can eventually turn a normal cell into a cancer cell.[4] In this scenario, it's easy to understand that cancer is a disease of mitochondrial metabolism.

## The Metabolic Theory of Cancer

Every paper and discussion of the metabolic theory of cancer begins with a description of what is referred to as the Warburg effect. Since this is key to your understanding of the science behind the ketogenic diet, let's look at the origins of this observation.

On some level, we're all familiar with how fermentation works. That's the process responsible for turning cabbage and milk, for example, into more gut-friendly foods such as sauerkraut and yogurt. It's relatively simple to bring about. You introduce a bacterial starter culture to a food, cover it to prevent contamination, keep it warm, and *voilà*. You've just fed the bacteria with the sugar in that food, which allows the bacteria to multiply. As the bacterial colony grows, the available sugars are rapidly fermented.

## Dr. Otto Warburg, Nobel Laureate

Otto Warburg was a prominent German biochemist of the early twentieth century who had a special interest in the metabolism of cancer cells. He observed that cancer cells increase their rate of glucose fermentation even in the presence of oxygen. In an email exchange with Dr. Seyfried (March 2017), he summed it up this way:

> Warburg's theory was based on his findings that all cancer cells have some defect in their ability to use oxygen to obtain energy through mitochondrial respiration. As a result, cancer cells relied more on fermentation than on respiration to obtain energy in order to compensate for their defective respiration. The reliance on fermentation even in the presence of sufficient oxygen was referred to as the Warburg effect.

> This fundamental shift in cancer cell metabolism, "the Warburg hypothesis," formed the basis of Dr. Seyfried's theory that cancer is primarily a mitochondrial metabolic disease that can be targeted by reducing the supply of fermentable fuels.

Fermentation is a primitive process that meets a bacterium's simple needs for energy. But in humans, fermentation by itself usually contributes relatively little to overall energy production. Yet as Warburg observed, cancer cells behave differently than normal cells: They become increasingly dependent on the fermentation of glucose within the cytoplasm of the cell for cellular energy. This differs from normal cells, which produce the majority of cellular energy within highly specialized organelles known as *mitochondria*. This switch in the fate of glucose within a cell may be the first indication that something has gone terribly wrong with cell function. If that cell survives and multiplies into a group of dysfunctional cells that are able to bypass immune system surveillance, we now have a malignant tumor.

As the tumor grows, it restricts the flow of blood containing oxygen and other vital nutrients. A cancer cell's ability to ferment glucose allows it to survive and thrive in a hypoxic (low oxygen) environment. This oxygen-starved state reprograms cell metabolism, promotes cell survival and proliferation, increases cancer's invasiveness, and stimulates the development of new blood vessel networks (referred to as *angiogenesis*) that serve to feed the tumor. A prime waste product of fermentation is lactic acid. This acidic waste is toxic, so it is quickly shunted to the microenvironment, the area immediately adjacent to the cell. Cancer thrives in this acid-inflamed environment, which leads to faster proliferation of cancer cells and acceleration of disease progression.

To add to the problem, dysregulated metabolism within cancer cells creates many more ROS molecules, which in turn inflict further damage to already dysfunctional mitochondria and lead to even more cellular disruption and disease progression (this occurs not only in cancer but in a whole host of other conditions as well).

This reliance on a more primitive way to fuel the cell's needs wouldn't make sense if I didn't mention that cancer cells ferment a lot of glucose, much more than what a normal cell would use. In fact, the rate of glycolysis in cancer cells is typically 10 to 15 times the rate in a normal cell. For that to occur, cancer cells need a way to allow more transport of glucose into the cell. They do this by increasing the number of glucose transporters and insulin receptors on the cell's surface. Remember that the next time you hear the term "glucose-avid" to describe cancer.

Recall that Warburg identified this process back in the first quarter of the twentieth century. In essence, his observation was the birthplace of the metabolic theory of cancer, and for a time, researchers worked to further explore this theory. But in the 1950s the discovery by James Watson and Francis Crick of the double helix structure of DNA derailed those explorations. Then, in the 1970s, the discovery of genetic mutations in the nuclear genome of cancer cells caused the pendulum to swing toward almost universal acceptance of the belief that cancer was a genetic disease.

With this shift in thinking, research efforts turned to identifying genetic mutations in DNA that could be linked to cancer initiation and progression. And, as is so clear from modern press releases, the medical and scientific community is still enamored with developing drugs that target these specific genetic mutations. So is the public. After all, who doesn't want to see a cure for cancer in a pill? In reality, though, decades of research and billions of dollars invested in this concept have produced little improvement in cancer outcomes. In other words, real people with real cancers are still dying from this disease.

Thankfully, not everyone jumped on board with the certainty that cancer was genetic in origin. And some very bright and talented researchers have been actively engaged in turning that ship around. To learn more about their discoveries and efforts, read Travis Christofferson's book *Tripping over the Truth*. In it

## Cancer as a Mitochondrial Metabolic Disease

In a paper published in the journal *Frontiers in Cell and Developmental Biology*, Dr. Seyfried describes intriguing research involving nuclear cytoplasm transfer experiments.[5] In these experiments, cytoplasmic hybrid cells, also known as *cybrids*, were created by transferring the nuclei of tumor cells into cells with normal cytoplasm. The result: cells that replicated and survived, despite having nuclei with mutated DNA. Other cybrids were created by transferring normal nuclei into tumor cells containing cytoplasm that displayed the Warburg effect (excessive fermentation of glucose). These cells also replicated, but the majority of them did not survive. According to Dr. Seyfried, "In summary, the information presented here supports the notion that cancer originates from damage to the *mitochondria* in the cytoplasm rather than from damage to the *genome* in the nucleus."

While I urge everyone to learn more about mitochondria, perhaps instead of approaching your study through the eyes of researchers, pick up a copy of science writer Nick Lane's book *Power, Sex, Suicide: Mitochondria and the Meaning of Life*. What a fascinating read! I came away from it even more in awe of what I view as "the improbability of my own existence."

you'll be introduced to the current leaders in metabolic theory: Dr. Thomas Seyfried, the pioneer, at Boston College, and Dr. Dominic D'Agostino, at the University of South Florida.

## The Inflammatory Response

The inflammatory response, a fundamental function of the immune system, is a normal and necessary part of life. It's the reason why head colds resolve in a week and paper cuts won't kill you, even though bacteria enter your body. When the inflammatory response is working properly, your immune system can quickly bring your body back into balance. But when it isn't working optimally, it stays turned on, overproducing inflammatory proteins called *cytokines*. Cytokines are essential to our immune defenses, as they direct activities that help target invaders for destruction. But overproduction of these proteins wreaks havoc in your body, leading to chronic inflammation, a prime driver of cancer and other chronic diseases. A wonderful and very welcome side effect of a well-planned ketogenic diet is that the presence of ketone bodies lowers the levels of inflammatory cytokines. When ketones are used for energy in place of glucose or fatty acids, normal cells produce fewer ROS. Cancer cells, however, have defects in their mitochondria that don't allow them to efficiently use the ketogenic pathway. Many cancer cells also produce less of the specific enzyme needed to utilize ketones for energy, further increasing their vulnerability to metabolic stress.[6]

*Immune surveillance* is the task of seeking out and destroying our own dysfunctional or damaged cells. When our immune system is doing its job, the process hums along smoothly. Occasionally, however, damaged cells adopt characteristics that allow them to fly under the radar, especially if our immune system's activity is compromised. Such cells may then collect even more mutations to aid in their survival, and this allows them to progress to full-blown cancer.

All cancer takes advantage of mutations that allow it to evade destruction by the immune system. The "fusion hybrid" hypothesis of cancer cell metastasis takes the process a step further with the speculation that infiltrating macrophages, a type of immune cell, reestablish themselves in locations distant from their place of origin. This contributes to an inflammatory cascade that can lead to rapid and uncontrollable progression of disease and a downward spiral in health. The more widespread the disease, the higher the degree of inflammation and the harder it is to restore balance. Radiation and many chemotherapy drugs are prooxidant therapies: that is, they work by overwhelming dysfunctional cancer cells, creating so much ROS that the therapy directly kills cancer cells. But there's collateral damage to neighboring healthy cells as well, and this collective damage contributes to widespread inflammation.

Chemotherapy, for example, targets cells that are replicating quickly (cancer cells), though unfortunately it also causes the death of the healthy fast-growing cells that line your digestive tract from "stem to stern" (mouth to anus). In turn, this disrupts your microbiome, which creates problems with appetite, digestion, and the absorption of nutrients. The conventional nutrition support offered by your oncology team is designed primarily to remediate these gastrointestinal side effects. When you consider that at least 70 percent of your body's immune defense arises from activity within the gut, you begin to get a clearer picture of the domino effect associated with conventional therapies.

Chemotherapy and radiation cause inflammation to skyrocket. That's why so many treatment protocols include pre- and post-treatment inflammation-suppressing steroid medications. Unfortunately, these medications also suppress immune function, a very undesirable side effect that lowers the body's resistance to everyday infections. Steroids also raise blood glucose levels, another detrimental side effect. Furthermore, some protocols also call for the use of prophylactic antibiotics. And, guess what? Antibiotics have side effects as well, including total disruption of your protective gut microbiome. (Vaginal flora are also indiscriminately killed, leaving women susceptible to infections that then require additional treatment.) Are you starting to see a pattern here?

I'm not suggesting that your choice of treatment is an either/or situation. In other words, you shouldn't have to choose between adopting alternative therapies, such as diet or nontoxic drugs, and receiving conventional care. In fact, most people I work with are successfully combining the best of both worlds, often with the help of integrative oncologists, to create their own personal protocols that appear to lead to better outcomes.

## Insulin Resistance Adds Fuel to the Flames

When over half your diet is made up of carbohydrate-containing foods, glucose is your body's primary fuel. A rise in blood glucose signals beta cells in the pancreas to secrete insulin, and a lot of insulin is needed to help move the glucose out of the bloodstream and into cells. Over time, persistently high levels of glucose and insulin can lead to insulin resistance. Put simply, your cells (particularly liver, muscle, and fat cells) become less responsive to insulin's constant knocking to let glucose into the cell. As a result, blood levels of both glucose and insulin remain high. Elevated levels of blood glucose and insulin are the markers used to diagnose diseases of insulin resistance, including prediabetes, type 2 diabetes, and polycystic ovary syndrome (PCOS). These markers are also associated with a higher risk of many cancers.

One mechanism that explains part of the role of insulin resistance in cancer is that insulin-resistant fat cells secrete inflammatory cytokines (including those involved in the immune response). This results in a chronic inflammatory state that damages cellular membranes and DNA while simultaneously altering normal mitochondrial activities, including molecular signaling and repair mechanisms, thereby opening more avenues for cancer progression.

When you adopt a ketogenic diet, you eliminate most dietary sources of carbohydrates. This shifts metabolism away from reliance on glucose as its primary fuel. A lowered blood glucose level also reduces insulin spikes, which in turn takes the brakes off of lipolysis, the breakdown of fat. As a result, the body shifts to burning fat for fuel. Some of the by-products of fat metabolism (in the absence of dietary carbohydrates) are converted to energy molecules known as ketone bodies. Ketone bodies burn more efficiently than either glucose or fatty acids and generate far fewer ROS in the process. In fact, studies have shown that ketones, even if ingested as a supplement, can lower many markers of inflammation, including some inflammatory cytokines that are associated with cancer progression. This has global benefits that help quench the flames that fuel cancer. Another bonus of this shift: Over time, your cells can regain much, if not all, of their original sensitivity to insulin.

## Targeted Therapies

Until recently, most anticancer drugs were chemotherapies designed to kill rapidly proliferating cells; as noted, they have significant impact on normal

### Protein Kinase Inhibitors' Impact on Glucose Metabolism

When I first learned of the impact of protein kinase inhibitors on glucose metabolism, I immediately questioned if this might be one of the mechanisms that led to a response to its use in the treatment of cancer. A review paper published in the Society for Endocrinology journal *Endocrine-Related Cancer* described a subset of people with both cancer and diabetes who experienced lower blood glucose as a side effect of broad-acting kinase inhibitors.[7] Treatment with these drugs allowed these individuals to lower the amount of insulin they needed. We know that both insulin and its associated hormone insulin-like growth factor, type 1 (IGF-1), drive cancer growth, so doesn't it make sense that this insulin-lowering effect might be one of the reasons why these drugs have an impact on cancer? If so, doesn't it also make sense to adopt a ketogenic diet as an adjunct to cancer treatment?

I also came across a study published in the journal *Cell Death and Disease* in which pancreatic adenocarcinoma cells that survived treatment with the protein kinase inhibitor axitinib (Inlyta) showed a sharp increase in the rate at which they used glucose, which also resulted in a rise in the acidification of the tumor microenvironment.[8] As mentioned earlier, this acidification contributes to inflammation and cancer progression.

cells as well. This has made the promise of "targeted therapies" in cancer treatment understandably seductive, but there are significant limitations and drawbacks to consider. In contrast to outright cellular destruction, protein kinase inhibitors, a class of drugs that includes some of the newer therapies for cancer, block certain enzymes associated with the progression of specific cancers. Drugs in this class include afatinib (Giotrif), which interferes with a growth factor receptor (epidermal growth factor receptor, EGFR) in non-small cell lung cancer, and bevacizumab (Avastin), which blocks activity of vascular

## Destroying versus Harnessing Your Immune System

As it stands right now, medicine is still heavily reliant on traditional interventions designed to poison cancer. In his book *Tripping over the Truth*, science writer Travis Christofferson describes the work of doctors who were researching the therapeutic potential of "war gas" (nitrogen mustard). In the mid-1940s the compound was injected into laboratory mice, confirming that it had a significant impact on lymphoid tumors. The next step involved administering nitrogen mustard to a man with advanced non-Hodgkin's lymphoma. Miraculously, he improved. This signaled the beginning of the age of chemotherapy.

This and other early chemotherapy drugs did indeed kill cancer cells, but there was so much collateral damage that people often died of the treatment rather than the disease. Today's chemotherapies are generally less toxic but still result in damage to the body that may be nearly impossible to remediate. Many people who undergo traditional chemotherapy care develop chronically low blood counts, along with an impaired ability to fight off even the most benign diseases, such as the common cold or seasonal flu. This is especially true of older adults.

The most exciting and potentially beneficial development in conventional medicine lies in the research into therapies that use the body's own immune system to aid in detecting and destroying cancerous cells. Although the early work seems promising, researchers are also discovering that these therapies can trigger the development of autoimmune diseases.[9] For this and other reasons it will take years, if not decades, to refine this approach. Added to this challenge is the crushing cost of access to these new therapies.

endothelial growth factor A (VEGF-A), a growth factor that is overexpressed in many cancer types. Although these anticancer drugs cause less inflammation than chemotherapy and radiation, they are still associated with significant short-term side effects. Long-term side effects are not yet fully understood; one paper (described in the "Protein Kinase Inhibitors' Impact on Glucose Metabolism" sidebar, page 9) notes endocrine-related side effects, including impaired thyroid function, bone metabolism, and adrenal function. However, most interesting in the context of this book, these drugs are often associated with changes in glucose metabolism. This includes both hyper- and hypoglycemia. This side effect may be an independent factor influencing outcomes, but to the best of my knowledge it has not yet been investigated.

While protein kinase inhibitors are designed to block specific metabolic pathways in cancer (and a few other diseases), they do nothing to address the root cause of disease. Cancer is very heterogeneous, which means that within any group of cancer cells some will *not* have defects in the targeted pathway and thus will be unaffected by a drug that works with such specificity. Cancer cells are also very adept at evolving and mutating to adapt to new conditions.

Another limitation of protein kinase therapy and other current targeted therapies: With few exceptions, highly aggressive cancer cells often resemble undifferentiated stem cells. That is, they develop characteristics that interfere with the cellular activities that normally keep cell growth and proliferation in check. This is what allows them to survive and thrive. To date, no drugs utilized in conventional cancer care have successfully cured cancer by targeting cancer stem cells.

That could change as a result of Dr. Seyfried's research using a preclinical mouse model. His current results show that targeting glucose and glutamine *simultaneously*, as he does with "press-pulse" therapy, is an integral part of an extremely effective and relatively nontoxic metabolic therapy that targets cancer cells' primary energy pathways while enhancing the energy efficiency of normal cells and tissues: a win-win approach in the management of cancer! This very important work is described in detail in Dr. Seyfried's and his colleagues' must-read paper in 2017 in *Nutrition and Metabolism*.[10]

# CHAPTER 2

# "Show Me the Evidence"

The practice of Western medicine is "evidence-based," and there is a recognized descriptive hierarchy in the various levels of proof that oncologists use to develop their practice guidelines and treatment protocols. If you do not have a science background, you will need to get up to speed with how to evaluate the quality of what you find online.

## Levels of Evidence

There is a good chance that when you started your online search for information, you were drawn to the kinds of information that are not traditionally viewed as scientific evidence: personal reports, mostly anecdotal in nature, or blog posts in which people report their personal data and experiences. Although you cannot draw conclusions from this type of information, it is valuable in that it can provide you an overview of options—alternative as well as conventional. This is a good thing if you can learn to discriminate between testimonials that are not based on facts or science (e.g., those used to support such approaches as the Budwig Diet and the Asparagus Cure). No matter how many people testify to cures, there is no credible reason to believe that either cottage cheese, flaxseed oil, or asparagus has curative properties. There are other legendary dietary cures as well, none with any science behind them; still, they create so much confusion that they need to be addressed, which I do in chapter 6 ("Comparing Keto to Other 'Anticancer' Diets," page 81).

Part of the confusion stems from the fact that people with cancer often (understandably) equate the much-desired though often misleading phrase "no evidence of disease" with the medically specific term "cure." However, "no evidence of disease" simply means that the tests used didn't *detect* anything. For example, a CT or MRI or ultrasound may reveal no evidence of a previously detected tumor mass. Importantly, however, failure to identify a tumor mass using these technologies does not rule out the presence of microscopic cancer cells—even if they exist in large numbers. But this may not be adequately explained to patients. The unfortunate result is that patients often conclude that the finding "no evidence of disease" on a scan or other test means they are free of cancer. Likewise, if they are told they are "in remission," this is also not a statement of cure; at best, these individuals can hope that the disease does not become active again or reemerge in another location.

However, despite these drawbacks, personal stories combined with the observations of doctors and researchers can serve a broader purpose if they provide information and data that can be used to develop research questions and protocols for rigorous testing. That's what happened with the ketogenic diet for epilepsy and what is now happening with the ketogenic metabolic therapy for a number of chronic conditions, including cancer.

In the oncology world, the least significant "level of evidence" involves peer-reviewed and published case studies or case series (multiple case studies with a single theme that are compared and contrasted in one paper). However, these are never used as the basis for making conventional treatment recommendations, and your oncologist will most likely show little interest in these reports.

As of this writing, there are a number of case studies suggesting that a ketogenic diet implemented as an adjunct therapy may improve outcomes over standard therapy alone in the treatment of cancer. Many of these studies include such objective data as lab results, radiographic images and reports, and blood glucose and/or ketone measurements. Although the number and diversity of these studies are growing exponentially, they are still too limited in scope to apply to the general population of individuals with cancer.

Still, these types of reports may be what piqued *your* interest in the ketogenic diet. These stories can be very compelling, especially if you can relate to them personally, as I did in the case report of two children with brain tumors who were put on a ketogenic diet in the mid-1990s. The lead researcher, Dr. Linda Nebeling, looked at the change in glucose uptake by tumor tissue and found that it decreased by over 21 percent in both children in just 8 weeks.[1] That, together with the safety data on the diet, was what gave me permission (essentially, "What have we got to lose?") to try this with my own son. But case studies in general have far too many confounding variables that can provide alternative explanations for the observed results. Baseline status and other individual differences also play a huge role here. Two people diagnosed with the same cancer, both following the same diet and maybe even taking the same supplements, are likely to have very different health histories and very different immune system responses, making it extremely difficult to compare apples to apples when evaluating their outcomes. Nevertheless, case studies are often intriguing and may lead researchers and even a few medical professionals to consider new theories.

"Preclinical data," as I mentioned before, are important in building the base for proposed studies in humans. This usually involves compelling animal model research, such as Dr. Seyfried's finding that in a mouse model of glioma, animals fed a calorically restricted ketogenic diet survived longer than their counterparts that were fed unlimited amounts of either the ketogenic formula or a standard mouse chow.[2] Or the subsequent work from Drs. Seyfried's and D'Agostino's labs that showed a mouse model of metastatic disease benefiting from a synergistic combination of ketogenic diet, ketone supplementation, and hyperbaric oxygen therapy.[3]

## Evidence-Based Medicine

Just a few short years ago, the ketogenic diet was not even on the radar as an adjuvant therapy for cancer. Now it's very likely that your oncologist is aware of the buzz, but you can still expect to hear this: "There's no evidence to support the use of a ketogenic diet." From the perspective of your oncologist, who may accept the results of clinical trials as the only adequate proof, this is true. He or she is willing to wait until the ketogenic diet has survived the gauntlet of clinical trials and popped out intact on the other side, complete with a set of clinical guidelines for its use. Although I fully expect this to happen, I know that even in the best of circumstances it will be decades before the ketogenic diet is a generally accepted evidence-based adjunctive therapy for cancer. But even meeting this high standard is certainly no guarantee that ketogenic diet therapy will be implemented as an anticancer therapy within the context of conventional care. There's a precedent here: Although there is clear evidence that the ketogenic diet is a safe and efficacious treatment for intractable pediatric epilepsy, and that quality of life is often better for children on the diet, most neurologists remain skeptical and dismissive. Are you OK with sitting back and waiting for acceptance that may never come? Or are you a person with cancer who doesn't have the luxury of time to see how this plays out?

It should be reassuring on some level to learn that the ketogenic diet has already cleared the first hurdle in cancer, clinical trials of feasibility and safety that answered the questions "Can this be done?" and "Can this be done safely?"[4,5] Recruitment to phase 1 trials is currently underway, but there are issues with achieving the participant enrollment numbers that are needed to proceed, partly because these trials are being conducted at small institutions, not multicenter big-name treatment hospitals. Looking to the future, administering phase 2 and 3 studies to examine the efficacy of ketogenic diet therapy will be even more challenging. These types of trials cost pharmaceutical companies millions if not billions of dollars to complete and come with the expectation of huge financial rewards if ultimately they lead to the patenting of a new drug or therapy. But who will fund advanced diet trials when there is no lure of potential profits? How lucky that you don't need to enroll in a clinical trial to whip up a keto meal in your own kitchen!

So, then, what path forward does the ketogenic diet have within the scientific community? Preclinical (animal model) research has looked at the effect of the diet as stand-alone therapy, while more recent research in both animals and humans has combined the diet with conventional treatments such as radiation and chemotherapy, as well as with such metabolic alternatives as ketone esters and hyperbaric oxygen. Studies to date have suggested that the ketogenic diet works synergistically with these other therapies.

Another line of inquiry is to look at the effect of combining the ketogenic diet with commonly prescribed and comparatively safe and inexpensive drugs, such as the blood glucose–lowering medicine metformin. In theory, the combination therapy would be more effective than either one on its own. In science, however, we can't simply speculate our way to a conclusion. When such questions are raised, research is designed to test the validity of the hypothesis.

Sometimes the answer may seem obvious, especially when it comes to alternative therapies. For example, an *anti*oxidant therapy, such as intravenous (IV) glutathione, would be expected to be incompatible with a *pro*oxidant therapy, such as high-dose IV vitamin C. In essence, the effect of one would cancel out the other. Most savvy practitioners are not going to suggest that they be administered together. However, predicting whether a certain combination is going to help or hurt is often not as clear-cut as this.

Science is data-driven, and that's generally a very good thing. After all, you wouldn't want your oncologist to base your treatment plan on what she or he had just read in a press release or single patient testimonial. Unfortunately, however, science can "throw the baby out with the bathwater" when it neglects to consider *any* information that hasn't been verified in clinical trials. Mainly because research moves at such a crawl, a wave of willing individuals have begun to conduct their own personalized trials.

A personalized trial can be thought of as a way to evaluate the clinical results and outcome of a specific treatment plan scientifically in a single individual. By convention, the number of individual subjects in a clinical trial or particular treatment arm is designated by the letter $n$. Ten subjects in a group is referred to as an "n of 10" (n=10); 500 subjects is an "n of 500" (n=500), and

## The Most Famous "N-of-1" Study

Edward Jenner, an English country doctor practicing in the late eighteenth century, observed that milkmaids who had contracted the cowpox virus (through transmission from an afflicted cow) seemed immune to smallpox. He decided to test his theory. His method was highly unethical by today's standards: He deliberately infected a child with the cowpox virus, waited for the child to recover from the disease, and then inoculated him with the smallpox virus. Jenner's n-of-1 trial was extremely risky, but, thankfully, the child didn't become ill. Jenner was then able to convince others that his theory was correct and that his method would work on a larger scale. He went on to develop the vaccine that has saved the lives of millions.

Today, Jenner's n-of-1 trial would be unthinkable, and in general trials of this type that accrue one-of-a-kind data don't generate much interest outside of the blogosphere. In fact, even data compiled from *thousands* of n-of-1 trials would not be sufficient to change practice in the oncology world.

Before moving forward with your own ketogenic diet n-of-1 trial, be sure to look over the list of contraindications and limitations in chapter 4 ("Considering Contraindications," page 39). Even if you think you are a good candidate, you should discuss your diet decision with your oncologist or other health care practitioner before you begin. Please seek professional oversight!

so on. Conclusions about the trial are drawn from the statistical extraction of evidence based on the number of individuals participating. But could we be missing something when we fail to rigorously evaluate the data resulting from the clinical treatment of a single individual subject? In fact, clinical trials of single individuals have become known as "n-of-1" trials, and "n-of-1" data are increasingly recognized as important sources of preclinical evidence needed to drive treatment decisions.

## CHAPTER 3

# "Show Me the Science"

I n chapter 1 you learned about the Warburg effect, Dr. Otto Warburg's observations that cancer cells utilize glucose differently than normal cells and that they use a *lot* of it. No reasonable researcher or oncologist will dispute that point. Now let's dive a little deeper into the science—at first, just enough that you'll understand *why* what you eat can make a difference when facing a disease as complex as cancer. Without this fundamental information, you would be hard-pressed to explain to anyone why you chose *this* plan over all the other diets that claim to be "anticancer."

## Cancer Thrives on Glucose and Glutamine

Cancer thrives on fermentable fuels. Study after study has confirmed this. A well-planned ketogenic diet restricts cancer's access to its preferred fuel sources, glucose and to a lesser degree glutamine, while providing abundant energy to healthy cells. That makes evolutionary sense given that early humans wouldn't have survived unless they had a backup system for those times when food was in short supply. Your body will respond to carbohydrate restriction similarly to how it responds to fasting or starvation: by flipping a metabolic switch that allows stored fat to be used as fuel.

The body's ability to switch fuels also explains why a well-planned ketogenic diet is uniquely positioned to interrupt not only the flow of glucose but also the supply of other cancer-promoting fuels, including glutamine. Furthermore, as you will learn, a ketogenic diet and other strategies that mimic starvation can compromise the very existence of diseased cells, which helps restore the normal cellular signaling that is responsible for putting the brakes on cancer. The players in these molecular signaling pathways have names like mTOR (mechanistic target of rapamycin), IGF-1 (insulin-like growth factor, type 1), SIRT1 (Sirtuin 1), AMPK (AMP-activated protein kinase), and others that at this point in your journey may seem more like secret code than a diet outcome. No worries: You don't

## Glutamine: Another Fuel Driving Cancer

There is no question in any researcher's mind that cancers cells use glutamine as an energy source, allowing cancer cells to survive and thrive, even in hypoxic (low oxygen) tumors. In fact, as the disease progresses, healthy cells are often destroyed by their cancerous neighbors in order to meet their ever-increasing demand for glutamine (much like a burglar ransacking his own neighborhood). Although this problem can't be addressed by diet alone, there are some actions you can take. See chapter 12, "Rein in Your Protein," page 199, for details.

need to understand these pathways to reap the benefits. Please understand that while this nutritional strategy is an extremely powerful tool, changing your diet is not going to cure your cancer. In fact, let's not talk cure; instead let's focus on long-term management with the added benefit of other improvements in health.

## Introducing Ketogenic Metabolic Therapy

A new term—"ketogenic metabolic therapy"—has recently been proposed by a group of researchers and clinicians who want to emphasize the use of a

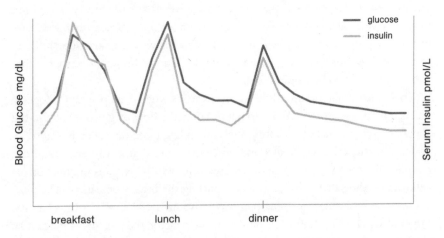

**Figure 3.1.** Typical 24-hour glucose/insulin spikes associated with a standard diet of 3 meals over 12 hours.

ketogenic nutritional intervention as an antineoplastic (anticancer) strategy.[1]
This new paradigm exploits cancer's metabolic cravings for glucose and other
fermentable fuels. In direct contradiction to this stands the conventional
dietary advice from the American Cancer Society, which recommends that
individuals with cancer eat whatever tastes good: "Use ice cream as a topping
on cake."[2] *Really?* If that advice makes sense to you, then you might as well
stop reading this and go out for some Ben & Jerry's. But if you're still with
me, read on for more guidance on how to adopt the ketogenic diet alongside
your other treatments. If you already have a handle on the science behind the
ketogenic diet, then this section can serve as a summary.

Let's start with one of the most damaging nutrition myths of our time:
namely, that our bodies need a continuous supply of carbohydrates supplied
by the foods we eat—45 to 65 percent of our total calories. That is simply not
true! Most of the people who regurgitate this "conventional wisdom" don't
understand that this is only an *opinion* that has been repeated so often that
it is accepted as the truth. In fact, even the very mainstream manual *Dietary
Reference Intakes*, published by the Food and Nutrition Board of the Institute of
Medicine (The National Academies Press, 2005), acknowledges that a combination of gluconeogenesis and ketone bodies is sufficient to meet the brain's
energy needs even in the total absence of dietary carbohydrates.

Consider this: Abundant sources of sugars and easily digestible carbohydrates have been the dietary default for only a tiny part of our overall history as
hominids. As you can see in figure 3.1, a standard diet that derives the majority

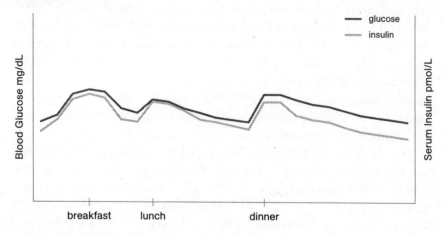

**Figure 3.2.** Typical 24-hour glucose/insulin spikes associated with a ketogenic diet
of 3 meals over 12 hours. Ketogenic diets minimize spikes in glucose and insulin.

of calories from carbohydrates (sugars such as glucose, fructose, sucrose, and lactose) results in "spikes" (rapidly occurring large increases) in circulating levels of both glucose and insulin—not just occasionally, but as a pattern that repeats itself many times over the course of a day. From an evolutionary standpoint, this is neither normal nor desirable!

## What Goes Awry with Glucose Metabolism?

Each of us knows that we must eat in order to survive, but there's no consensus on what constitutes the ideal diet. Despite what you may now believe, there is no single diet that best fits everyone's needs, just as there is no universal shoe size. Human cells are exceedingly complex and have compartmentalized many of the activities needed to sustain themselves. Specific genes—for example, the one that codes for the enzyme lactase—influence our ability to digest certain foods—in this case, lactose—but, as you will learn in the pages that follow, food itself can change the *expression* of some of these genes: that is, the messages that control vital activities at the cellular level. Even if you already eat what you feel is a very healthy diet, cancer is a game changer and what might have been a good plan for you before you developed this disease may no longer serve you well.

As stated previously, the fermentation of glucose fuels cancer's ever-increasing energy needs. When blood glucose levels are high (which they are after a carbohydrate-dense meal), beta cells in the pancreas begin pumping out insulin to help move glucose from the bloodstream into the interior of cells. Glucose molecules need transporter proteins to facilitate their movement across cell membranes, and many of these proteins are activated by insulin. (Exceptions include GLUT1 and GLUT3, two transporters found in brain tissue, which are *not* dependent on the presence of insulin.) Cancer cells have *up to 10 times* the normal number of insulin receptors embedded in the cell membrane. No wonder so much glucose can be made available to them. Levels of IGF-1, a hormone associated with cancer progression, rise along with insulin. IGF-1 can bind with the same receptors as insulin and with a similar effect, thereby contributing to the pro-cancer molecular activity in the cancer cell. This is obviously *not* a healthy scenario!

Once inside the cytoplasm of the cell, each glucose molecule is split into two molecules of pyruvate in a process known as *glycolysis*. In *normal* cells, most of the pyruvate then passes into the cell's mitochondria (cellular powerhouses), where it is efficiently oxidized to generate energy. In *cancer* cells, however, since the mitochondria are damaged and dysfunctional, more pyruvate remains in the cytoplasm, where it is fermented instead of oxidized for energy. (This process is described in detail in chapter 1, "The Metabolic Theory

of Cancer," page 3). Fermentation produces lactic acid, or lactate—which threatens cell survival—so it is quickly transported out of the cell, where it acidifies the surrounding microenvironment. (This acidification contributes to inflammation, a major promoter of cancer dissemination.) Most lactate then makes its way to the liver, where it is converted back into glucose and returned to the bloodstream. Here we have an example of how changes at the cellular level, including alterations in genetic expression, can control both the number of glucose transporters on cell membranes and the amount of glucose that's processed by fermentation in the cytoplasm versus oxidation in the mitochondria. Now let's look at how we can turn that ship around by shifting from a predominately carbohydrate diet to one comprised chiefly of fats.

## The Shift to Ketosis

On its own, this book is not going to change oncology practice. But what it *can* do is help you to become better informed about the disconnect that exists between science and practice and reduce the number of obstacles you may encounter as you move toward a ketogenic diet. To that end, you should first be aware of the effect of the "genetic disease" filter and perspective on the thinking of cancer specialists, even brilliant ones. For example, Drs. Matthew McGirt and Alfredo Quinones-Hinojosa, both outstanding neurosurgeons, have published several papers in which they link hyperglycemia (persistently high blood glucose levels) to a poorer prognosis for patients with brain cancers.[3,4] But that same strong link between glucose and cancer isn't limited to brain tumors. In fact, if you were to search PubMed, the NIH's online repository for biomedical literature (www.ncbi.nlm.nih.gov/pubmed/), using the keywords "hyperglycemia" and "cancer," you'd find over 3,230 peer-reviewed and published papers. So why hasn't conventional oncology practice caught up with the science yet? Partly because of the widespread belief that the glucose level can't be lowered enough to make a difference, but also (I suspect) because no one wants to be the first to lay their credentials on the line in what is likely to lead to a confrontation with colleagues. Instead, practitioners are willing to stay the course, waiting patiently for a silver bullet that will cure cancer. But as I've said before and will say again many times, most people with cancer don't have the luxury of time. So let's look at how ketogenic metabolic therapy—essentially, a different mix of foods you already know—can stand in for treatments that are still just pipe dreams.

Most likely our ancient ancestors didn't give much thought to missing a meal or two, but in today's world that can feel like deprivation. Understand that your body will perceive the switch to ketosis as starvation—this will require strong commitment to your plan to get past that initial bump in the road. Ketosis begins with a short fast or a significant drop in carbohydrate intake that pushes your body's metabolism to find other fuel sources. Carbohydrate restriction results in predictable metabolic changes that will continue to meet the specific needs of each organ and tissue. Let's walk through the process.

## Step One

In the first step of the shift to ketosis, a drop in blood glucose levels greatly reduces the need for insulin secretion. In turn, low glucose levels stimulate the secretion of insulin's opposing hormone, glucagon. Glucagon stimulates the process of *glycogenolysis*, the breakdown of glucose stored in the liver as glycogen. Each gram of glucose provides four calories, so glycogenolysis is capable of liberating approximately 100 grams (400 calories) of this stored glucose.

We also store glucose as glycogen in muscle tissue. In most individuals, muscle glycogen consists of 400 to 500 grams of glucose (1,600 to 2,000 calories), but the glucose can be utilized only by the muscle tissue in which it is stored, so it never enters the bloodstream. In essence, muscle glycogen serves as a reserve fuel tank for those times when our muscles need a burst of energy to flee from that saber-toothed tiger or chase down lunch.

## Step Two

Once the liver's glycogen stores are mostly depleted, typically within 18 to 24 hours after the last carbohydrate-containing meal, the liver (and kidneys) will ramp up activity in yet another metabolic pathway, *gluconeogenesis* (literally, "making new glucose"). Yes, we *can*—and *do*—make our own glucose! This is another of those marvelous adaptations that keep our metabolism humming along despite inevitable swings in our food supply. But gluconeogenesis is not triggered only by periods of starvation. Whenever glucose levels drop too low, hormones are activated to jump-start the process, just like a furnace clicks on when the temperature drops below a certain preset level. This happens many times throughout the day and during the course of a normal night's sleep (as long as you haven't eaten too close to bedtime).

When stimulated to produce glucose, the liver and kidneys use a smorgasbord of substrates and precursors—that is, molecular bits and pieces of nutrients—that can be cobbled together to form glucose. (A ketone researcher once told me that the liver could make glucose from rubber bands. That's a "stretch," but still a great way to communicate the versatility of this pathway.)

## A Closer Look at Gluconeogenesis

It's very important to expand on the role of gluconeogenesis because you will often read or hear misinformation about degradation of muscle mass as a side effect of ketogenic diets. This is very misleading and points to a poor understanding of the ketogenic diet as compared to fasting or starvation. Let me set the record straight now: When raw materials are in short supply, as they are during the first few days of a fast or when beginning a ketogenic diet, it is true that the liver will respond to signals that in turn initiate the breakdown of muscle tissue. Those precious amino acids are then either reconfigured into needed proteins or used to make glucose. However, after the first few days of the ketogenic diet, gluconeogenesis relies mostly on the glycerol backbones from triglycerides (more on this shortly), so the reliance on muscle tissue for building blocks eases up. (Don't make the mistake of replacing carbohydrates with a lot of protein—the excess will be converted by the liver to glucose. This can actually keep your body reliant on glucose even after you have started to burn fat.)

Let me add that some amount of muscle tissue breakdown is totally normal—actually, it's *absolutely essential* to building muscle mass in both athletes and weekend warriors. Stress to muscles stimulates protein synthesis, which leads to the creation of new muscle. Aren't our bodies fascinating!

Lactate, amino acids, and the glycerol backbones from triglycerides can all be converted to glucose—we'll get to that shortly!

## Step Three

By itself, gluconeogenesis can't keep up with our body's energy needs (and doesn't even begin to address the energy needs of our big brains). But once again, our bodies have a reliable workaround, one that anyone who has been on a weight-loss diet is sure to love: When we need more energy, the next in the series of metabolic shifts flips the switch to our auxiliary fuel tank—fat! Now, we can aggressively break down both the triglycerides stored in adipose tissue (fat cells) and the triglycerides we ingest as fats.

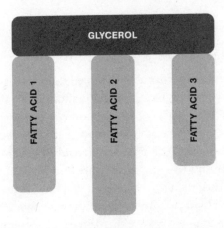

**Figure 3.3.** Simple Schematic of a Triglyceride Ester. Triglycerides are made up of three chains of fatty acids attached to a glycerol backbone.

## Think of a Hybrid Engine

In today's world it's hard to imagine our species experiencing frequent and lengthy disruptions in their food supply. In modern times and in affluent nations like our own, interruptions have been reduced to a very short window, usually limited to a few hours while out running errands or being stuck in a meeting. While even today's short disruptions may cause feelings of hunger, thankfully we all have an auxiliary fuel tank with the capacity to power us past many missed meals.

"Hybrid engine" is a great way to describe the flexibility of our backup energy systems. Normal cells really do operate like tiny hybrid engines: They are metabolically flexible, meaning that built-in signaling mechanisms allow them to seamlessly integrate fuels from a variety of different sources. Knowing this, it's easy to understand how a shortage of dietary carbohydrate results in both the endogenous (internal) production of new glucose and the breakdown of fats into free fatty acids and ketone bodies. As I've said before, this makes evolutionary sense. Fortunately, the accumulated mutations in cancer cells render them less metabolically flexible, allowing them to be targeted through this change in diet.

Triglycerides are made up of three chains of fatty acids bound together by what's referred to as a "glycerol backbone." Enzymes strip off this backbone, releasing the fatty acids into the bloodstream, which carries them throughout most of the body. Fatty acids are readily taken up by tissues that metabolize them for energy through the process of fatty acid oxidation. Under normal physiological conditions, the heart and skeletal muscle prefer fatty acids over glucose as they are a much more dependable source of fuel. This makes sense when you consider that all but the most compromised among us have enough stored fat to support us through weeks to months of total starvation.

But here's a drawback that needs yet another workaround: Not all cells can use fats for energy. One big drawback is that fatty acids can't be used to meet the brain's energy needs. Most of their chains are too large to be transported across the picky blood-brain barrier, a semi-permeable protective interface consisting of specialized endothelial cells with uniquely tight junctions lining the blood vessels that lead to the brain. The blood-brain barrier plays a critical role in blocking passage of large molecules, including potentially harmful toxins as well as many drugs (including those that kill cancer cells). In addition to brain cells, cells that lack mitochondria, such as mature red blood cells and lens tissue, also cannot use fatty acids for fuel.

So if fatty acid oxidation can't fill the energy gap, particularly the needs of the brain, what's the next fuel to step up to the plate? Ketones! Finally, we arrive at ketogenesis, one of the most exquisite of all the adaptations and the only one that can fuel our big brains when dietary sources of glucose are in short supply. Ketones are one of the small, water-soluble molecules that are synthesized from the accumulation of breakdown products of fatty acid oxidation and, to a lesser degree, the conversion of certain amino acids. Not very sexy, but who cares?

Ketones are an amazing form of energy, especially for the brain. For example, when your neurons are running on ketones, you are less likely to experience those gaps in brain function that we often refer to as "brain fog." Ketones are also neuroprotective and neurotherapeutic—in simple terms that means they protect your brain cells.[5] Dr. Jong Rho, a prolific researcher and keto-for-epilepsy advocate at the University of Calgary, has written extensively on this topic. And Dominic D'Agostino, PhD, at the University of South Florida, is investigating how ketones, even in supplement form, might be used in preventing seizures in Navy SEALs, the members of military special operations teams who rely on "rebreathing" apparatus during their underwater missions. In a personal email (March 2017), Dr. D'Agostino noted, "Ketone supplementation in the form of ketone esters was originally developed for enhancing warfighter performance and further development and testing are ongoing for

## Red Blood Cells:
## A Unique Indicator of Blood Glucose Status

As red blood cells mature, they maximize their oxygen-carrying capacity by squeezing out their mitochondria, allowing more room for hemoglobin. As a result, mature red blood cells become totally reliant on the fermentation of glucose for energy. Using glucose as its sole energy source literally runs red blood cells ragged in just a few months, resulting in a high turnover rate. Within the cell, glucose binds with the protein in hemoglobin in a process called glycation. The higher the level of glucose in the cell, the more glycation occurs. That's why the level of glycated hemoglobin (better known as hemoglobin A1c, or HbA1c) can be used to evaluate the average amount of glucose present in the bloodstream over the previous three or four months (the typical life span of a red blood cell).

Checking the level of HbA1c is part of routine diabetes monitoring; an elevated HbA1c indicates poor glucose control. High HbA1c is also associated with a number of conditions that commonly occur alongside diabetes, such as cardiovascular disease, neuropathy, retinopathy (damage to the retina), and nephropathy (damage to the kidney). When endocrinologists note a rise in HbA1c, they will alter the mix of drugs or, in patients with advanced type 2 diabetes, may even prescribe insulin to help remove excess glucose from the bloodstream. Treating signs of an illness, however, does nothing to address the underlying cause. What a high HbA1c level *should* do is wave a red flag in the face of anyone who has a glucose-loving cancer. Instead of encouraging insulin to push more fuel into greedy cancer cells, why not try a more common-sense approach? Compromise the supply by cutting back on the foods that are the richest source of dietary glucose. This makes so much sense that it's amazing to me that the medical community targets the test result (high blood glucose) rather than its cause, particularly when the mechanism here is so clear.

Although you may want to use HbA1c levels as a marker of your own blood glucose control spanning the past three months, you won't get an accurate reading if your red blood cell counts are low, as is typically true of most people undergoing conventional treatments that kill cancer cells by creating a lot of ROS.

that application." In fact, many people I know now refer to ketones as a "super-fuel," and elite athletes, not just Navy SEALs, are using ketone supplements to enhance their performance.

There are three types of energy substrates commonly referred to as ketone bodies. All are produced by the liver and, to a lesser degree, by the kidneys:

- **Acetoacetate** is preferentially taken up by muscle tissue and oxidized for energy. The brain also uses acetoacetate for energy.[6,7] With keto adaptation, most acetoacetate is converted ("reduced") to beta-hydroxybutyrate, primarily by liver and muscle tissue, and returned to circulation.
- **Beta-hydroxybutyrate** (βHB) is produced in almost equal proportions as acetoacetate. As the body adapts to ketosis, interconversion of acetoacetate and βHB favors the production of βHB, a preferred fuel for heart, muscle, and brain tissue.
- **Acetone** is usually produced from the spontaneous breakdown of acetoacetate. Only a small amount of acetone undergoes reactions that allow it to be used for energy. Most of it is simply eliminated from the body and is responsible for fruity-smelling "keto breath."

The ketogenic pathway represents a stunningly sophisticated adaptation not only to periods of prolonged fasting or even starvation, but also to the voluntary restriction of carbohydrate intake.[8] (Think: ketogenic diet.) This makes sense from an evolutionary standpoint; otherwise, we would have died off as a species the first time our food supply fell short of our immediate needs. This adaptation allowed our brains to stay sharp even during periods of minimal or no food availability.

Starvation does indeed stress tumor tissue, and it also helps to weed out other aberrant and dysfunctional cells. But starving yourself is obviously not a sustainable long-term solution to managing your cancer. Thankfully, a calorie-restricted ketogenic diet, used alone or in combination with periods of fasting, mimics many of the same benefits found in starvation, including the abundant production of ketone bodies. (More details are provided in chapter 7.)

Ketone bodies are produced in specialized liver cells and also, to a lesser degree, in the kidney. Interestingly, the liver cannot use ketone bodies for its own energy needs; instead, they are exported to the bloodstream and distributed throughout the body. Unlike fatty acids, these small molecules easily pass the blood-brain barrier and are readily taken up and utilized as energy by most normal neurons. In fact, after a short period of adaptation, ketones can supply up to 70 percent of the brain's energy needs. But even in the presence of ketones, tumor tissue must remain reliant on glucose and glutamine, most likely because abnormalities in the number, structure, and function of cancer cell mitochondria prevent tumor cells from efficiently metabolizing this alternative energy source. (After all, our evolutionary adaptations to starvation states did not include activities unrelated to survival, such as feeding cancer cells!)

Research suggests that ketones may also help to slow cancer progression for reasons unrelated to their ability to meet energy needs, including their favorable influence on genetic expression in a number of cancer-promoting and cancer-inhibiting pathways. For example, ketones help in the reduction of inflammation, yet another example of an adaptation that doesn't favor cancer cell survival.

As I mentioned earlier, the shift to ketosis impacts cancer cell metabolism and compromises cancer cell function (including the generation of energy), leaving them more vulnerable to therapies that put even more pressure on their faulty metabolism. Keeping protein intake low but adequate limits the amount of excess amino acids that can be converted to glucose through gluconeogenesis or utilized directly for energy. (Much more on that in chapter 12, "Rein in Your Protein," page 199).

Maintaining low levels of protein intake also beneficially inhibits a metabolic pathway known as the mammalian (or more recently, "mechanistic") target of rapamycin, abbreviated as mTOR. Bodybuilders like activity in this pathway because it's associated with building muscle mass. Unfortunately, mTOR is overactive in most cancers, where instead of stimulating the synthesis of muscle it stimulates the rapid growth and proliferation of cancer cells. Reining in protein intake slows activity in this pathway. Downregulating mTOR by restricting protein has been identified as a nutritional strategy in managing cancer.

Genetic expression in other pathways, even those with mutations, is altered by the presence of ketones as well. They include (but certainly aren't limited to) the inhibition of:

- vascular endothelial growth factor (VEGF)
- epithelial growth factor receptor (EGFR)
- histone deacetylase (HDAC)
- angiogenesis

Simultaneously, there are also epigenetic changes in the pathways associated with improved cellular health, such as SIRT1, AMPK, and P13K. The net effect can be a slowdown in cancer progression. Who wouldn't appreciate the value of altering gene expression, especially since that is one of the goals of "targeted therapies"? Unfortunately, these therapies usually target only a single pathway, and let's not forget that they all have side effects. (I'm not suggesting that you abandon all consideration of these drugs—but I do want to make you aware of some of their limitations.)

## Nutritional versus Therapeutic Ketosis

Nutritional ketosis is generally defined as a metabolic state in which the ketone body βHB is present in the blood at a level between 0.5 and 5.0 mmol/L.[9] This represents the body's normal physiological response to a very-low-carbohydrate diet. If levels drop below this threshold, people are no longer in a ketogenic state. Levels above 5.0 mmol/L are not usually seen in adults except during fasting, intense exercise, or ketone supplementation in keto-adapted individuals.

Recently nutritional ketosis has worked its way from the research on metabolic health and human performance into the keto blogosphere. In my opinion, this has a downside: Too many people believe that you can reap all the benefits of ketosis without having to make significant dietary changes by simply adding a ketone supplement that boosts blood levels of βHB to that 0.5 mmol/L threshold. I urge you *not* to buy into this hype! Although these supplements do provide some benefits, an extremely important part of your keto-for-cancer plan is the elimination of sugars and other sources of easily digestible carbohydrates.

If you've read any of Dr. Seyfried's work or have heard anecdotes based on his research, you may already have encountered these terms: therapeutic ketosis, therapeutic zone, and glucose ketone index (GKI). Therapeutic ketosis describes the use of diet for cancer with the goal of maintaining high levels of ketones (greater than 3 mmol/L). Research has yet to confirm if even higher levels of ketones, such as those that may be reached through ketone supplementation, may be therapeutic as an adjunct therapy in cancer or in neurodegenerative diseases.

Dr. Seyfried and his colleagues have outlined a way to assess the likelihood that glucose and ketone levels are in a proportion (or index) that he defines as "the therapeutic zone." Details on calculating and monitoring this are included in chapter 16 ("Monitoring Your Glucose Ketone Index (GKI)," page 306). For now, it's enough to know you may gain the most therapeutic benefit when blood levels of glucose and ketones are roughly equal to one another. But as is true with all therapies, there are many exceptions to the rule, and I view the GKI as a movable target that should be personalized to meet each person's unique needs and circumstances.

## Beyond the Basic Science

I just presented a simplified explanation of how keto diets "starve" cancer of glucose and insulin while providing ketones to healthy cells as an alternative energy source. That's an important first step in understanding why the ketogenic diet for cancer caught the eye of cancer researchers, and maybe that's all you're ready for right now. But as I mentioned earlier, the diet's full impact on cancer can't be explained in such simple terms. In order to read about and understand the science behind ketogenic metabolic therapy, you will first need a basic framework that describes mitochondrial energy production. Assuming that very few of you have had much, if any, exposure to cellular biology—cellular energy metabolism in particular—I will try to break down this heady topic into bite-sized pieces. In addition, check the resources section for where to find more information, including diagrams and lectures that will aid in your understanding of energy metabolism.

## Cellular Energy Production

If you've already left the simplistic "starve cancer" in the dust and begun to dig deeper into the more sophisticated science behind the ketogenic diet, you have come face to face with phrases like "inhibits mTOR," or "upregulates AMPK" or "reduces markers of inflammation." What I present here is somewhere between these two extremes. Please know that you don't need to understand why it works in order to adopt the diet any more than you need to know how your computer translates digital information in order to send an email. But I'm hopeful that you are interested in what you might get out of a quick read of the simplified science that I present here. After all, why not meet the major players, particularly those that are intricately tied to the ketogenic metabolic management of cancer? These key terms and concepts keep popping up in the literature, and they'll soon begin to make a lot more sense if you can first develop your foundational knowledge.

So let's start our mini science lesson with the simple cell. Human cells are varied in appearance. Muscle cells, for example, bear little resemblance to liver cells or red blood cells. Even so, all of the cells in the human body are made up of the same basic parts; they're just organized differently to meet some very specialized requirements. Each cell contains a nucleus as well as a number of other very specialized organelles (literally, "small organs") that are suspended in the cytoplasm of the cell. The cytoplasm is more than just a fluid bath—it is also the site for certain metabolic activities, such as glycolysis.

## Old Habits Die Hard

Science evolves quickly, but the practice of medicine—and nutrition—lags behind by decades. This is unfortunate, but understandable given human nature. Imagine how hard it is for people who have spent a lifetime building a reputation for excellence in their field to encounter a new finding that doesn't fit neatly into the framework of their beliefs. As an example, even the most recent editions of the premier textbooks for graduate-level nutrition courses persist in viewing ketosis as either an adaptation to starvation or an aberrant and dangerous medical condition (diabetic ketoacidosis). At most, these books may offer a sidebar on low-carbohydrate diets, but the editors of these textbooks have yet to incorporate all the new information into the main body of their work.

In my view, the real tragedy is that these textbooks are being used to educate the next generation of nutrition specialists, women and men who are likely to become clinicians in conventional care settings. It's painful to watch the old guard go to such extremes to protect their turf. Even worse, this failure to incorporate new findings is anti-science and counterproductive to the advancement of ideas that may help us more effectively address current epidemics of many chronic diseases, including cancer.

I experienced this first-hand during my own nutrition education. My undergraduate nutrition classes adhered to the "balanced diet" dogma. Even at the graduate level I was still taking quizzes with questions such as "True or False: Glucose is the primary [or 'only'] source of energy for the brain and central nervous system." Of course I had to answer "true," even though I knew this wasn't the correct answer. After all, I had this amazing little guy at my side who was living proof that brains, even damaged ones like his, could thrive on ketones.

Although most of my peers and instructors never got on board, a few of my professors were bright critical thinkers who were open to what I brought to the table. I've often wondered if the information I shared with them changed what they taught to the next wave of students.

Included among the organelles are the mitochondria—powerhouses of the cells where the bulk of cellular energy is generated. Mitochondria are exquisitely adapted to their role as the primary energy producers, but they perform other vital functions as well, such as controlling programmed cell death (apoptosis) and sending and receiving messages to and from the nucleus. This signaling function is essential to the health and longevity of the cell (and is absent in cells without mitochondria, such as red blood cells, which have a short life span). The prevailing theory is that long ago mitochondria originated as the result of a single event in which a bacterium was engulfed by another bacterium. The two organisms entered into a symbiotic relationship in which the engulfed organism surrendered its autonomy in exchange for protection and nourishment by its "host" cell. That theory is supported by the fact that mitochondria have retained a portion of their own original DNA, an abbreviated set of genetic instructions that allow them to repair and multiply independent of instructions from nuclear DNA. To keep it clean and simple, mitochondrial DNA is passed down only on the maternal side.

Now let's look at two of the most important energy-producing pathways.

## Glycolysis

In chapter 1 you learned about glycolysis as it relates to the Warburg effect, the phenomenon of cancer cells increasing their rate of glucose fermentation even when oxygen is available. By this point you may understandably be thinking that glycolysis is a horrible thing. But let me stress here that it's not glycolysis itself but rather the increase in fermentation *even in the presence of oxygen* that is the problem in cancer.

Normal glycolysis is *anaerobic* (meaning no oxygen is involved), and the glucose involved in normal glycolysis is not usually fermented. Instead, it's prepared for further metabolism (referred to as *oxidation*) within the mitochondria of the cell. This produces energy along with water and carbon dioxide as the end products. Glycolysis in normal cells starts with the transport of glucose (derived either from digestion or from gluconeogenesis) to cells via the bloodstream. Meanwhile, insulin facilitates the increased production and selective placement of glucose transporters on cellular membranes to allow glucose to enter the cytoplasm of the cell. But upon entry into the cell, that molecule of glucose can't be utilized immediately for energy. Instead, it must first be cleaved (split in half) by a series of enzymatic reactions in preparation for the real work that needs to be done.

Two of the early steps in glycolysis require energy. This is provided in the form of two molecules of adenosine *tri*phosphate (ATP). (ATP molecules are often referred to as "the currency of energy" because they store energy in the form of phosphate groups that can be used to power cellular activities.) In glycolysis, two molecules of ATP each give up one of their phosphate groups, which reduces them to molecules of adenosine *di*phosphate (ADP). In essence, the "tri" in *tri*phosphate is reduced to the "di" in *di*phosphate.

In the next series of reactions, four ADP molecules each *gain* a phosphate group, to yield a total of four ATP molecules. So, four ATP in the "plus" column minus the two ATP used in the "minus" column results in a net gain of two ATP molecules. In addition to the energy produced through the net gain of ATP molecules, each molecule of glucose has now been converted to two molecules of pyruvate. (Are you still with me? If not, that's OK. You can always come back to this later.)

The act of glycolysis also "recycles" nicotinamide adenine dinucleotide hydride (NADH), a very important molecule. NADH is a coenzyme, a class of small molecules that help enzymes do their job. The "H" in NADH represents a

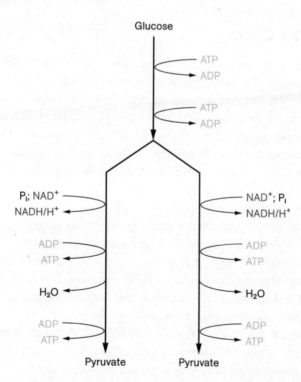

**Figure 3.4.** Glycolysis. The conversion of glucose to pyruvate in the cytoplasm of the cell.

positively charged atom of hydrogen, also known as a proton. Protons are crucial to the process of bonding the phosphate group that converts ADP to ATP.

In a normal cell, a small portion of pyruvate stays in the cytoplasm and is quickly fermented to lactate (a form of lactic acid). But the bulk of this newly formed pyruvate has a different fate: It's transported into the mitochondria, the cellular energy powerhouses, where it undergoes an incredibly complex series of reactions that yield 15 times the energy that was produced by glycolysis in the cytoplasm. This means that for each single molecule of glucose that enters the cell, mitochondrial activities are able to produce at least 32 molecules of ATP, compared to merely the 2 molecules of ATP that were generated in the cytoplasm. Considering that each of the overwhelming majority of cells in your body has anywhere from dozens to thousands of mitochondria, you can begin to appreciate how much energy can be produced. (Recall from earlier in this chapter that unlike normal cells, cancer cells ferment glucose in the cytoplasm; in other words, much of the pyruvate formed from glycolysis remains in the cytoplasm, where it undergoes fermentation into lactic acid.)

## The Krebs Cycle

The Krebs cycle has many functions, but for now let's focus on its role in producing energy. The cycle begins when pyruvate (the molecule produced during glycolysis), fatty acids (from the breakdown of fats), or ketone bodies (from biosynthesis or exogenous sources) cross the mitochondrial membranes and enter the mitochondrial matrix, where each can be converted to molecules of acetyl-CoA. In the first official step of the Krebs cycle, each molecule of acetyl-CoA combines with a molecule of oxaloacetate (an organic compound) to form a molecule of citrate.

Those of you with a biochemistry background may already know that acetyl-CoA delivers a high-energy acetyl group to the Krebs cycle. The first step in the cycle combines acetyl-CoA with oxaloacetate to form citrate. Successive steps generate energy, release $CO_2$, and recycle intermediates that can then serve as electron donors in the electron transport chain. But don't worry if you're not at this level of understanding. As I said, my intent is to expose you to the process, not to overwhelm you with details.

Each reaction in the cycle flows smoothly into the next, with little net change in the number of ATP molecules. What's more important is that Krebs cycle intermediates, those compounds needed to sustain the reactions, are regenerated with each turn of the cycle. Another important activity is the *reduction* (gain of an electron) of $NAD^+$ to form NADH, the "electron donor"

## Cellular Respiration

The mitochondrial process of creating energy in the form of ATP molecules, referred to as *cellular respiration*, starts with a merry-go-round of reactions that go by various names, all referring to the same process:

- citric acid cycle
- tricarboxylic acid (TCA) cycle
- Krebs cycle (after Hans Krebs, the scientist who first described it)

For simplicity's sake, I'll use the term Krebs cycle throughout this book. (To fully appreciate why the process is called a "cycle," take a look at the diagram in figure 3.5.)

Another component of cellular respiration, also found in the mitochondria, is the *electron transport chain*. The two processes in combination comprise a system that is exquisitely efficient at creating energy.

Overwhelmed? So was I. It's my intent to provide a simplified explanation of an extremely complex process. Figure 3.5 shows a basic schematic illustrating the relationship between the two processes, but please be assured that this is for reference only. There is no expectation that you understand every chemical reaction!

you were introduced to in glycolysis. Another key proton donor, flavin adenine dinucleotide (FAD), also gains an electron in the Krebs cycle, converting it to $FADH_2$. Now take a few deep breaths as we move on to the final phase of mitochondrial energy production.

# The Electron Transport Chain

The electron transport chain is where the bulk of energy production actually takes place: The positively charged protons generated during the Krebs cycle are pushed from the mitochondrial matrix into the intermembrane space (an area between the mitochondrion's two membranes), while the electrons remain in the interior. The result is a buildup of a positive charge (proton gradient) in the inner membrane space. This difference in electrical charge across

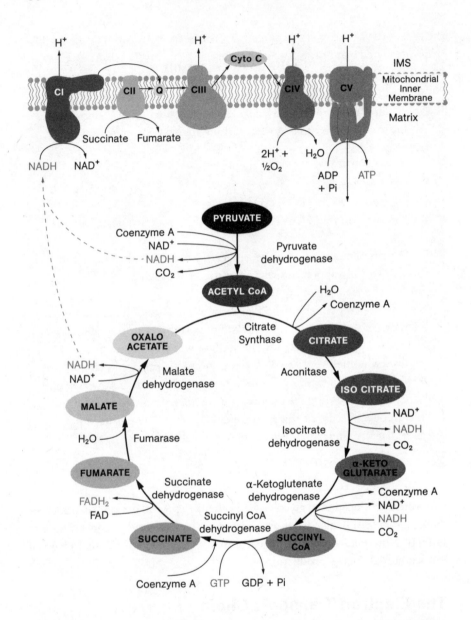

**Figure 3.5.** Mitochondrial Energy Production: The Krebs Cycle and the Electron Transport Chain. The lower portion of the diagram depicts the enzymatic reactions of the Krebs cycle. The upper portion shows the components and energy-generating activities of the electron transport chain. This simplified diagram shows pyruvate (derived from glucose) as the sole precursor of acetyl-CoA. However, fatty acids, ketones, and even some amino acids can also undergo conversion to acetyl-CoA. No matter the source, all acetyl-CoA enters the first step of the Krebs cycle.

the inner membrane of the mitochondrion is instrumental in causing the flow of positively charged protons back into the matrix. But to do this, they must pass through special protein pores in the membrane that act like tiny turnstiles. Each click of the turnstile (actually, ATP synthase) uses the force of the proton's movement to attach a phosphate to a molecule of ADP, thus forming a molecule of ATP. Oxygen ($O_2$) in the matrix combines with the protons (as hydrogen) to form water ($H_2O$). How amazing is that!

As noted previously, this is just a quick overview of what is actually an incredibly complex process. If it's any comfort to you, only a tiny percentage of the people on this planet really understand the intricacies of this system (and I'm not one of them). The two critical takeaways: (1) The electron transport chain is where the majority of the energy is produced, and (2) this process can get very messy. Moving electrons around has fallout in the form of highly reactive molecules that can damage the cell. In cancer, we've got a problem when those molecules are oxygen, in the form of ROS.

Mitochondria have had eons of experience in dealing with these highly reactive molecules, and healthy mitochondria produce enough of their own antioxidants to quench free radicals. In cancer, as in many other metabolic diseases, inefficiencies in the system, including electron leakage, result in the production of more ROS than the mitochondria can effectively manage. Unfortunately, fermentation makes cancer cells more tolerant of ROS, creating chaos not only within the cell but system-wide. According to Dr. Seyfried, diminishing the availability of fermentable fuels removes the cancer cells' protective antioxidant shield, making them more vulnerable to therapies that induce oxidative metabolic stress.

I hope you learned something from this quick tour. I invite you to revisit these pages as you develop your framework to better understand ketogenic metabolic management. For those of you who want to dive even deeper into the science, I highly recommend a series of online lectures developed by medical student and engaging speaker Andrey Kopot (www.aklectures.com/subject/biochemistry).

# CHAPTER 4

# Is the Ketogenic Diet Right for You?

The good news is that most people *can* adopt a ketogenic diet! At first it may seem quite overwhelming, and you may have no idea what you can eat. Let me simplify it for you:

1. Cook up some meat, chicken, fish, or eggs.
2. Make a salad and/or prepare some delicious non-starchy vegetables.
3. Include condiments, grated cheese, and flavorful seasonings and spices.
4. Do you have some favorite nuts or nut butters? We can certainly work with that!
5. Add fat. Lots of it! Choose healthy fats, and ditch the inflammatory oils.
6. Repeat three times a day.

That's it. Don't overthink this. If you enjoy salmon and asparagus, or beef and broccoli, then you're all set. Here's the catch (you *knew* there would be one!): To reach ketosis, you will be eliminating a lot of the foods that are probably staples in your current diet. Out goes sugar in any of its forms, both obvious (in cookies) and sneaky (in canned tomato sauce). You'll also give up those inflammatory grains—in fact, I encourage everyone, keto or not, to rid their diets of wheat, corn, and oats. Eliminate starchy vegetables. This means potatoes, of course, but also sweet potatoes and cooked carrots. Keto diets do not include legumes or much in the way of fruits. Dairy fats (butter, ghee, heavy cream) can be part of the plan, but some dairy products, such as milk, are out; others, such as hard cheeses, can be enjoyed in small amounts. And of course you'll be eating plenty of good, healthy fats. That's the basic plan. So read on if you're willing to make these changes.

## Considering Contraindications

Before you commit to a ketogenic diet, it's essential that you look objectively at your current situation and weigh its possible benefits against potential risks. Let's look at some of the most common exclusions and limitations. It's a small but important list: In fact, it consists mainly of genetic disorders that would interfere with your body's ability to utilize fats as fuel. Because these disorders cause major problems very early in life, it's very unlikely that you would have reached adulthood without a diagnosis. A more complete description of these conditions can be found in the book *The Ketogenic and Modified Atkins Diets*, coauthored by the ketogenic diet team at Johns Hopkins Hospital.[1] If you know that you have one of these genetic disorders, you should definitely NOT begin this diet:

- a primary (i.e., inborn, not acquired) carnitine deficiency
- a fatty acid oxidation pathway defect
- pyruvate carboxylase deficiency
- porphyria (usually inherited, but possibly acquired)

The following list of "relative contraindications" is much broader, and if one or more of these apply to you and you decide to proceed with the diet anyway, you may require specialized medical and nutritional oversight. In other words, you may still be able to implement the diet, but it's essential that you have a supportive and readily available keto-savvy team before you begin. Here they are:

1. You are currently either pregnant or lactating.
2. You are considering implementing this diet for a child.
3. You are unable or unwilling to restrict alcohol intake until after you are keto adapted.
4. You have:
   - either primary or metastatic liver cancer
   - elevated liver enzymes (high enough to suggest liver damage)
   - a history of a surgery that affects the structure or function of your gastrointestinal tract (e.g., esophageal surgery, a Whipple procedure)
   - type 1 diabetes
   - type 2 diabetes that is poorly controlled or for which you take a medication that puts you at high risk for ketoacidosis (e.g., an SGLT2 inhibitor, such as canagliflozin [Invokana])

- a history of gastric bypass surgery (or currently have a lap band)
- intractable constipation as a side effect of painkillers (opiates)
- difficulty swallowing
- slowed gastrointestinal motility due to neurological impairment or neurodegenerative disease
- gallbladder obstruction or a history of pancreatitis
- heart disease (including an elongated QT interval or a rhythm disorder)
- renal disease
- short bowel syndrome
- cachexia due to cancer (which needs intense management)
- red flags in your bloodwork (high or low values) that suggest underlying metabolic issues or impaired immune function

It's often difficult to predict if the challenges you're facing are just a bump in the road or significant enough to stop you in your tracks. Be realistic in the assessment of your situation and seek medical advice from members of your team.

Understand that some people experience only mild side effects from chemotherapy or other anticancer treatments, while others have difficulty coping with nausea, vomiting, or diarrhea. On its own, a chronic bowel disease (such as Crohn's disease or ulcerative colitis) won't prevent you from starting the diet, but if your symptoms are not well controlled, or if the only way you can get through the day is with a bland diet of easily digestible carbohydrates, then you may want to rethink moving to keto right now. On the other hand, if your only gastrointestinal symptom is uncomplicated gastroesophageal reflux disease (GERD), then you may be happy to learn that this may improve with a ketogenic diet (despite the frequently given advice that cutting out fatty foods will improve your GERD symptoms).

Other health issues, such as kidney stones or gout, usually don't preclude embarking on a ketogenic diet, though you should work closely with a practitioner who can monitor both symptoms and treatment (if any is needed). If you do have a personal or family history of kidney stones, discuss prophylactics (such as potassium citrate) with your doctor before you start the diet. For those of you without a gallbladder, it may ease your mind to know that you certainly can adopt a ketogenic diet. All of these issues are discussed in more detail in chapter 15 ("Challenges Introduced by Other Chronic Diseases," page 277).

In some cases medications may need to be monitored or adjusted. Examples include drugs used to treat high blood pressure (including diuretics), diabetes drugs (including those noted previously), steroids used to control inflammation (such as prednisone or dexamethasone), and opiates used for pain relief (such as hydrocodone or fentanyl). Hormones used to treat thyroid disease may cause a rise in morning glucose levels, and some people prefer to switch to overnight dosing. But as with all medications, talk to your doctor before you make any changes.

If you currently have malabsorption problems, or you have little to no appetite, those issues should be addressed by your team before implementing a ketogenic diet. Also, if you are on the path to recovery but are still at too low a weight, or at risk of losing weight because of known side effects of your treatment, then you must be followed closely by a clinical nutritionist. (Expect to hear that you need to eat a "balanced diet" or drink "nutritional" shakes to increase your calories using easily digestible carbs.) Under these circumstances, you should first gradually increase your intake of fats while simultaneously removing foods with added sugars. If you can hold your weight steady, then you may be able to slowly transition to a ketogenic diet over a period of several weeks. Again, it's best to do this with guidance—preferably from a keto-savvy nutrition specialist.

On its own, use of a feeding tube is not a strong enough reason to dismiss the diet. There are commercially available keto formulas, but many people who have tubes prefer to blenderize their meals instead. In fact, it's often easier to keep to your targets this way; meals can be prepared in batches well in advance, then frozen for future use. I cover this option in chapter 15 ("Blender Ketogenic Diets," page 287).

Unfortunately, disease progression can make it very difficult to lower your blood glucose levels. A large tumor load produces a lot of lactic acid, which contributes to the worsening of disease. Remember, too, that lactate is converted by the liver and sent back out into the bloodstream as glucose. Disease in the liver itself can also directly and indirectly interfere with the many metabolic pathways, such as gluconeogenesis, that are controlled by this organ.

Vigorous exercise is not recommended during the early weeks of the diet. It's best to become keto-adapted first so you can run on ketones instead of glucose. For more information read chapter 17 ("The Benefits of Moderate Exercise," page 315).

Even if you're a good candidate and decide to commit to the diet, there is no guarantee that you'll be able to lower your blood glucose levels to the therapeutic zone described in chapter 3. That said, please understand that even if you can't reach your intended goal, blood glucose that is *lower* and *steadier* than it was before you adopted a ketogenic diet is still an improvement over continuing with a diet that repeatedly causes spikes in your glucose and insulin levels.

I can't emphasize enough what a deleterious effect inflammation or injury has on blood glucose levels, whether caused by cancer or its treatment. The same goes for external stressors, such as poor sleep, fatigue, anxiety, or feeling overwhelmed by what's happening in your life. All of these can lead to a rise in your stress hormone levels, which in turn stimulates your liver to make new glucose. Take a look at chapter 17 ("Reduce Stress!," page 311) for some advice about how to cope.

## Commitment to the Ketogenic Diet

Far and away the most common reasons people find themselves unable to continue with the ketogenic are not due to any problem with the diet itself, but rather due to either a physical or logistical challenge. These can be grouped together under labels such as side effects of cancer treatment (typically nausea, vomiting, constipation, diarrhea, loss of appetite) or quality of life issues (fatigue, depression, loss of hope, financial worries), or physical or logistical limitations (lack of support, challenges in acquiring keto foods, limited ability to prepare meals, cognitive impairments).

Be prepared to experience "keto flu" (a treatable malaise). Also understand that you may feel deprived in giving up foods that aren't part of the keto plan, or experience tolerance issues as you begin to increase the amount of fats and oils. If you don't understand the basic science behind the diet, you may be vulnerable to pseudoscience that compromises your commitment to the diet by promising a cure. Also, not having enough resources to create new and interesting meals can lead to boredom with the plan. Lastly, it can be very challenging to stick to a keto diet if you have a history of eating disorders or if you rely on carbohydrate-laden comfort foods during stressful times.

A cancer diagnosis overflows into all areas of your life, at least temporarily. You may already be dealing with more than you can handle at home or at work; cancer just adds to the chaos. There are more demands on your time, especially if your treatment is complex or involves downtime for surgeries, and simply managing your appointments takes time and energy. Lucky you if you have a dedicated caregiver as well as support from family and friends.

As I mentioned earlier, there are a few chronic diseases involving the gastrointestinal tract that create obstacles to adopting a high-fat, low-carbohydrate plan. There are also a number of issues that pop up surrounding food allergies, aversions, or intolerances. Self-imposed limitations—veganism, for example—can complicate compliance or compromise nutrition.

Last but certainly not least, you need to look long and hard at your social and emotional circumstances before you begin, as these can also have a huge impact on commitment and adherence. Some of these issues can be dealt with by asking others for help or accepting help that's offered to you. If accepting

## A Special Note for Vegetarians and Vegans

Most keto consultants and coaches will not work with clients who want to keep to a vegetarian or vegan diet. I felt the same way until one of my clients expressed the deep desire to keep to her vegan pattern because of her strong belief that it was unwise to consume any animal products. I agreed to help her with the diet, but I asked her to sign a disclaimer. I wasn't convinced that she could take in all the nutrients she needed without consuming any animal products at all. I also set another condition: She would need to come up with her own meal plans. She rose to the challenge and did amazingly well with her vegan diet for five years, at which point she decided to include some fish in her plan. Now, six years following her cancer diagnosis, she has joined the ranks of the elite group of "long-term survivors" of glioblastoma multiforme, a very aggressive form of brain cancer that carries a median survival of just 14 to 16 months. It's my belief that part of her amazing cancer outcome may be due in part to her minimal protein intake (still adequate given her lean body mass). In my experience, people with brain cancer have better outcomes if they keep protein intake low. I'll go into the possible reasons for that in chapter 12 ("Rein in Your Protein," page 199). With strong support from her husband, my client has done an excellent job of covering all the nutritional bases with little need for supplements (she requires only vitamins $B_{12}$ and $D_3$, choline, and minerals).

All this aside, if you are following a vegan plan for perceived health benefits rather than for ethical reasons, then please reconsider your decision. The ketogenic diet is easier to follow if you don't layer on an additional set of demanding dietary restrictions.

My experience with this client changed the way I view vegan and vegetarian diets. Now when I speak before a group, I make sure to mention vegan (and vegetarian) options, with the caveat that these may not be appropriate for everyone's situation, such as those who are recovering from surgery or treatment, or those with higher than normal protein needs due to greater lean body mass. All things considered, though, if you do choose to remain vegan, understand that your food choices still need to be keto-friendly and that maintaining adequate protein intake while keeping carbs low will require extra work on your part.

help is difficult for you because of your role as "the strong one," then all I can say is, please try to move beyond this. There's no need to go it alone. People want to help, and you can direct them to what you need most. In other words, you can gently guide them away from preparing comfort foods like lasagna or carb-heavy casseroles and let them know that what you *really* need is help with shopping or cleaning or running a few simple errands.

## Make Peace with Your Plan

What if you agree with the science behind the diet and you are almost certain that you want to give this a try but are not quite ready to commit to all these changes? You may ask, is there any benefit to going part of the way; for example, by just eliminating added sugars from the diet? Honestly, while that is certainly a good first step, I doubt that it will make a significant difference as it relates to your disease. Cancer cells don't care where they get their sugar. A heaping serving of potatoes or a glass of orange juice will keep them just as busy as a chocolate bar—maybe even more so! If you can't fully commit to all

### Does "Yeah, But . . . " Sound Familiar?

*"Yeah, but* it's my birthday, and my daughter always bakes me a cake."

Think about this. Is the tradition more important to you or to your daughter than your life? Let me make clear that "yeah, but" thinking isn't fixed by finding a replacement in the treasure trove of low-carb substitutes for traditional carb-centric goodies. Instead, look forward to forging new family traditions for birthdays and other celebrations. In our family, we chose experiences—such as a soak at our favorite hot springs—over food.

Here's another one that I hear way too often: *"Yeah, but* my husband/kids would be lost without potato chips." The real issue here is why you believe you need to keep these foods in your home when they could easily sabotage your efforts. Your spouse can keep snacks at work or elsewhere, and your kids will find plenty of opportunities to score poor-quality foods outside your home. Instead, take pleasure in the knowledge that you are modeling healthy habits and that everyone will benefit from the new foods you stock in your cupboard and fridge.

the changes required of a ketogenic diet, then yes, clean up your diet by eliminating added sugars and refined starches. You may feel so much better that you will then gladly take on the rest of the plan! Another approach, assuming of course that you get rid of sugar and starch, is to add another nutritional strategy, such as traditional calorie restriction or intervals of fasting. (Read more about these options in chapter 7.)

The bottom line is that if you believe that you can commit to a ketogenic diet for at least three weeks—enough time for most people to get up to speed with the changes—then it's time to get started. But if you can't keep the "yeah, but" out of the story you tell yourself, even for just a few short weeks, then don't give the diet another thought, as you have already put up a barrier between you and any chance for success with this intervention.

## A Word to Caregivers

You caregivers are on the front line. You're already doing a million and one things for your loved one, so it's only natural that adding yet another change,

### Is Your Loved One on Board with These Changes?

A while back I read a series of online posts written by a woman who adopted a ketogenic diet at the urging of both her doctor and her husband. As I scanned her blog, I realized she had never personally embraced the diet and was following it simply to please others. Her posts were filled with details of her "cheats and sneaks," how she missed the sweets that were part of her social life, and how sad it made her feel to pass up sandwiches and settle for salads. I wish I could have reached out and told her that she was free to eat what she wanted, with no guilt.

I get many requests for guidance from caregivers, family, and friends of people with cancer. My first and most important question is always the same: "Is your loved one on board with these changes?" At times I've been asked to convince a loved one to adopt the diet. I gently explain that my role is to educate, not coerce. So even if you are sure that your loved one is making a mistake by not embracing the diet, please respect that decision and continue to provide your love and support in all the other ways you can.

especially a complete dietary overhaul, may seem overwhelming. Sit back and take a breath. I offer you the same advice that I do to people going it alone: Take it one step at a time. Moving forward with these changes at a sustainable pace is more likely to lead to success than piling on the workload to the point that you are too physically and mentally exhausted to meet even the basic needs of your loved one. Bring this up with the oncology team. They can direct you to a number of social services that can lighten your load.

At the other end of the caregiving continuum, recognize that even if you are personally sold on the ketogenic diet, and are ready and willing to help with all aspects of meal planning and preparation, your loved one may not be equally enthusiastic. Remember, this diet must be *their* choice, not *yours*! When they are in control, their commitment will be stronger and they will be better equipped to weather the transition than if they feel pressured into complying simply to make you happy.

## When the Person with Cancer Is Your Child

My personal experience with adopting this diet for my son has made me a passionate advocate of implementing the diet for children, although not without significant caveats. There are certainly many childhood cancers—such as brain tumors, neuroblastoma, and Ewing's sarcoma—that are well suited for *adjuvant* ketogenic diet therapy. (As a reminder, adjuvant means that the diet would be implemented alongside a standard oncology protocol.) Some parents are reluctant to bring up the subject of the ketogenic diet with their child's oncologist, but this is an absolute must, as a rigorous ketogenic diet needs both medical and nutritional oversight. It also needs to be flexible enough to meet your child's changing health and nutrition needs over the long term. Even less rigorous forms of the diet should not be undertaken without support and monitoring. And of course, don't expect perfection—both you and your child will surely make occasional missteps.

There are some situations in which a ketogenic diet may not be an appropriate adjuvant therapy. Treatment protocols that include high doses of corticosteroids given over extended periods of time stimulate the appetite and raise blood glucose. Both factors complicate adherence to the diet and lower the therapeutic potential. Childhood leukemia and other cancers may also involve stem cell treatments that require long hospitalizations under very carefully controlled conditions. I can't imagine any of today's hospitals accommodating a request for a ketogenic diet under these circumstances, as there are specific protocols that need to be followed during treatment and recovery.

## Raffi's Gingerbread House

Raffi was constantly confronting challenges, sometimes from unexpected places. One Christmas season his physical therapist decided it would be a great idea for him to make a gingerbread house. Knowing the limitations of his diet, did she choose cardboard and papier-mâché? No, she kept it authentic: gingerbread, frosting, and a variety of sugary treats for added "curb appeal."

Raffi was rightfully proud of his creation, and I was caught between a rock and a hard place. How could I take his work of art away from him? Somehow I deluded myself into thinking that our long talk about how to sidestep temptation would keep him on the straight and narrow for a day or two, after which time I could move the house to the mantle and out of reach. Of course I was wrong, and my poor kid ended up consuming a sizable portion. I'm sure it did no permanent harm, but I was very upset by how badly Raffi felt about this lapse—as though it was a failure on his part. I knew differently and reassured him that we all make mistakes. Live and learn.

## Another Dietary Therapy: Intermittent Fasting

In 2016 a group of researchers at the University of Texas Southwestern Medical Center published the results of a study using mice with various types of leukemia to look at the effect of several dietary restriction patterns on the course of their disease.[2] In the mouse model of acute lymphoblastic leukemia (ALL), the mice that underwent six cycles of intermittent fasting (fasted one day and fed the next) showed very few remaining cancerous cells at seven weeks. And, as expected, the disease progressed in the well-fed "controls" (mice with ALL that were fed normally). It takes some effort to work through the dense science in this paper, which was published in the journal *Nature Medicine*, but you can read the highlights in a press release posted on the web-based medical news service Medical Xpress (www.medicalxpress.com).[3] Granted, this is preclinical data, but it gives a boost to those who believe as I do that *diet does matter*.

In working with parents implementing this diet for their sick child, I've found that one of the biggest challenges parents have is getting beyond the feeling that they are depriving the child of foods or food traditions they clearly enjoy. Plus, as a parent, you want your child's life to feel as normal as possible. After all, didn't life already make a massive and devastating shift at the moment of diagnosis?

Years ago one mom told me that even if a ketogenic diet might help her young teen with medulloblastoma, she would be reluctant to make this change. In her words, how could she deny her daughter her favorite ice cream for breakfast? Now, because there are a lot of very keto-friendly treats to help get kids on board with the diet, families no longer have to make such tough choices. In the years since that mom expressed her reluctance to change her daughter's diet, I've worked with many families facing a myriad of challenges, and I'm so glad there are now more tools in the toolbox. Of course, I like to see that dependence on sweet treats lessen over time—in both children *and* adults—but let's use a few "training wheels" (see below) to get kids and families started down the right track.

These days when I am working with a child, my first step is to find out what foods or situations are going to need those training wheels. Creating special replacement foods has other benefits as well: These treats are a perfect way to introduce high-fat foods into the diet before pulling out the carbohydrates,

## The MaxLove Project

I urge parents of children with cancer to connect with the MaxLove Project, a volunteer-based advocacy group for families with children facing a myriad of life-threatening illnesses. Cofounders Audra DiPadova and Justin Wilford, Max's parents, are strong advocates for healthy, whole-food diets, including keto. Audra is a trained culinary artist, and she has created some amazing kid- and keto-friendly meals that she shares on the MaxLove Project website and Facebook page. Their materials use positive language when discussing the changes required by the diet with families: "Who *wouldn't* want delicious keto ice cream or yummy strawberry cupcakes with buttercream frosting for breakfast? Use those foods like training wheels." What a great analogy! Siblings can be drawn into being more supportive here, too, if these new sugar-free treats are to become a part of everyone's day.

which helps limit the amount of weight loss often seen when making a more rapid shift to ketosis.

Now let's turn to one of the greatest challenges facing families: teenagers. As many parents of teens already know, adolescents present their own unique set of challenges that will undoubtedly affect their adherence to a ketogenic diet. Moving toward independence often means preferring to hang out with friends instead of family, which translates to spending less time under your watchful eye. Work with them. You might be surprised to learn that they are quite content to slide the topping of a slice of pizza onto a plate and toss the crust if that means they can join their friends for a night out. Of course, fast-food pizza is far from an ideal meal, but you are not looking for perfection here. Help keep them accountable for their choices by using objective measures, such as ketone blood testing. Be careful here—you don't want to become known as the food police. Instead, use every opportunity either to congratulate them on their good choices or to suggest ways they might want to handle a similar situation in the future. Keep your language positive, as this will keep the family stress level from climbing when you are dealing with a lapse.

If you are parenting a child with cancer, it might help you to view the decision to start your child on the ketogenic diet just as you would any of the other decisions you make on their behalf. For example, would you let your child opt

## My Doctor Says the Diet Is "Too Difficult"

Too often, one of Raffi's doctors told me that, even though we were able to pull off this miracle for our son, the diet is "too difficult" for most people to undertake. Let me assure you, the diet is a *walk in the park* compared to what my son was forced to endure from the moment of his diagnosis. My response to this kind of flawed thinking is this: "No, the diet wasn't difficult. What was difficult was sitting in the waiting room while Raffi was in surgery and not knowing what we would be left with at the end of the day."

So, despite what you might hear from those who aren't living in your personal hell, if you want to give it a trial, you get to decide for yourself: "too difficult" or that breath of fresh air that your family so desperately needs? Make it *your* choice.

out of a surgery even if it was clearly necessary? Certainly not. Of course, you should always discuss any change in diet with your child's medical team. Listen carefully to what they say as well as what they don't say, and read between the lines. Remember: Conventional oncologists are not taught nutrition in medical school, so it's not a foundational consideration for most of them. Seek input from integrative practitioners whenever possible; they'll undoubtedly be more open to the idea of a therapeutic diet. If the only resistance to making these changes is the oncologist's own perception that the diet is too difficult, remember that they haven't walked in your shoes, so they can't truly comprehend what "difficult" means.

## The Power—and Responsibility—of Shared Decision-Making

Is your health care team willing to engage in what the American Cancer Society defines as shared decision-making?[4] In this model, your care provider fully involves you in the decision process by sharing information about treatment options (including what to expect if you elect no treatment) and fully informs about the likely immediate and long-term side effects of any suggested treatment. In turn, you inform the provider about your preferences and concerns and are free to ask any and all questions you may have. You may even request copies of research papers or results from clinical trials that have guided your doctor's recommendations. This is especially important if there is no clear consensus or guideline for "best practice" for your cancer. You and your doctor then arrive at a plan together. This is more empowering for you, but also requires that you assume personal responsibility for the decision, no matter the outcome. (Incidentally, I highly recommend that you obtain a second opinion outside of the network that employs your primary oncologist.)

You may believe that you have little choice in such decisions. Too often I hear comments like these:

"My doctor won't allow me . . ."
"I was told that I can't . . ."
"I have to . . ."

In fact, no doctor can prohibit you from making lifestyle changes or force you to receive treatment against your will. Seek care from those who support you in your personal journey toward better health. Learn what to expect from your

(continued on page 54)

## Common Questions and Concerns about the Diet

When I first meet with a client, I expect to be asked a lot of questions. Many of these are specific to the individual situation, but there are a few that come up in almost every conversation. Let's spend a moment addressing the most common questions and concerns.

### Q: MY DOCTOR SAYS, "DIET DOESN'T MATTER; EAT WHAT YOU WANT."

It is distressing that conventional medical training offers virtually no education in nutrition. Instead, oncologists rely on standard diet dogma. A prime example: The recently updated US Dietary Guidelines for 2015–2020 (published jointly by the US Department of Health and Human Services and the US Department of Agriculture) suggest we "limit added sugars to less than 10 percent of calories per day" (the equivalent of about 12 teaspoons of table sugar). These added sugars are above and beyond the sugars already found in the grains, starches, fruits, and milk that make up over half of the standard diet in the United States. If you believe that this amount of sugar is part of a healthy diet, then you shouldn't waste your time reading this book!

### Q: MY DOCTOR DOESN'T WANT ME TO LOSE WEIGHT.

Weight loss in people with cancer may be due to disease progression, side effects of chemotherapy drugs, or some other combination of conditions that erode health. Unintended weight loss is a red flag that is often associated with poorer outcomes. Your doctor may also be concerned about cancer cachexia (wasting syndrome). However, if you are at or above a normal weight and have other characteristics of a good candidate for a ketogenic diet, then some weight loss in the context of a well-planned diet may allow for quicker keto-adaptation and potentially better disease management. Track your weight and consult with a keto-savvy nutrition specialist. (Again, oversight is essential if you are nutritionally compromised!)

### Q: WHAT IS "KETO-ADAPTATION"?

Before you can begin to reap the benefits of ketosis, your body must adapt to the series of metabolic changes that accompany a sustained shift to ketosis. These changes include an increase in the production of enzymes needed to metabolize fats and ketones, along with an increase in the number of transporters needed to move ketones across cellular membranes. Other changes include those that help maintain glucose homeostasis—switching from dependence on insulin and glucagon to other signaling mechanisms that act primarily to stimulate glucose production by the liver. Ketosis happens within days, whereas keto-adaptation takes weeks to months.

Dr. Jeff Volek, an expert in the field of low-carb nutrition, has written and lectured extensively on this topic. You may want to view a video of his 2013 presentation at the Institute of Human and Machine Cognition. (I've included a link to it in the resources section.) His talk is not specific to cancer, but it will help you get up to speed quickly with what it means to be keto-adapted.

I should point out that becoming keto-adapted does not guarantee that you have overcome all pre-existing metabolic issues. Some, such as insulin resistance, may linger, although it should improve considerably. Other metabolic issues may arise from endocrine disorders that don't respond to ketogenic metabolic therapy, such as problems caused by pituitary tumors.

Q: IS A HIGH-PROTEIN DIET DANGEROUS?

There is no need to ponder this question with regard to the ketogenic diet, since protein intake on this diet is lower than protein intake on a standard diet.

Q: WHO WILL MONITOR MY HEALTH STATUS?

If you are undergoing treatment, your medical care team or naturopathic doctor is already engaged in some form of monitoring, such as blood testing and routine radiographic scans. Ask your team to add a few specific blood tests, such as those for vitamin D and HbA1c (described in chapter 16, "What Laboratory Tests to Order, and Why," page 299). You may also want to monitor immune function, specific tumor markers, and markers of inflammation. If your current team is not on board, ask another health care provider to order these tests.

## Q: WHAT WILL HAPPEN TO MY CHOLESTEROL LEVEL?

First, you need to look at the separate components that make up "cholesterol." A rise in the level of low-density lipoprotein (LDL, also known as the "bad" cholesterol) may occur, but this is often temporary and/or accompanied by a corresponding rise in protective high-density lipoprotein (HDL, the "good" cholesterol). Including more omega-3 oils (such as fish oil) and increasing your fiber intake may help limit the rise in LDL. But should this number even concern you? Most heart disease specialists now acknowledge it is the *oxidation* of LDL—not elevated LDL itself—that leads to chronic inflammation, the primary driver of cardiovascular disease. Well-formulated ketogenic diets reduce inflammation. Ketogenic diets also typically lower triglyceride levels, which may be more indicative of cardiovascular health than LDL.

If you are concerned about your lipid levels, discuss the risks and benefits of the diet with your doctor. Also, ask for a nuclear magnetic resonance (NMR) or other type of advanced lipid test that can distinguish between LDL types (pattern A—larger, lighter particles—and pattern B—smaller, denser particles that are believed to be more atherogenic).

In my opinion, addressing your cancer usually takes precedence over a slight rise in cholesterol!

## Q: I CAN'T AFFORD ORGANIC FOODS, ESPECIALLY MEATS AND DAIRY. ALSO, I CAN'T SPEND A LOT OF TIME PREPARING SPECIAL MEALS. IS THE KETOGENIC DIET STILL AN OPTION FOR ME?

You bet! The first step is commitment to changing your diet pattern by cutting way back on carbohydrates. This will have the intended metabolic effect. Over time, you can improve food choices and learn healthier meal preparation techniques. Remember, you're in it for a lifetime!

This list of questions is far from complete! You are invited to add to the database of questions by sending them to me using the contact form on my website (http://www.dietarytherapies.com/contact.html).

conventional oncology team and understand that by and large their tools are surgery, chemotherapy, and radiation. There's no room in their world for alternative medicine and little consideration given to the value of complementary therapies. (Of course, that shouldn't stop you from working with an experienced integrative oncologist along with your conventional team!)

Instead of curing the disease, successful treatment in all but the most aggressive cancers is now defined as "five-year survival" or "no evidence of disease" (otherwise known as remission). This change in wording is deceptive, as many people assume that achieving remission represents a cure. (In fact, how many of you reading this book have passed that five-year milestone, only to learn that your cancer has recurred?)

## Does Self-Advocacy Play a Role in Cancer Survivorship?

Clearly, self-advocacy matters in how well one survives even it doesn't significantly impact how long one survives. Those who relinquish control may experience more depression and feelings of hopelessness. This can blind them to options that might improve survivorship. In every type of cancer, there are verified reports of people who survive even the most dire prognoses. They are the outliers, and their successes are just a footnote in conventional oncology, often because there is no scientifically valid way to analyze retrospectively why they survived. But their existence is a clear reminder that statistics don't dictate outcomes, so why shouldn't you believe that you, too, will join the ranks of the survivors?

I once asked a 30-year survivor of ovarian cancer what she thought she had done differently. She replied, "Well, 22 different things." I then asked her what she thought had helped her the most. "I don't know. Maybe all of them. Maybe none of them," she answered. She is one example of someone who didn't sit back and accept her doctor's belief that her cancer was not survivable. (For more stories of hope, read *Radical Remission*, by Dr. Kelly Turner.)

Dr. David Servan-Schreiber, author of *Anticancer: A New Way of Life*, was a long-term survivor of brain cancer. He was also a medical doctor. As such, he enjoyed improved access to self-directed care and colleagues' acceptance of his self-advocacy. You deserve this advantage as well!

## Defining Wellness

MedlinePlus, a source of online health information published by the US National Library of Medicine, defines *wellness* as "the quality or state of being in good health especially as an actively sought goal."[5] This definition is a good start in that it gives a nod to the importance of lifestyle, but, in my opinion, it is still too limiting. For example, even the frail elderly who aren't in "good health" can make great strides toward wellness despite physical limitations that prevent them from attaining that higher standard.

The National Wellness Institute's model of wellness, on the other hand, is more inclusive: "Wellness is an active process through which people become aware of, and make choices toward, a more successful existence."[6] The key words here are "more successful existence." In other words, wellness is defined on a continuum. In this model, physical wellness encompasses one of six dimensions. The other dimensions of wellness include social, intellectual, spiritual, emotional, and occupational. Do you see yourself on this continuum?

It's understandable that your prognosis may prompt you to want to focus solely on curing your disease. To that end, you may right now be considering some combination of surgery, radiation, and chemotherapy—along with a host of complementary and alternative therapies. This degree of disruption in your life may be all that you feel you can reasonably handle at the moment, but I urge you to look ahead, past your illness and on to wellness. Like most directions you go in life, you arrive at points where you have choices to make. So here are a few ideas about where to start:

- What stress relievers can promote your emotional wellness?
- What activities can reinforce your emotional strength and resilience?
- What lifestyle changes will move you toward fulfillment?
- How can you improve your social connections with family, friends, and community?
- How will you move closer to your own *personal* definition of wellness?

How you live your life should grow in importance despite (or maybe because of) your disease. Look for every opportunity to move toward wellness.

## Defining Success

I always like to ask people, "What are your goals in adopting this diet?" But I also believe that it's important for each individual to look within and ask themselves other questions as well: Are you positive and upbeat, or fearful and anxious? Do you believe that you have, or can find, the right tools to put you on the path to wellness? Or are you fearful that you aren't doing enough? Are you hopeful? Or are you worried that any and all efforts may be in vain? *This is very personal.* Your idea of success may hinge solely on whether or not you achieve a cure, while

## Debunking the Myth of Consensus

It can be daunting to begin the ketogenic diet if you believe that there are better answers elsewhere. As one of my clients stated, "You come up against this wall of experts and you have to believe that they know what they're doing." While such a perspective is understandable, the experts' certainty is not a guarantee of your success, however you have chosen to define the term. It's not even an indication that there is true consensus among the experts in their own field. (I learned that one the hard way.) What this means in the real world is that you choose your own path and deal with uncertainties as best you can. This is the trade-off you have to make in exchange for empowerment and self-advocacy.

After we were hit with the devastating news of the utter failure of Raffi's initial chemotherapy protocol, the so-called "gold standard" treatment for his tumor type, my husband and I were reluctant to simply go along with any future prescribed treatments. So of course we were cautious when his oncologist stated that radiation now was his only option. We knew that irradiating the thalamus of a six-year-old child was a last resort, given that it would doubtless degrade and then stall completely Raffi's executive functioning and expressive language. Despite that, we made the long trip to the pediatric hospital to discuss this option further. When we arrived, the same oncologist then told us that the radiologist was unwilling to proceed with this treatment because the tumor was too large and the margins were too infiltrated. Without missing a beat, he then suggested that we start Raffi on a new chemotherapy drug, one he had previously mentioned as not being effective for our son. *Two strikes!*

By this point, a year and a half into this journey, I had joined several parent forums and knew that *no one* was having success with that particular drug. Add that to the statistics indicating that Raffi had at

another person in a similar situation would accept living comfortably with their disease for a few more months or years. What I really hope to see included as part of any answer to my question is the desire for a better quality of life. That desire is what kept us continuing with keto long after our initial success. The least a 5 percent chance of developing leukemia as a result of this drug (possibly even more given that he had a genetic anomaly, Poland's syndrome, that already put him at risk of developing the disease). When I expressed my concern about sparking a new cancer, the oncologist's reply (which I can only assume sounded reasonable to him) was, "But it's a *treatable* form of leukemia." *Strike three!* It was obvious to us that Raffi needed a new primary oncologist.

I composed a short paragraph describing Raffi's situation and emailed it to all twelve members of the Pediatric Brain Tumor Consortium, an elite group of pediatric oncology specialists practicing at hospitals that were deemed the very best at treating his disease. Only seven of the twelve members offered us the courtesy of a reply. Remarkably, only two of them gave us the same recommendation, the drug that Raffi's oncologist had insisted was his best option. The other responses ranged from a blunt "Let him go" to the most aggressive surgical option possible.

So where does "consensus" fit in? Well, obviously, it doesn't. When you hear a phrase like "tumor board consensus," what you *really* need to understand is that this so-called consensus may, in fact, be the opinion of just one person, especially if that person has the highest status and most influence and the other members of the board are silenced. Since the board needs to present a unified front, you will never know what the dissenters think. This is yet another reason why I urge everyone to seek a second and third opinion, even if you like your team or fear that you may offend them. Get over it. Second opinions are part of their world. Without a doubt, they themselves have provided second opinions that are not in keeping with another hospital's findings. Of course, conflicting opinions put you in the position of having to decide which way to turn. But that's your right—and your responsibility—if you want a say in your health care decisions.

diet gave Raffi the time to live his life, away from hospitals and oncology clinics. And those added years allowed us to build a treasure trove of memories.

Your thoughts and feelings color how you approach the journey ahead. They also have a major impact on the decisions you make and how you prioritize your actions. You may believe (or at least hope) that the answer is out there and all you need to do is to connect with the right people, people who have traveled the same path. But the reality is that your journey is unique, even if your situation appears similar to someone else's. That's why it's so important to separate yourself from the herd. Only then can you begin to think on your own and make decisions based on what you want out of life, with the understanding that no conventional treatment or alternative therapy works for everyone, just as no single diet has the desired effect every time.

So how will you judge the "success" of this diet? Some of that depends on your personality. You might use subjective measures, such as comparing how you feel after following the diet for several months to how you feel now. Or maybe you are drawn to using more objective measurements, such as looking for improvements in blood markers of your disease or positive changes seen in your scans. Ideally, in my view, you'll choose to use a combination of both.

# CHAPTER 5

# Understanding the Origins of the Ketogenic Diet

I f you ask the general public to describe the ketogenic diet, you'll get a variety of answers. Those who follow celebrity news will point to dramatic weight loss. People with diabetes may be focused on the buzz about the metabolic benefits of lowering their carbohydrate intake. And individuals from the elite fitness world are rapidly latching onto the enhanced performance of low-carb and ketogenic athletes, especially in cycling and running endurance events. As I've mentioned already, the diet as we know it today originated nearly a century ago as a therapy for intractable epilepsy in children. Before we dive deeper into the nuts and bolts of the diet, let's take a closer look at the diet's origins.

## History of the Diet: Fasting and Ketosis

The development of the ketogenic diet as a medical treatment has a long history, beginning with observations made long ago about the benefit of fasting as a treatment for various diseases, including epilepsy. However, it wasn't until the first few decades of the twentieth century that physicians in clinical settings began to put fasting into practice as a therapy. In 1921 Dr. H. Rawle Geyelin, an endocrinologist, presented evidence at a medical convention that fasting not only resolved epilepsy but also improved cognition that had declined as the result of seizures. Two Harvard physicians who attended this conference were intrigued enough by the findings to conduct fasting experiments of their own and discovered that improvement in seizure control in their patients was associated with the metabolic shift to using stored fat for energy. However, it's important to state the obvious: Although the benefits of fasting were fascinating observations, starvation was not a solution. As soon as people resumed a normal diet, their problems returned. Thankfully, a better long-term approach would soon become available.

## The Dire State of Diabetes Care

There is no doubt that the discovery of insulin was a lifesaver for people with type 1 diabetes, an autoimmune disease that destroys the insulin-secreting beta cells of the pancreas. In fact, the story of Elizabeth Evans Hughes, one of the first children to receive insulin injections, reads like a novel. Elizabeth was 11 years old when she was diagnosed with what was known then as juvenile diabetes. She was placed on the only treatment available at the time: basically, a starvation diet. Three years later, in 1922, she was near death when Canadian medical scientist Frederick Banting discovered a way to provide diabetic patients with insulin. Elizabeth's politically powerful family intervened on her behalf, and soon she was one of a very select few who received regular insulin injections. Almost immediately, she started to regain weight and strength, and she went on to live a full life.

Type 2 diabetes, which used to be called "adult onset" diabetes, is now distressingly common, even in adolescents. Unlike type 1 diabetes, this type develops over time, usually due to increasing insulin resistance accompanied by the loss of beta cell number and function. Type 2 diabetes responds amazingly well to treatment with dietary

Rollin Woodyatt, an independent researcher who studied carbohydrate metabolism, was the first to observe that ketone bodies—essentially by-products of breaking down lipids—were present in the body under three specific conditions: fasting, starvation, or very-low-carbohydrate intake. The observation that ketones are present in *fed* as well as *fasting* states moved further exploration in a groundbreaking direction as early as the 1920s.

Researchers outside of the epilepsy world had also noted the potential therapeutic effects of a ketogenic diet, this time as a dietary therapy for diabetes. In 1918, Dr. L. H. Newburgh and his colleague Dr. Phil Marsh, physicians and clinical investigators at the University of Michigan Medical School "dared to ignore the belief concerning the danger of fat in the diet of diabetics" and proceeded to promote a calorie-restricted high-fat, very-low-carbohydrate diet for what was then termed "diabetes mellitus."[1] Although this change in diet made perfect sense, any consideration given to limiting carbohydrates was discarded shortly after a new discovery, insulin, became widely available in the 1930s.

therapy, yet most health care practitioners fail to acknowledge this. Instead, type 2 diabetics are often advised to increase their intake of "healthy" whole grains, fruit, low-fat dairy products, and starchy vegetables, and to consume sugar "in moderation."

Tragically, the disease inevitably progresses in those who follow this misguided advice, and it is common for people with diabetes to suffer from blindness, cardiovascular disease, neuropathies, limb amputations, and renal failure. In addition to lowering quality of life, diabetes carves years off of life expectancy. In response to the growing market for products, pharmaceutical companies have ramped up research on an ever-increasing number of profitable drugs and devices. Do you see anything wrong with this picture?

In my view the world would be a better place if the American Diabetes Association returned to its early and unbiased advice to eliminate most carbohydrates from the diet. It would also be refreshing if the Academy of Nutrition and Dietetics, the umbrella organization for registered dietitians, would align its advice with the research that clearly shows better glucose control and overall better outcomes in those who adhere to low-carbohydrate diets.

Also, in the 1920s, Dr. Russell Wilder of the Mayo Clinic took an interest in research on fasting and went on to develop a *very* high-fat, *very* low-carbohydrate diet that pushed the body into producing large amounts of ketone bodies. He speculated that ketones were somehow protective in brain tissue and tested his theory on a group of young children debilitated by epilepsy. At the time, the only available antiseizure drugs were bromides and phenobarbital, both of which were deemed unsafe for children. Wilder's "ketogenic diet," as he called it, succeeded in eliminating or reducing seizures in many of the children. Furthermore, he observed that seizure control correlated to a large degree with blood ketone levels: The more ketones present, the more likely it was that the child would experience a therapeutic effect. Essentially, his ketogenic diet had mimicked the metabolic benefits of fasting while keeping the children well fed.

This was an amazing leap forward for the diet (or so you'd think). But even with evidence of success in treating such a devastating condition, the ketogenic diet was nearly discarded mid-century in favor of drug therapies,

## Charlie Abrahams's Story

Jim Abrahams, founder of The Charlie Foundation, describes his family's experience with their son's epilepsy as a living nightmare. In 1993, 20-month-old Charlie was experiencing hundreds of seizures a day, and over the course of the previous year had failed to respond to countless drug therapies. He also underwent brain surgery—all to no avail. Jim learned about the ketogenic diet through his own research and brought the information to his son's doctor. Initially the doctor held fast to the belief that they should continue with different combinations of drug therapies until all possibilities had been exhausted, even though Charlie's disabling seizures were close to destroying his physical and neurological health (with psychological impacts that extended to every member of his family). This is a textbook case of a protocol taking precedence over common sense . . . but don't get me started!

Despite this lack of support from Charlie's team, Jim and his wife, Nancy, made the fateful decision to take Charlie to Johns Hopkins Hospital, where he was started on the ketogenic diet under the watchful eye of the hospital's experienced keto team. Within days Charlie was seizure-free and soon off the medications that had kept him in a zombielike state. Soon he was making progress toward developmental milestones that he had not been expected to reach.

Jim's view of following the diet, in his own words: "A walk on the beach, compared to drugs, surgery, continued seizures, and progressive retardation." Now I wouldn't want to mislead you by suggesting that adhering to the ketogenic diet is easy. But I can tell you that it's far, far harder to sit helplessly by as your precious child suffers progressive and often irreversible damage.

beginning with the introduction of phenytoin (Dilantin) in the late 1930s. The travesty: Pharmaceuticals and surgery are still the only options presented to patients by the majority of neurologists, even when the cumulative effects of uncontrolled seizures include impairment of cognition and degradation of quality of life for the entire family.

To this day, prejudice against the ketogenic diet persists, as most doctors believe that the diet is too difficult to follow or too unpalatable for widespread use. This is exactly what we were told, even after our son's amazing experience on the diet. But our story is far from unique.

Despite this near-total abandonment, a small but dedicated group of pediatric specialists at Johns Hopkins Hospital—led by Dr. John Freeman and dietitian Mildred Kelly—continued to implement the diet. Few families were aware of this option, and consequently only a few children each year were treated until it was given new life in the 1990s when the parent of a child with epilepsy, desperately searching for a way to save his son, stumbled across a description of the diet in an old medical text. Jim Abrahams and his wife Nancy then took their son Charlie to Johns Hopkins, where the family's nightmare ended shortly after Charlie was placed on the ketogenic diet (see sidebar). In awe of this result (and understandably angry that this option had not been suggested earlier), Jim and Nancy founded The Charlie Foundation, a nonprofit organization that to this day continues to advocate for research and dissemination of knowledge on the use of the diet for epilepsy and other neurological disorders.

## Daring to Challenge the Diet Dogma

The mid-nineteenth century brought the first challenges to the "balanced diet" model, which states that it is medically necessary to provide over half of total calories in the form of carbohydrate-containing foods. In the 1860s, William Banting self-published his "Letter on Corpulence, Addressed to the Public."[2] Banting was a member of England's elite class and, like a growing number of his peers, he became obese and developed a number of related health issues starting in his thirties. His physicians recommended diet and exercise regimens, tonics, and spa treatments, none of which improved his health. At the age of 64, a new physician consultant advised him to cut out sugar and starches. Banting lost weight and his health improved dramatically, and his success led to the publication of his pamphlet. The treatise was so popular that it was reprinted and distributed throughout Europe and the United States, and those who followed his plan became known as "Banters." (You can read more about William Banting's fascinating story on the Weston A. Price website.[3]) However, this unorthodox approach to diet was met with a great deal of criticism from the medical community. The prevailing belief, not grounded in science, was that wheat-based "farinaceous foods" were a *necessary* component of a healthy diet.

The William Banting debate was revived in the early twentieth century as explorers traveled to the far reaches of the northern hemisphere and observed that aboriginal diets were very dissimilar to those of the Western world. These populations were generally healthy and relatively free from conditions such as heart disease, cancer, and diabetes, diseases that were becoming quite prevalent in the Western world.

In 1928, Arctic explorer Vilhjalmur Stefansson, dedicated to confirming his observations linking the Inuit diet to their apparent robust health, undertook an Inuit-style meat-and-fat diet, which he began under clinically controlled conditions at Bellevue Hospital in New York City. After several weeks, the dietary habits of Stefansson and another subject were then kept under close scrutiny by paid observers for the balance of the year. Despite predictions that he would develop scurvy and other diseases related to nutritional deficiencies, he remained healthy throughout. These findings were documented in a paper published in 1930 in the *Journal of Biological Chemistry*.[4]

A paradigm shift occurred in the 1970s, when the ketogenic diet gained a much wider audience with the publication of Dr. Robert Atkins's bestselling book, *Dr. Atkins' Diet Revolution*. In his clinic Atkins, a cardiologist, had observed the beneficial effects of carbohydrate restriction in weight loss and popularized a low-carbohydrate diet based on progressive "phases."[5] Carbohydrate restriction was the centerpiece of the plan, with carb intake limited to 20 (net) grams per day. Atkins set no specific limit on protein, fat, or total calories. The diet was very effective, at least in the short term, and soon his name was a household word. Of course, Atkins's plan didn't align with the standard dietary recommendations at the time (or today), and its instant popularity further incensed the conventional medical and nutrition community, uniting them in universal resistance to what they viewed as a dangerous fad running counter to their belief that weight-loss diets should be low in fat and restricted in calories.

The work of Atkins and other low-carbohydrate advocates was further eroded by a new wave of scientists and doctors with a strong bias toward low-fat diets, including vegan patterns. They came out in force to prove their point, even if it didn't align with the research. Their names became well known, even outside of the nutrition community: Ancel Keys, Dean Ornish, and T. Colin Campbell. By cherry-picking studies and manipulating the data, they pressed on with their mantra that it is fat—not sugar—in the diet that directly contributes to deposition of fat in the body and in arteries. This bias got a huge boost in 1977 when the US Senate Select Committee on Nutrition and Human Needs, led by Senator George McGovern, published recommendations for the *Dietary Goals for the American People*: Low fat, high carb, moderate protein. Then, as now, the science dictating these guidelines was flawed and hotly debated, but it didn't take long before the guidelines were accepted nearly globally, first in the United States and then abroad.

# Comparing Standard, Low-Carb, and Keto Diets

In the standard diet (sometimes referred to as either a Western or Standard American diet), carbohydrates make up more than half of the total calories consumed, much of them coming from grains, starches, and added sugars. Fat intake is generally less than 35 percent of calories; and protein makes up the balance. In contrast, a keto-for-cancer diet limits calories from carbohydrate to an average of 6 percent of total. With protein kept low (but adequate to meet the body's needs), the amount of fat in the diet rises to over 80 percent of calories.

There are several popular versions of low-carbohydrate diets. However, these differ in important ways from a classic ketogenic diet; mainly, they are lower in fat and more liberal in carbs and protein. This can still shift metabolism to burning fat as fuel, certainly an important goal in weight loss, but there is often no attempt to educate people about the additional health benefits offered by raising ketone levels and improving food quality. Also, low-carb diets on their own are not likely to have as potent an effect on limiting glucose availability to tumors or inhibiting cancer-promoting pathways as a therapeutic ketogenic diet. I've listed some of these diet variations here along with brief descriptions.

## Nutritional Ketosis

As you might recall from chapter 3 ("Nutritional versus Therapeutic Ketosis," page 29), the threshold for nutritional ketosis is a blood level of βHB at or above a threshold of 0.5 mmol/L. Nutritional ketosis has generated a great deal of attention and excitement in the fitness world, but beyond that it has also shown great potential to spur weight loss, reverse insulin resistance (in

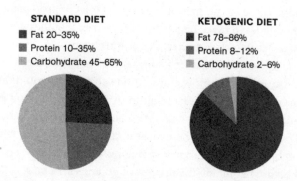

STANDARD DIET
■ Fat 20–35%
■ Protein 10–35%
▨ Carbohydrate 45–65%

KETOGENIC DIET
■ Fat 78–86%
■ Protein 8–12%
▨ Carbohydrate 2–6%

**Figure 5.1.** Macronutrient Distribution as a Percentage of Total Daily Calories. These graphs represent typical ranges for standard and ketogenic diets; individual patterns may vary.

diabetes and polycystic ovary syndrome), and improve cognition. Some people (myself included) view nutritional ketosis as an anti-aging strategy. In most cases, the plan may initially include calorie restriction, which often enhances the positive outcomes (e.g., more weight lost, reversal of diabetes), especially in those who are overweight at the start.

However, some people's interpretation of the ideal plan allows for too much protein, usually due to the assumption that extra protein will stave off the loss of muscle mass. But unless you're a bodybuilder or an extreme athlete, there is no requirement for a 12-ounce steak to help you build or retain muscle. And for those with cancer, keep in mind that more protein than what's needed can stimulate cancer-promoting pathways as well as interfere with blood glucose control. Remember what feeds into gluconeogenesis? Amino acids! Our bodies don't have much capacity to store amino acids. Once the "amino acid pool" in cells is full, the excess is diverted to the liver, where it's converted into glucose. This extra glucose can replenish your liver glycogen stores as well as stimulate your pancreas to secrete insulin. Insulin moves glucose into cells, including cancer cells. Insulin also dampens fat burning, switching off the conversion of fats to ketones. This makes good evolutionary sense: If your body can meet energy needs without tapping into its reserve fuel tank, it can save that supply for the next time you miss a meal.

## The Atkins Diet

As noted earlier in this chapter, the Atkins diet is a low-carb plan primarily aimed at those who want to lose weight (and weight loss is generally associated with improved health). In phase 1 (Induction), net carb intake is kept at or below 20 grams per day, and there is no requirement to divide that amount equally between meals. Atkins provides a list of acceptable Induction foods (which does not include nuts and seeds). There are no specific guidelines for fat or protein intake, but few people eat enough fat to make up for the carb calories that they cut.

Despite detractors' claims that the Atkins plan is a kidney-damaging, high-protein diet, years of research suggest that most people who follow the diet don't consume significantly more protein than they would on a standard diet. The combination of carb restriction and a calorie deficit jump-starts weight loss, and—since the diet also has a diuretic effect—the sheer number of pounds lost in the first few weeks can be exhilarating for people who have tried and failed with other weight-loss programs. But most people stay at phase I for only a few weeks before beginning the process of adding carbs back into the plan.

The main drawback for those of you who want to maintain either nutritional or therapeutic ketosis is that those who follow Atkins's plan may not achieve the low glucose levels seen with more rigorous adherence to a ketogenic diet. Also, ketone levels typically decrease over time in Atkins dieters, even if they maintain a low-carbohydrate intake. Some of this is due to the impact of taking in more protein than what is needed for repair and maintenance.

## The Modified Atkins Diet

What is now known as the Modified Atkins is a version of Atkins's plan that was developed and promoted by Dr. Eric Kossoff, an epileptologist at Johns Hopkins Hospital. He was responding to the growing demand for a simpler ketogenic plan, one that doesn't require children to be hospitalized or to fast during initiation of the diet and doesn't expect families to carefully pre-plan each meal. The modified plan is also more user-friendly for adolescents and adults, few of whom are compliant to the restrictions imposed on younger children. In this version, carb intake is still low—initially, 10 to 15 net grams of carbs per day—and while raising fat intake is encouraged, there are no specific guidelines for either fat or protein. In the epilepsy world, Kossoff's version of a ketogenic diet is still viewed as a medical therapy and, as such, must be overseen by a team of specialists that include (at a minimum) a neurologist and a registered dietitian.

The Modified Atkins is a good alternative to the ketogenic diet for people with cancer who cannot (or will not) plan meals or weigh their foods. Although they still need to track net carbs, the more relaxed approach to planning makes it easier for families to dine out and travel. (In fact, the Modified Atkins is a good choice for those with cancer while they are away from home or at other times when they have less control over meal preparation.)

Over a decade of experience with the Modified Atkins has shown it to be a safe and efficacious alternative to classic ketogenic diet therapy in epilepsy.[6] In 2016 a team of researchers at Johns Hopkins School of Medicine published a paper in the journal *Epilepsy and Behavior* that detailed a five-year study of the benefits and challenges of therapeutic ketogenic diets, including the Modified Atkins. The authors concluded that the study provided evidence that these diets are feasible, effective, and safe as long-term therapies in adults.[7] These conclusions are reassuring for those who question the safety of keeping carbohydrate intake low for an extended period of time.

Various studies of the Modified Atkins diet have shown that blood glucose levels range higher and ketosis is not as strong when the ketogenic diet is liberalized in this way. These revisions have only a minor effect in adults on the diet for epilepsy, which is balanced out by higher rates of compliance to the plan. However, in adults utilizing the diet for cancer management, these higher glucose and lower ketone levels are not likely to be as therapeutic as those induced by a more rigorous ketogenic diet. Still, the Modified Atkins may still be a better choice than the classic ketogenic diet for those with compromised health status or complex medical conditions that prevent them from adhering to a more exacting plan.

## Mitochondrial Health

Simply put, healthy, well-functioning mitochondria are essential to maintaining a person's health throughout the lifespan. We are learning that *what* and even *when* you eat have a profound impact on mitochondrial health, and ketogenic metabolic therapy is emerging as one of the most powerful non-drug approaches to correcting the underlying cause of many diseases, including cancer.

### Alzheimer's Disease and the MEND Protocol

Most of us have been brainwashed into believing that there's nothing to be done to reverse the cognitive decline that accompanies Alzheimer's disease. Put aside for now what you've heard about genetic markers, plaques, tangles, and tau, and focus instead on the root cause: impaired cerebral glucose metabolism. In fact, because of this commonality with types 1 and 2 diabetes, many within the research community are beginning to refer to Alzheimer's disease as "type 3" diabetes.

Current drugs, such as memantine, have been shown to impede progression of the disease, but they do nothing to reverse it.[8] But what if instead the brain's reliance on glucose as its primary fuel was decreased by replacing glucose with ketones? Ketones are readily metabolized by most brain cells, and studies have shown them to be neuroprotective and neurotherapeutic as well. This could amount to a win-win-win in the effort to combat Alzheimer's disease!

The MEND protocol (MEND is an acronym for metabolic enhancement for neurodegeneration) was designed to study the effects of changes in diet and lifestyle on symptoms of mild cognitive impairment and early Alzheimer's in a small group of older adults. Interventions included lowering the intake of grains and refined starches, adding medium-chain triglyceride (MCT) and coconut oils,

We've come a long way in our understanding of mitochondrial pathways in just a few decades. Remember that explosion of information gathered from the Human Genome Project? At first we were led to believe that certain gene mutations such as *BRCA* in breast cancer cemented our fate, but there were always a few people who had these mutations that didn't fall prey to disease. Now it's increasingly clear that, for most of us, mitochondrial health is determined by more than just the code that is written in our genes. Instead, it is strongly influenced by epigenetic changes. What do you eat? Do you smoke? How many and what kind of stressors do you live with? What illnesses have you had over your lifetime? How healthy is your gut? All of these factors—and many more—can influence how your genes interact with the environment.

What actions and environments move you toward cellular health? And which nudge you further down the path of declining health and chronic

optimizing sleep, and reducing stress through mind-body practices. Subjects could pick and choose from a smorgasbord of these and other options that each by itself would have little total impact on disease but taken together did appear to move the needle in the right direction for a majority of participants.[9]

Combination therapies rather than single-agent miracle cures, have proven to be the solution for long-term management of many other diseases as well, most notably HIV-AIDS. Here, the development of the successful protocol was not made within the context of a conventional medical model that tests one drug or therapy at a time in clinical trials. In fact, that model initially hindered progress but was ultimately overshadowed by a public patient-driven movement that combined scientific research with political activism.

What makes all this even more exciting is that the potential to improve mitochondrial health is not dependent on developments within the pharmaceutical industry. Instead, it is already within your grasp. Our current tools may not be perfect, but as the MEND trial demonstrates, it is hugely important to prioritize results over protocols. (For a deeper dive into the enormous potential of ketogenic diets for the treatment of this neurodegenerative disease, read Amy Berger's *The Alzheimer's Antidote*.)

disease? Those are the basic questions asked by researchers in the emerging field of epigenetics, and to date we have explored only the tip of this iceberg. An even newer subspecialty—nutrigenomics—focuses on how macro- and micronutrients influence gene expression.

Research in both of these areas is surging ahead at a rapid clip, partly because of the scientific discoveries that highlight the role of mitochondria in metabolic health, but also because we are facing epidemics of many metabolic disorders for which, like cancer, we have no pharmacological cures. If the financial burden of treating type 2 diabetes isn't sufficient to sink our health care system, we must also contend with the destructive and resource-sapping effects of rising rates of Alzheimer's disease

So what is the point of this digression from the discussion of cancer? Mainly that the underlying cause of so many diseases, adult cancers included, has its roots in the dysregulation of mitochondrial function. And treatment can be simple: Address the root cause and you can change the course of the disease. I'm extremely interested in the research here because it has enormous implications—not only for our understanding of metabolic and neurodegenerative diseases, but also for our understanding of what we now believe to be "normal" aging. Instead of focusing our efforts solely on extending our lifespan, what if we also looked for ways to extend our *healthspan*, so that we can look forward to pedaling at top speed as we go off the cliff instead of limping blindly toward it?

Aging is inevitable. So why do I believe that a low-carb or ketogenic diet may be beneficial for those who are moving past their "biological imperative"? (By that I mean those of us who are no longer biologically essential to the continuation of our species, although I hasten to add that we still have enormous contributions to make that extend way beyond the survival of our offspring.) Emerging research is not yet conclusive, but it is pointing in the direction that diets low in sugars, low in proteins, high in healthy fats, and controlled in total calories may be most helpful in extending healthspan for those of us past mid-life. Fine-tuning the mechanism that preserves function by tapping into fuels other than glucose is one benefit, since it reduces the otherwise inevitable development of some degree of insulin resistance, even in those of us who don't develop diabetes. Ketogenic metabolic therapy may also hold one of the keys to healthy aging through the regulation of genetic expression.

As of this writing, I'm actively tracking the areas of research described above, and I'll happily share what I'm learning in my next book. Until then I'll keep you as up to date as I can on my website. There, I'll also try to simplify the science behind aging as I've tried to do here for cancer. I'll also post papers and links to books and other resources that I believe are putting us on the right track.

# CHAPTER 6

# Diet *Does* Matter!

Macros matter.

Food quality matters.

Meal timing matters.

Fasting matters.

Micronutrients and minerals matter.

Hydration matters.

**DIET MATTERS!**

It's nearly unimaginable to me that these truths aren't as hardwired into us as our drive to eat. That said, I don't have to look too far back into my own past to see how little attention I paid to what I ate, especially since I was one of those fortunate people who wasn't carrying any extra weight. Raffi's cancer diagnosis (followed by failed therapies) was my wake-up call. As rough as that was, I'm now sharing what I've learned over the past decade with as many people as I can. You can thank my son, Raffi, for that!

## Beginning the Diet Discussion

There are several predictable responses you are likely to hear as you broach a discussion of the ketogenic diet with your medical team—and maybe even your friends and family. Understand what they are and be prepared to offer some reassurance. Let's start with the classic, which I've already discussed to some degree.

## "Diet doesn't matter; eat what you want."

If you believe this assertion, you wouldn't be reading this book.

## "There's no evidence."

*What most people, especially busy doctors, are actually saying here is, "I'm not interested in what you found on the internet."*

That's it in a nutshell. What's important to remember is that they are *not* stating that there is evidence that it *doesn't* work, or even that they view it as harmful. It's simply not on their radar yet.

## "You'll lose weight."

*It's true; the ketogenic diet can be very effective for weight loss.*

If weight loss is beneficial for you right now, for example, if you have other health issues that are tied to carrying excess weight, then you'll be moving in the right direction by losing a few pounds, especially in the first few weeks and months of the diet. Cancer cells will be stressed by limiting specific nutrients, while healthy cells will respond by cleaning up their act—literally—by improving the signaling pathways associated with better mitochondrial health. However, if you don't have an ounce of extra weight to spare, there are several weight-conserving approaches to the ketogenic diet that will be a better choice for you. I discuss these regimens in detail in chapter 7.

## "You'll get kidney stones."

*Yes, people who follow a classic ketogenic diet, including children with epilepsy, do have a higher risk of developing kidney stones.*

First, understand that everyone who follows a ketogenic diet should stay well hydrated! That's the simplest way to lower your risk of getting kidney stones. If you have a history of kidney stones and have been advised to stick to a diet low in oxalates, be aware that some keto-friendly foods, such as spinach and almonds, are high in oxalic acid. Oxalates can bind to calcium and form very painful crystals in the kidneys. However, other factors also contribute to crystal formation, such as the type and amount of calcium and other minerals in your diet. We'll address this later in chapter 15 ("Challenges Introduced by Other Chronic Diseases," page 277).

If you do have a personal or family history of kidney stones, be proactive. Talk to your renal specialist about ways to manage the risk (for example, by adding a prescription potassium citrate, which helps to alkalinize the urine). This simple change to the protocol initiated by the keto team at Johns Hopkins Hospital has significantly reduced the incidence of kidney stones.[1] (Don't make this decision without consulting a doctor first as there are many scenarios in which supplementing with potassium may be a poor idea.)

## "You'll develop gout."

*High uric acid levels are associated with gout and certain types of arthritis.*

Yes, I expect to see a rise in uric acid levels early in the ketogenic diet. In fact, it's puzzling if I don't see this increase in the first month or so. To sum up the science, the rise in this compound occurs because uric acid competes with ketones for excretion in the urine. In most cases, no action on your part is required, and with keto-adaptation, uric acid returns to pre-diet levels. More great news: I haven't seen anyone develop gout or gout symptoms as a result of the temporarily high uric acid levels. Nevertheless, just as with kidney stones, it's important to be proactive by bringing up this possibility with your doctor before you start the diet. (I've included an interesting sidebar on gout in chapter 15, "Challenges Introduced by Other Chronic Diseases," page 277). If you'd like to learn more about this and other biochemical changes associated with the adoption of a ketogenic diet, I highly recommend Stephen Phinney and Jeff Volek's book, *The Art and Science of Low Carbohydrate Living*.

## "You can't follow a high-fat diet if you don't have a gallbladder."

*Even without a gallbladder, you will continue to make bile, which will then randomly trickle into the duodenum.*

The purpose of the gallbladder is to store and concentrate the bile salts that are then secreted into the duodenum of the intestine in response to a meal containing fats. Bile salts, phospholipids (found in lecithin), cholesterol, and bilirubin have a specific job each, but the main purpose of bile is to emulsify dietary fats that have been acted on by pancreatic lipase, a fat-digesting enzyme. The combined effect aids in the digestion and absorption of fats. A small percentage of people who have had their gallbladder removed experience some post-surgical symptoms, such as nausea or diarrhea, but the majority adapt without any special accommodations. Still, many of the people I work with express concern about what may happen if they eat a high-fat diet. All I can say is the fear far outstrips the reality. I suggest easing into the diet without an initial fast. Gradually add fats, preferably in whole-food form (such as macadamia nuts, avocado, or flaxseed) or incorporated into a salad dressing (with an emulsifier, such as non-GMO sunflower lecithin). Some people supplement with high-lipase pancreatic enzymes. Others choose ox bile or herbal choleretics (bile stimulants), but I generally don't recommend these until you've tried other options. Also, be sure to work with a practitioner who knows the ins and outs of herbs and botanicals. Remember, many of these are potent medicinals.

Another way to circumvent the fat digestion issue is to include MCTs, particularly caprylic acid (C8), as a supplement to the diet. MCTs bypass normal fat digestion; instead, they diffuse through the intestinal membrane and into the capillary bed of the hepatic portal vein. They are then transported to the liver, where they are converted directly to ketones and sent back out into circulation. Let me also note here that coconut oil, though often promoted as "rich in MCTs," is only about 14 percent caprylic acid (C8) and capric acid (C10). What makes it "rich" is its high lauric acid (C12) content. Some of that is diverted to the liver, but the bulk undergoes normal digestion. (Keep in mind that lauric acid has other benefits that make it an important addition to the diet, such as its antiviral, antifungal, and antimicrobial properties.)

## Know Your Priorities!

Recently I worked with a young man who had a high-grade brain tumor. He shared the results of a lipid test that showed a slightly elevated LDL along with very favorable triglycerides and HDL. He reported that his doctor was, in her words, "alarmed" by this change. She wanted him to start on a statin drug right away. At this same appointment, however, she reiterated to him that she expected him to succumb to his cancer within a few months.

Obviously, he was shaken by this reminder of his dire prognosis, but now he was also concerned about this news regarding his cholesterol. Honestly, did she really believe that this young man was going to succumb to heart disease in those next few months? I pointed out to him that her comment was ludicrous and, yes, insensitive, and that she had added to his already heavy burden. The kindest explanation I could offer for the remark was that perhaps this was one small area where she felt that she had some control over an outcome.

I'm not here to call doctors out on this. There's no point in that. Instead, I offer it as an example of the need for you set your own priorities.

## "A high-fat diet will raise your cholesterol."

*Emerging research suggests that it is triglycerides, not LDL, that contribute to the development of heart disease and related conditions, such as obesity, type 2 diabetes, and stroke.*

Most people do see a temporary rise in total cholesterol, which may stay elevated for a few months to a year. But "cholesterol" by itself is a catch-all term—it includes both LDL (generally referred to as "bad" cholesterol) and HDL ("good" cholesterol). Although you may see a rise in LDL, your protective HDL may also rise, keeping the ratio within the "normal" range. Lipid tests also note triglyceride levels, and high triglycerides are increasingly seen as a major risk factor in heart disease. If your triglyceride level is currently high, it is very likely that on the diet you will see an almost immediate drop to mid-range or lower.

Still, if you believe that a rise in cholesterol will spark a debate with your team, please talk to your doctor about your concerns and consider going beyond the standard lipid panel to get a closer look at the actual size and number of LDL particles with an advanced lipid test, such as the NMR LipoProfile.[2] You may want to add tests for high-sensitivity CRP (but this is of limited benefit if you have systemic inflammation from cancer or an autoimmune disease). When the pressures of a cancer diagnosis have lightened up, you may even want to have an arterial calcium scan to identify arterial calcification. Although none of these tests are perfect, the overall picture may help you decide whether you're going to prioritize efforts to lower your LDL number.

## "You can't stop your body from making glucose."

*Of course you can't stop your body from making glucose! Nor would you want to. Remember the critical role that gluconeogenesis plays in regulating energy metabolism? If not, look back at chapter 3 ("The Shift to Ketosis," page 21).*

Given the amount of glucose produced through gluconeogenesis, it's no wonder that this statement comes up often, not just from doctors who are refuting use of the ketogenic diet, but also from people with cancer who are teetering on the edge of commitment. After all, if cancer thrives on glucose and your body can make it so freely, then why should you consider eliminating it from your diet? The answer: The ketogenic diet keeps blood glucose lower and steadier than a standard diet. But the diet is about so much more than simply starving cancer of glucose. It also has a profound impact on the pathways associated with progression of the disease.

## "If a diet worked, I'd read about it in the professional journals."

*Research on the ketogenic diet for cancer has made it into many professional journals, including those read by oncologists, but that's no guarantee that your doctor will be interested in diet therapy.*

Word is getting through despite this roadblock, and I am starting to see much less resistance from oncologists as long as they can be reassured that you are not planning to forgo conventional care in favor of a stand-alone diet. Remember that you need to listen to their concerns, but if their lack of support is based solely on a lack of curiosity on their part, then the ball's in your court.

## What Your Oncologist Doesn't Know about Nutrition

I wish I had a dollar for every time an oncologist has told one of my clients that "diet doesn't matter; eat what you want." Understandably, this dismissive statement has a huge impact on resolve and morale. "After all," you might ask, "don't these experts know best what will help me beat my disease?" The answer is, yes and no. Yes, within the scope of their practice, they have knowledge of and experience with which drugs and therapies are approved for your cancer. But a resounding No! when the topic turns to diet. Believe me: You don't have to be an expert in nutrition to know more about it than most oncologists! Most medical schools and residency programs devote a scant 20 to 25 hours total to any discussion of nutrition, and this usually never includes an in-depth analysis of the effect dietary therapy can have on disease. Instead, suggested lifestyle changes, such as "eat less" and "exercise more," are given lip service. Of course, this approach is reinforced continuously by flawed national nutritional guidelines and, unfortunately, heavily reinforced by bias and the status quo.

Given the dearth of nutrition information provided to medical practitioners in training, it is no surprise that patients are often disappointed that their doctor "wasn't the least bit curious" about the ketogenic diet, even when they have gone through immense effort to gather relevant research papers and develop a list of vetted resources. My clients don't understand why sharing this information is so often met with a blank stare or an empty "Thanks," accompanied by body language that says "I'm still not interested." An entrenched paradigm is just that—and these doctors are not going to be influenced by what you bring to the table.

Understand, though, that this flippant "diet doesn't matter" attitude on your team's part can be used to your advantage. Using their logic, if "diet doesn't matter," then they should not have a problem with you adopting a ketogenic

## Finding an Integrative Oncologist
## Who Will Support the Ketogenic Diet

Why do I suggest an integrative oncologist? Well, given the constraints of the health care system, it's not likely that you will find much support for nontraditional adjuncts, those therapies offered as "add-ons" to conventional care. If you have the financial means to look outside the box, you will find some highly trained and very experienced people, mainly integrative medical doctors (MDs and DOs) or naturopathic doctors (NDs). Naturopathic doctors who are fellows of the American Board of Naturopathic Oncology (you should see the FABNO credential listed after their name) have had extensive training on protocols, including the ketogenic diet, using an "evidence-*informed* approach" that, unlike conventional evidence-*based* medicine, incorporates information from clinical observation.

Knowledge is em-*power*-ment! Dr. Nasha Winters, FABNO, and Jess Higgins Kelley share what they have learned in their book, *The Metabolic Approach to Cancer: Integrating Deep Nutrition, the Ketogenic Diet, and Nontoxic Bio-Individualized Therapies.*

There are a growing number of integrative oncologists who are waking up to the power of ketogenic metabolic therapy. I've included a few names in the resources section and will maintain an updated list on my website as well.

Do your search wisely. If a practitioner guarantees a cure or suggests that you should abandon conventional care and sign on to their proprietary (and often outrageously expensive) treatment plan, then continue on with your search. Similarly, if all they can offer are testimonials, and they can't produce any peer-reviewed science to back up their claims, I strongly advise you to see what you can find out about them as practitioners as well as what you can learn on your own about the treatment options they are suggesting.

diet. Expect your oncologist to either drop the topic (most expedient for them) or feel compelled to produce a reason why you shouldn't move forward with the diet (typically, one of the statements covered in the preceding pages, to which you now know how to respond).

## Troubleshooting for the Future

Would you like to share your oncologist's reaction to the diet? Then send me an email via my website. I'll address as many of your responses as I can.

What are other possible reasons your doctor may not be even slightly curious about diet? Perhaps he or she just doesn't have the time or interest to devote to learning about new concepts. It's also possible that your doctor may have limited communication skills, another topic that is inadequately addressed in most medical schools. Yes, there are situations in which poor bedside manners may have to be overlooked, especially if you believe that your doctor is your lifeline, but communication is so critical to your well-being that at least one member of your medical team must be a skilled and empathetic listener. (Integrative oncologists could fill that role if your conventional team doesn't.)

Also be prepared mentally to deal with the continued lack of interest from that same "diet doesn't matter" doctor *even when they personally witness your amazing response to treatment*. This can feel like a real kick in the pants! You may want to follow up this dismissal by asking if your response to the cancer treatment was exactly what they expected, or better. Even if they admit that it is better than expected, don't hold your breath for them to attribute any part of your success to the ketogenic diet or any combination of other complementary or alternative therapies you've chosen. This is unfortunate but understandable, given that there is no way for them to validate that any given deviation from the standard of care was responsible for your success.

## The Key Is Communication with Your Team

After reading all of these potential negatives associated with beginning the diet discussion, you might be thinking, "Why should I even bother?" In fact, multitudes of studies and surveys show that only a small percentage of patients initiate any discussion of adjuncts or alternatives, including dietary supplements, with their doctors. But even if you believe it will be uncomfortable, make the effort to begin the diet discussion with your doctor. It's important that your team is aware of your plans, and your interaction here is likely to provide insight into how you can expect to be treated as you move

### Raffi's "Amazing Response" to Keto

My son's "amazing response" couldn't be attributed to anything *but* diet since he was no longer following a protocol expected to elicit even a minor response. His oncologist conceded that the diet was, in fact, working for him and even added, "There will be other Raffis," with the caveat "—but this diet isn't for everyone." As I mentioned earlier, Raffi's endocrinologist, too, felt obliged to offer his opinion that the diet was "too hard" for most mortals, even though he had nothing as effective to offer in its place. Is it any wonder that I am so determined to get the word out that (1) yes, there are other Raffis; and (2) no, the diet is not out of the reach of most people? At its worst, it's inconvenient, but that becomes a non-issue if you're rewarded with an "amazing response" of your own.

forward. You will also learn if your doctor has valid medical concerns that need to be addressed before you decide to adopt a ketogenic diet. If these concerns seem disingenuous, off-target, or downright ridiculous, then take the time to seek out a second opinion. In fact, any time that you are faced with a life-changing decision, you owe it to yourself to get that second opinion. You may be hesitant to seek this out for fear of alienating or offending your oncologist or surgeon, believing that could result in poor care. I see this as an *enormous* red flag! If you are fearful of stepping on toes this early in the game, then it's almost a guarantee that you are not (yet) comfortable with self-advocacy (or, if you are the caregiver, that you are not comfortable advocating for your loved one). Let's separate fact from fear. Fact: If your doctor is thin-skinned, this will certainly interfere with open communication. It's best for you to learn that early on.

Now let's look beyond the merely impatient doctors and zoom in on those who present unacceptable barriers to communication by using bullying and intimidation. These tactics are intended to shut down communication and keep you on track by discouraging any discussion outside of the planned standard of care. Condescension, shouting, smirks, and eye-rolling are rude, disrespectful, and unprofessional, yet they all occur all too often. It's devastating to have your attempts at meaningful dialogue belittled and dismissed in this manner. It also speaks *volumes* about what you can expect from this doctor in the future. If you do encounter unacceptable behavior, the simplest action is to transfer responsibility for your treatment to another physician in the same group, as long as the same culture doesn't extend to the entire team. Oncology nurses are my go-to here, as they deal with these physicians on a daily basis and are acutely aware of individual strengths and biases. Don't expect nurses to volunteer this information, unless you ask them for help; then they are often more than happy to point you toward a more suitable match (as long as you keep them out of the discussion of why you are making this change).

It's also important to truly understand that if you are a good candidate for the ketogenic diet, you don't need your doctor's permission to start any more than you need permission to eat a bag of potato chips. Diet is a choice. Your oncology team will still be there to treat you with whatever surgery, drugs, or radiotherapy is part of the medically approved standard of care. That usually includes monitoring your progress with physical exams, bloodwork, and scans, which you can use to track the impact of the diet.

A word to the wise: If you decide not to accept a proposed treatment plan, your oncology team has no obligation to keep you on as a patient. After all, their reimbursement is based on the services they perform, and services are tightly constrained by diagnostic insurance codes and without their participation you will need to independently obtain the tests you will need to monitor your health. In some cases, the tests can be ordered by another doctor (usually your primary care provider or integrative oncologist). You may have to pay out-of-pocket for part or all of this testing.

## A Bright Light on the Horizon

More and more often, clients will tell me that their doctor (usually a surgeon) was very enthusiastic when they mentioned the diet. This prompts the question, "If he's so supportive, why didn't he bring it up with me from the start?" Simple: It's the culture. Your oncologist is breaking the code if he or she mentions a therapy outside their practice. But if *you* are the one to bring it up, then the doctor is free to offer an opinion. Another positive sign: I've heard some oncologists, even those who don't appear to support the diet directly, now saying to their patients on the diet, "Whatever it is you're doing, keep it up." That's music to my ears!

Fortunately, there's a potential workaround here. As long as your oncologist has reason to believe that you will eventually move forward with *some* part of their plan, then it may be possible to keep yourself in their loop. I'm certainly *not* suggesting that you lie to them—that undermines trust and respect—but you do have the option to express your concerns about the rush to treatment, opting instead to mull over any decision regarding your care.

## Comparing Keto to Other "Anticancer" Diets

If you are reading this book, you already believe that diet *does* matter—not only for managing your disease but also as a way to move toward better health. You don't need medical experts to confirm the power of food; just look around you for the proof. What is less clear is the science behind *which* dietary patterns might be most therapeutic. To date, most of what we know about the disease-remediating potential of ketogenic metabolic therapy comes from animal model research, case studies, and anecdotal reports. There remain many unanswered questions.

Within the keto world there are different approaches to the diet, each geared to a slightly different scenario. For example, "best practice" for an estrogen-sensitive breast cancer may mean that you remove dairy from your diet due to the estrogen metabolites found in dairy fats, while best practice for brain cancer may focus instead on using diet and other strategies to lower the availability of amino acids that can fuel brain tumor tissue. Another consideration: If you are newly diagnosed and otherwise healthy, you may be able to pack a bigger punch with a short fast that jump-starts your shift to ketosis, but if your health is already compromised by your disease, it might be wiser to ease into a ketogenic plan to sidestep some of the transition effects (such as unintended weight loss). I'll be discussing these options in more detail in the next chapter.

For those of you who are just starting with chemo or radiation, or are recovering from surgery, your plan needs to be individualized to accommodate side effects of treatment, including medications, changes in taste or tolerance to food in general, digestive issues, and a host of other factors that should be considered when developing your ketogenic plan. Also, the degree to which you use calorie restriction or any variation on fasting should be dynamic, with frequent assessment to be sure that the plan is still meeting your needs. (Learn more about these protocols in chapter 7.)

The guidelines outlined in this book reflect the best of what is known at this moment, but this knowledge is evolving even during the writing of this book! (For updates, visit my website.)

I've already made my case for why you should consider a ketogenic diet, calorie restricted if possible, as an adjunct therapy for cancer. Now let's turn our attention to some of the other diets that claim to be anticancer.

## David Servan-Schreiber's *Anticancer: A New Way of Life*

Dr. David Servan-Schreiber was a neuroscientist who learned he had brain cancer in the early 1990s. He underwent standard care but added specific foods, supplements, and lifestyle changes to his personal protocol. He succumbed to his disease in 2011 but the changes he made (and his connections within the medical community) are most likely what helped him to survive for 19 years past his diagnosis. His poignant memoir, *Anticancer: A New Way of Life*, offers both hope and a practical place to start in making dietary and other lifestyle changes.[3] His diet was not ketogenic; in fact, the ketogenic diet was not yet on the horizon for use in cancer when he was first diagnosed. Although he acknowledged that cancer feeds on sugar, and he understood that insulin and IGF-1 contribute to cancer progression, he didn't go far enough in eliminating (rather than just limiting) glucose-laden foods. I often wonder if he would have revised his thinking based on the evidence we have now that supports the use of ketogenic metabolic therapy.

## The Budwig and Gerson Diets

There is an abundance of hype and a lot of pseudoscience surrounding these two diets but none of it holds up to scientific scrutiny, especially when you consider what we know about the processes that drive cancer. Mixing quark or cottage cheese with flaxseed oil (Budwig) may be soothing and satisfying but it isn't going to cure your cancer. Neither will taking in all your nutrients as juice (Gerson), even if you believe you are preserving enzymes and megadosing with antioxidants. Again, there's *no science* to support that either of these diets is a cure for cancer, and if you are directed to papers or trials, you'll see that these are not peer-reviewed research. Of course, the Internet is replete with testimonials touting both of these diets as a cure for cancer but these personal stories are certainly not proof of effect. My opinion: These diets may stall progression briefly if they shift your eating pattern away from poor-quality foods or a standard carbohydrate-heavy diet, but the effect seen by some people may be explained by the fact that they inadvertently restrict total calories (see the benefits of that in chapter 7, "Caloric Restriction without Malnutrition," page 94). Unfortunately, these diets are at best a short-term approach that will do little to alter the long-term course of your disease.

## Plant-Based Diets

Proponents of plant-based diets (vegan plans) have a strong online presence that pushes back against those who believe that it is more normal and natural for us as humans to consume animal protein. The controversies and conspiracy theories on both sides create a whirlwind of confusion. Add that to the passionate support from some prominent people, including T. Colin Campbell and Dean Ornish, who rely on cherry-picking data to arrive at persuasive arguments that favor their personal bias. No wonder so many people come away with the view that there must be something terribly wrong with being an omnivore! The real benefit here may be that fervent veganism, it is important to remember, is part of a *total lifestyle* that limits exposure to environmental toxins, reduces stress, places value on physical activity, and improves overall food quality. And yes, veganism presents an ethical argument against the use of any products—foods included—that are sourced from animals. Vegans who adhere to a whole-foods diet—in other words, no processed or packaged foods—most likely practice caloric restriction, though often it's unintentional. (Have you noticed that virtually all of the leaders in this movement are leaner than the general public?)

I do believe that whole-food organically sourced diets, including vegan diets, may be beneficial in *preventing* cancer, but once you are diagnosed with the disease, the emphasis needs to shift toward *treatment*. Veganism does *not* rescue people with cancer. I know this because I've worked with many ardent vegans with progressive disease. Controversies aside, understand that you can choose to adopt a vegan low-carb plan, which is a variation of classic keto. It just takes more work: more understanding of how to meet your nutritional needs, more time spent sourcing foods, more modifications in how you meet your protein and other nutrient needs, and more restrictions on dining out.

You will also benefit mentally and physically by following healthy lifestyle practices, such as meditation, yoga, stress reduction, and maintaining a healthy environment (physical, social, emotional). *All* of these factors can enhance the bigger anticancer picture. So if you are already a practicing vegan and your heart thrives on this lifestyle, there is *absolutely no requirement* for you to start eating animal products. However, I strongly recommend that you track your nutrient intake using Cronometer so that you can supplement the nutrients that are lacking in a plant-based diet.

One more important consideration: If you've adopted a vegan diet because you're convinced that meat is bad for you, then rethink that decision. Meat, like fat, has been unfairly vilified. Most studies involving red meat draw their conclusions without considering food quality or portion size. Who would argue that there are no health consequences to a steady diet of fast-food burgers? On the other end of the continuum, where are the studies looking at health effects, good or bad, of keto-sized portions of meat from well-nourished grass-fed livestock raised on organic pastures?

## The Mediterranean Diet

There are benefits to a Mediterranean pattern over standard American fare, such as the use of olive oil in place of corn or soy. But there is no statistically significant evidence at this time that the Mediterranean diet is associated with a lower risk of cancer, or that it improves outcomes in those already diagnosed with the disease. That makes sense given that most people who self-identify with the Mediterranean plan take in a substantial amount of their diet (45 to 65 percent) as carbohydrate in the form of whole grains, starchy vegetables, sugary fruits, and high-sugar dairy. The plan also allows for foods with added sugars. In sum, it retains too many of the problems seen in standard diets, such as the propensity to develop insulin resistance and weight gain over time due to the cumulative impact of glucose/insulin signaling and insulin resistance. Those are factors that are indeed *strongly* linked to the development of certain cancers as well as a host of other diseases.

## The Paleo Diet

"Paleo" plans are created around foods assumed to have been eaten by our Paleolithic hunter-gatherer ancestors. The Paleo world is huge and diverse, but most plans exclude all grains, legumes, and dairy, as well as most vegetable oils. They emphasize high-quality meats and fish as well as whole-food sources of sugar and starches, such as fruits and root vegetables. Nuts and seeds provide a high percentage of the fats and oils. Added sugars are allowed as long as they come from "natural" sources, such as dates or coconuts.

For many, a Paleo plan is a great start toward a high-quality whole-foods way of eating, and for some, it's a way of life as well. People familiar with a Paleo diet have a much easier time transitioning to keto (though they do miss the fruits, berries, and Paleo bars). Look deeper into Paleo, and you'll find that there are some low-carb and even ketogenic variations (such as the Wahls Paleo Plus plan promoted by Terry Wahls for people with multiple sclerosis, an autoimmune disorder). But keep in mind that most Paleo followers are not limiting the amount of protein they eat, and this is important to do when you have cancer.

## The Alkaline Diet

The popularity of this diet is based on a misunderstanding about the connection between acidic environments and cancer progression. Yes, it's a fact that cancer thrives in an acid environment, but this relates only to the *microenvironment* of the cancer cell—the space immediately beyond the cell membrane—which is acidic primarily due to high levels of lactic acid, a by-product of glucose fermentation produced by the cell itself. (You might recall that lactic acid is toxic, so it is quickly shuttled from the cell into the extracellular fluid.) This acidity isn't neutralized by a diet of ash-producing foods, as the alkaline diet proponents suggest. In fact, we wouldn't have survived as a species if the pH in our blood or extracellular fluids could be greatly altered by our food choices. Why? Because fundamental metabolic activities, such as enzymatic reactions and protein synthesis, can occur only within a narrow pH range maintained by a complex system of internal buffers and changes in $CO_2$ concentrations. In contrast, *urine* and *saliva* pH can shift easily between acid and alkaline. Urine that is either too acidic or too alkaline raises the risk of kidney stones. If you're

### Keto for Cancer: Not Simply a Leap of Faith

I understand that for many people the switch to a keto diet is a leap of faith, usually prompted by a suggestion from a loved one, by reading about it online, or by listening to "I cured my cancer" testimonials. Of course, you are hopeful that a change in diet will stop this dark disease in its tracks. But faith in the plan needs to be buttressed by the science behind the diet. Otherwise, you would be tempted to give equal credence to *all* diets that claim to be anticancer, eventually hopping from one diet to the next in your search for a cure.

I'm often asked for a rebuttal to *this* criticism or an explanation of *that* testimonial, but I always bring it back to the science. Yes, in many ways we did take a leap of faith with our son, but it was only after doing a lot of homework and learning that the ketogenic diet was already evidence-based, in humans, for one purpose and that there was mounting preclinical evidence it would have a positive effect in cancer as well. So, trust your instincts, but only after you've trained your mind to recognize the difference between science and wishful thinking.

curious, you can use urine pH test strips to determine your urine pH, then take steps, such as adding a prescription potassium citrate, to raise your urine pH.

The acid/alkaline myth is so pervasive and dangerously distracting to everyone, including those with cancer, that I've added much more information about it in chapter 14 ("The Acid/Alkaline Debate," page 266).

## When Conventional Wisdom Is No Longer Wise

On its surface, the official compilation "Dietary Guidelines for Americans," updated in 2015, looks very similar to its predecessor. The macronutrient recommendations as a percentage of total calories are as follows: 45 to 65 percent carbohydrate; 10 to 35 percent protein; 20 to 35 percent fat. What has changed is the recommendation regarding added sugars: It's down to 10 percent of total calories from a former high of 25 percent.

You might ask, "If low carb is a healthier way to eat, why aren't we hearing that message from the government agencies entrusted with keeping us healthy?" Unfortunately, special interests reign! In his new book, *The Case Against Sugar*, science writer Gary Taubes shines a much-needed light on the tactics used by the politically powerful sugar industry that has successfully used paid industry shills to promote its agenda and obfuscate the science pointing to sugar's toxic effects. Other powerful groups and agencies, including the NIH and the US Department of Agriculture (USDA), have wasted decades of time and millions, perhaps billions, of dollars funding biased research that serves to reinforce the status quo. Why? Perhaps in part because the biggest and most influential stakeholders, such as members of the National Corn Growers Association and the American Soybean Association, are among the largest recipients of government crop subsidies. This insult is compounded by the fact that a handful of powerful, high-profile individuals have successfully stifled dissenting voices, even when the science supporting the dissenters' claims was clear. No dark conspiracy theory here; instead, their motives are completely transparent. Follow the money (and power) all the way to the present, and you'll easily understand the underpinnings of our flawed Dietary Guidelines.

Noteworthy authors are also challenging the conventional nutritional dogma. In his controversial book *Good Calories, Bad Calories*, Gary Taubes pecks away at the so-called research used by several influential people (led by Ancel Keys, the American physiologist known for promoting the belief in a relationship between dietary fat and cardiovascular disease). Keys and others used their personal biases and agendas to buttress the "diet-heart hypothesis." Nina Teicholz walks us further down this road in her bestseller, *The Big Fat*

## What You Need to Know about Corn

Corn growers have an agenda that is not in your best interest! I'm not suggesting that we banish all corn from our keto world, as that would be extremely challenging; just to be aware of where you might find it, so that you can make an informed choice about when to allow it in. Take a look:

- The United States federal government subsidizes corn crops, which in turn supports other industries , such as the manufacture of high-fructose corn syrup (HFCS), that are also not in our best interest.
- Corn is also the raw ingredient in the production of other corn-derived sweeteners, such as dextrose in all its forms.
- Corn is processed into animal feed that is very hard for some animals to digest. (NB: As of this writing, whole-grain corn is still listed as the first ingredient in Purina Dog Chow Complete, as well as in other Purina feeds.)
- Corn oil has an omega-6 to omega-3 ratio of 46 to 1, placing it at the top of the list of oils that are pro-inflammatory. This impacts the lipid profile of the animals that consume it. It's not just animals that are fed this garbage. Check your own food ingredient labels!
- Industry corn is a genetically modified (GMO) crop, which means it is laden with the pesticide glyphosate, a known carcinogen that burdens our environment with toxins.
- The glucose in corn is fermented in processes that yield many foods that we don't normally associate with corn, such as erythritol, a sugar alcohol. That's why it's important to look for labels that specify if it is non-GMO, or organic.
- Soluble corn fiber is added to many foods; again, this includes foods that many people on keto diets rely on daily, such as MCT powder. I mention this simply to create awareness.
- Corn is also fermented to make ethanol, touted as a renewable fuel. Ethanol production is another corn product that receives huge government subsidies.

This list represents just the tip of the iceberg!

## Pushing Back against Diet Detractors

The ketogenic diet has been disparaged by those who believe that a low-carb, high-fat plan limits intake of healthier foods. Let's look at a piece of "conventional wisdom" from Harvard Medical School's e-newsletter *HEALTHbeat*, which states that low-carb diets are unhealthy: "The lack of carb-rich fruits and vegetables is . . . worrisome because eating these foods tends to lower the risk of stroke, dementia, and certain cancers."[5] But where is the evidence that only carb-rich fruits and vegetables have this protective effect? Instead, why not conclude that these benefits can also be gained by eating fiber- and nutrient-rich non-starchy vegetables, such as broccoli or asparagus?

*Surprise.* Now, even the NIH is revisiting its stance on low-carbohydrate diets; it recently funded a study comparing low-carb and low-fat diets. (The conclusion: The low-carb diet proved superior at lowering body weight and *reducing* cardiovascular risk.)[4]

It is increasingly clear that diets high in carbohydrates drive up blood glucose and insulin levels. Cancer cells thrive on this bounty and in turn reprogram built-in mechanisms that would normally filter out and destroy defective, damaged, or cancerous cells. The research is compelling, and I am convinced that those among us who are sounding the alarm are on the right side of history.

# CHAPTER 7

# Fasting for Health

O ur bodies have evolved to handle a certain amount of toxins and stressors through activation of a healthy adaptive response known as *hormesis*.
(The concept of hormesis is perhaps most readily understood from Friedrich
Nietzsche's quotation: "That which does not kill us makes us stronger.") The
study of hormesis has health implications beyond the scope of this book and
has become a very active area of research in the "healthy aging" community.
It's also one of my personal interests and one of the reasons I practice what I
preach regarding the need for a paradigm shift in our dietary guidelines.

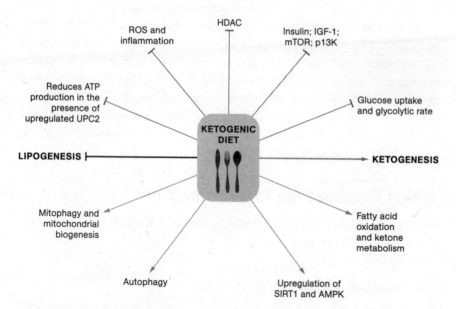

**Figure 7.1.** The ketogenic diet is about so much more than starving cancer of glucose. Truncated lines indicate cancer-promoting pathways that are inhibited through
diet strategies. Arrows indicate upregulation of healthy cellular activities.

## The Benefits of Fasting (and a Few Caveats)

All forms of fasting reduce glucose and insulin levels and improve insulin sensitivity. As a reminder, this results in lowered activity of IGF-1, a hormone associated with cell proliferation in many cancers. In fact, fasting during Ramadan has also been shown to lower the levels of pro-inflammatory cytokines, including IL-1β and IL-6, both known cancer promoters.[1]

During a fast, our cells find ways to economize on activities that normally require a lot of energy, such as cell growth and proliferation. They also step up their housekeeping activities by breaking down and/or removing accumulated garbage and recycling it into new building materials. This housekeeping is called *autophagy*; whereas *mitophagy* is the same activity directed at replacing mitochondria. In this process, damaged or inefficient cells and organelles are sacrificed for the greater good. This includes the dysfunctional mitochondria found in cancer cells.

Mitochondria are important not only for energy production but also for their role in directing cell activities such as apoptosis (cell suicide). They also control cell signaling pathways (such as mTOR) that are involved in cancer progression or pathways (such as AMPK) that help inhibit cancer. The metabolic theory of cancer presents a strong argument that dysfunctional mitochondria are the root cause of the initiation and progression of cancer.

Why is this important to a discussion of fasting? In a review article written by Noboru Mizushima, he states: "The most typical trigger of autophagy is nutrient starvation."[2] Here, the author is referring to brief breaks in the flow of nutrients to cells. I'm so convinced of the benefits of fasting that I bring up the topic with every one of my clients. Understandably, there's a great deal of confusion and uncertainty surrounding best practice, and it can be challenging to navigate through the data and opinions presented by researchers, bloggers, science writers, biohackers, and forum junkies.

## Which Fasting Plan Is Best for You?

It's likely that there is more than one right answer. Let's look at the most commonly considered options.

### Intermittent and Short-Term Fasts

These are my favorite fasts for people with cancer, and they come in many "flavors." In fact, I see benefit in these types of fasts for anyone who is interested in disease prevention and healthy aging.

## Water-Only Fasts

Many people choose to jump-start the ketogenic diet with a water-only fast lasting two or three days. This abrupt shift can feel harsh since you are straddling the line between reliance on glucose and the "new normal" of living on fats and ketones. Those who are already keto-adapted may also opt to fast for two or three days periodically. In this scenario, symptoms are much milder.

## Protein-Sparing Modified Fasts

These are not true fasts because they involve intake of lean protein. Protein-sparing fasts are popular with some people because they result in weight loss while sparing lean body mass. This is *not* a good choice for most people with cancer, however, because excess protein may drive disease progression. (Also, you need an obesity medicine doctor to monitor your health here.)

## Extended Fasts

There is evidence that long fasts promote greater autophagy; that is, they help clear the body of diseased cells or cellular components and dysfunctional mitochondria.[3] However, long fasts are stressful on the body and are not likely to be appropriate for you right now given that you will lose weight and muscle mass.

# Short Two- or Three-Day Fasts

Are you considering a short (two- or three-day) water-only fast? Fasting can jump-start ketosis and speed you past the side effects of the transition, allowing you to become keto-adapted in a shorter period of time. But there are some important considerations before you begin:

- First and foremost, you are responsible for the safety of any children in your home. I strongly advise against fasting under these circumstances unless there is another adult in the home who is ready to take over if you feel dizzy or light-headed.
- Even if you don't have children at home, I strongly advise against fasting if you have mobility or balance issues or a history of seizures. (Obviously, the diet can reduce or eliminate seizures in some people, but initiation requires supervision.)
- Of course, you shouldn't fast if you are pregnant!

## A Few Things to Know before You Fast

Do you identify yourself in any of these situations noted below? If so, it is essential that you seek advice from your health care team before you decide to fast.

- If you have a history of "sluggish" gallbladder or other gallbladder disease, a water-only fast may exacerbate the problem. Here, the risks outweigh the benefits.
- Also, if you are an older adult, are in active cancer treatment, or have not yet recovered from the effects of surgeries or cancer therapies, you should not fast for more than 48 hours. It may place too much stress on your system and lead to breakdown instead of repair.
- If you have a history of eating disorders, there is the potential pitfall that you may slip into a pattern of "feasting and fasting" that is actually closer to "bingeing and purging."

And please don't fall prey to every new post on fasting from your favorite biohacker or blogger. Although they may hold strong opinions, beware of overreach beyond what can be verified by the scientific evidence.

- A water-only fast is not a good option if you are already at a low body weight or nutritionally compromised.
- Fasting is also not a good option if you feel weak and shaky as a result of your disease and/or current treatments.
- If you take diuretics or blood pressure medications, you may need to adjust your dosages and add electrolytes to account for the water and electrolyte loss associated with fasting and the ongoing diuretic effect of the diet. Discuss this in advance with your doctor.
- If you have low blood pressure—or suspect that blood pressure may drop while fasting—you should discuss your plan first with your health care provider.
- Check with your health care provider before fasting if you have health conditions or diseases that may complicate a fast. These

include (but are not limited to) diabetes, thyroid disease, chronically low sodium levels, or cardiovascular disease. (Be aware, however, that your doctor may be totally unaware of the benefits of fasting or openly antagonistic to fasting under any circumstances.)

- It's best if you plan your fast during a time that involves very few responsibilities, such as during a break from work, or a weekend when another adult can care for your children.
- You may need to modify your fast if you have to work or drive. Consider bone broth or hot drinks, such as "Bulletproof" coffee (described later) with added fats or oils.
- While fasting, continue to take your prescribed medications!
- Test your blood glucose and ketones several times a day and record what you see.

## Pay Attention to Nutrients

Fasts and ketogenic diets present a few unique challenges in maintaining the adequate intake of nutrients, but before we dive into that discussion, I want to be sure you have an understanding of what tools you need to prevent malnutrition. The *least* valuable tool is also the one with which you may be most familiar: the US Food and Drug Administration's (FDA's) percent daily value ("%DV") used on the "Nutrition Facts" labels found on packaged foods and supplements. Unfortunately, the %DV on food labels is too limited in both scope and information to be much help to you in determining your nutritional needs. For one reason, only a select few nutrients, such as calcium and sodium, are included; for another, the %DV is based on a 2,000 calorie a day diet and must be adjusted up or down to account for variation from that standard. These percentages also don't account for any variations based on age, gender, or pregnancy or lactation status.

The Dietary Reference Intakes (DRI), developed through the collaborative efforts of a number of government agencies, are a better guide.[4] These tables are very complete; for example, they include detail on individual amino acids that goes well beyond simply listing protein, as in the %DV. This information is presented as the Recommended Dietary Allowance (RDA) of nutrients for nearly all *healthy* people, while acknowledging that the needs of certain groups will fall outside of these recommendations. If there is not sufficient evidence to develop an RDA, then an alternate guideline, Adequate Intake (AI), is used. (Another set of standards, called Tolerable Upper Intake Level, sets a maximum vitamin and mineral intake above which there may be adverse health effects, including toxicity.) All of these guidelines are explained in detail on the National Institutes of Health (NIH) Office of Dietary Supplements website.[5]

Why did I just walk you through this exercise? It's possible that you are either blissfully unaware of the potential adverse impacts of nutrient deficiencies or, on the opposite end of the continuum, naive to the adverse health effects of megadosing on certain supplements. If nutrient sufficiency hasn't been of concern to you in the past, understand that it is about to become central to your keto plan, especially if you are considering restricting calories. You'll learn how to do this in chapter 9.

## Caloric Restriction without Malnutrition

Caloric restriction (also called calorie or energy restriction) simply refers to a reduction in total calories. But it's crucial that you keep attuned to meeting your need for essential nutrients (e.g., vitamins, minerals, essential amino acids, and essential fatty acids). There are well-documented benefits to caloric restriction in delaying the chronic diseases associated with aging, and many of those benefits should apply to cancer as well. I've summarized these in the list below. (Note that most of the research I'm referencing here is from preclinical data in mouse models of cancer, though there is evidence from human studies as well.)

**Caloric restriction inhibits angiogenesis.** In many cancers, tumor tissue actually directs the development of new blood vessel networks to increase the supply of nutrients to cancer cells. This process is known as angiogenesis. It is well documented that restricting calorie intake suppresses angiogenesis.[6]

**Caloric restriction enhances apoptosis.** Apoptosis is the cellular process that normally directs the self-destruction of damaged or dysfunctional cells ("cell suicide"). Remember that a failure of apoptosis is one of the hallmarks of cancer.[7]

**Caloric restriction reduces chronic inflammation.** This anti-inflammatory effect also improves outcomes in hypertension, type 2 diabetes, coronary heart disease, stroke, and osteoarthritis.[8]

**Caloric restriction limits the availability of nutrients to the tumor tissue,** which in turn inhibits opportunities for cancer cell proliferation.[9]

**Beyond cancer, caloric restriction has been shown to extend the health and life span of a variety of organisms from yeasts to**

**rodents to primates.**[10] The language of science refers to the genes involved here as "highly conserved" across species.

**Caloric restriction enhances a cellular housekeeping process, known as autophagy,** which weeds out dysfunctional cells and restores healthy cellular signaling.[11] (Yoshinori Ohsumi was awarded the Nobel Prize in Physiology or Medicine in 2016 for his work in this field.)

Dr. Thomas Seyfried's landmark paper, "The Calorically Restricted Ketogenic Diet, an Effective Alternative Therapy for Malignant Brain Cancer," was published in February of 2007 in the online journal *Nutrition and Metabolism.*[12] This important research clearly shows that a calorically restricted ketogenic diet offers survival benefits in mouse models of brain cancer. Dr. Seyfried used two distinct brain cancer types and there were a total of six interventions in his study: (1) two groups fed normal mouse chow *ad libitum* (all-you-can-eat), (2) two groups fed a ketogenic diet *ad libitum*, and (3) two groups fed a ketogenic diet in calorie-restricted

## The Average Keto Diet Calorie Intake

I encourage most people with cancer to lower their net carb intake to 12 to 20 grams per day and reduce protein to 0.8 grams per kg of *ideal* body weight per day (or 1.0 gram per kg of lean body mass) unless their needs are higher due to malnutrition or recent surgery. The balance of their intake is in the form of fats. When feasible and safe, I suggest calorie restriction as well, but not to the extremes that I see with weight-loss diets. I usually set the lower limit at 1,200 to 1,500 calories for women and 1,600 to 2,200 for men, taking into account age, current weight, and activity level. A calorie-restricted ketogenic diet virtually guarantees that you will reach nutritional ketosis (blood ketones at or above 0.5 mmol/L), and most people who restrict calories are at or near therapeutic levels of both glucose and ketones (a 1:1 to 2:1 ratio of blood glucose to blood ketones). *Please understand that these are generalizations intended to provide an overview, but you need to work through the process in chapter 9 to determine if caloric restriction is appropriate for you.* Work with a keto-savvy nutrition professional to optimize your plan, and always listen to your medical team's input.

## A Deep Dive into Mouse Chow

Dr. Thomas Seyfried's paper offered data to support the conclusion that mice with cancer fed a ketogenic diet *ad libitum* did not fare as well as those that were calorie restricted. This was true even though both groups were fed KetoCal 4:1, a complete medical food developed primarily for children on the ketogenic diet as a treatment for epilepsy. KetoCal, though medically complete, was formulated at the time with hydrogenated soybean oil. Ouch! Three strikes against it: (1) Soybean oil by itself creates systemic inflammation; (2) *trans* fat from the hydrogenation process is a health disaster, causing damage to the lipid structure of cellular membranes; and (3) the oil was made from GMO soy, meaning that the soy crop had been treated with Roundup.

KetoCal 4:1 is about 90 percent fat. The mice fed *ad libitum* were getting full energy needs by converting this oil into ketones or by oxidizing it in normal tissue, such as heart and muscle, while the restricted mice were fed only enough KetoCal to meet 60 percent of their energy needs (40 percent calorie restricted). That means that the calorie-restricted mice needed to use both dietary (exogenous) and stored (endogenous) fats to meet their fuel requirements. So in theory, the lipid profile of their own body fat may have been less inflammatory than the KetoCal. This is just a thought, but this is how hypotheses for research come into being. (Note: KetoCal was recently reformulated using less inflammatory, non-hydrogenated oils.)

amounts. All of the mice underwent a procedure that established colonies of brain tumor cells. The mice fed normal chow were the controls in the study. The mice fed the two forms of the ketogenic diet served as the experimental groups.

Dr. Seyfried and colleagues observed in all the mice that levels of mito-chondrial enzymes that aid in metabolizing ketones were lower in the tumor tissue than they were in the surrounding normal brain tissue. This offered one explanation of why both groups of keto-fed mice lived longer than the controls. But the more intriguing observation was that the mice in the group that was calorically restricted lived *significantly* longer than either the control mice or the mice fed unrestricted amounts of the ketogenic formula. The calorically restricted mice had lower blood glucose levels and higher blood ketone levels

Let's look at other areas that deserve investigation. Would the results of this study have been different if the mouse chow had been formulated with mouse-friendly ingredients and a high-quality (e.g., omega-3-rich) source of oils? And what about the potential benefit from other forms of restricted feeding, such as feeding *ad libitum* one day and fasting the next? In a mouse model of acute lympho-blastic leukemia (ALL), this nutritional strategy resulted in a dramatic reduction in cancer cells. (See chapter 4, "Another Dietary Therapy: Intermittent Fasting," page 47.)

Dr. Seyfried reviewed this section of the book and stressed that it was important to make clear that there are fundamental differences between human and mouse metabolism. For example, the basal meta-bolic rate of humans is about seven times less than that of mice. Thus, the 40 percent caloric restriction in the mice he used in one study was roughly equivalent to a one- to two-week water-only fast in humans. Also, the mice in this study were young and healthy before they were implanted with glioma cells, whereas most humans diagnosed with brain cancer are mid-life or older and may have accumulated any number of chronic diseases.

These are just a few of the many reasons why we can't use pre-clinical data from mouse model research to draw conclusions about an effect in humans. Instead, this data can—and should—be used to develop hypotheses that can then be tested on human subjects.

than either of the groups fed *ad libitum*. Tumor microvessel density was also lower in the calorie-restricted mice (in other words, there were fewer blood vessels, which limited the transport of nutrients to the tumor). Dr. Seyfried concluded that both of these factors (vessel density and blood glucose levels) had reduced the amount of circulating glucose available to the tumor tissue, which, remember, was already compromised because tumor tissue was less able to utilize ketones for energy.

Interestingly, Dr. Seyfried has also speculated that the unintentional weight loss often experienced as a side effect of chemotherapy and radiation protocols may be what's driving the good initial response seen in some standard of care treatments. This begs further investigation. Weight is routinely tracked by all oncologists, so the data here would be readily available to any clinician curious enough to ask, "Does weight loss as a percentage of total weight at baseline correlate with outcomes in cancer?" Of course, there are far too many variables to arrive at a simple yes-or-no answer, but questions such as this one could lead to the development of new hypotheses to test in the context of future studies.

Generally, caloric restriction in humans consists of reducing caloric intake by 20 to 30 percent for the first month or so. Given all the possible variables, is it realistic to believe that all people with cancer who start a ketogenic diet should also restrict calories? My opinion: absolutely not.

There is one glaringly obvious limitation with caloric restriction: It is not sustainable over time. Taking in far fewer calories than you expend means that your energy needs will need to be met by accessing your fat stores. This has its limits. Also, mobilization of fat stores resulting in too-rapid a weight loss dumps a great many toxins and hormones into the bloodstream, possibly at a rate that is too high for your body to either detoxify or assimilate. Women in particular seem to have more hormone-related issues surrounding rapid weight loss. Another important consideration involving caloric restriction, especially relevant to people with cancer, is the potential it has to suppress immune system function.

Calorie-restricted diets may exclude adequate intake of needed nutrients. That's why you need to track what you eat to ensure that you are meeting the recommendations for all nutrients—in other words, consuming fewer calories but without risking malnutrition. The more restricted your plan, the more important it becomes to focus on the foods that are richest in nutrients. This takes some planning and most likely some nutritional supplementation as well. (I'll spell that out in chapter 14.)

The point is that the decision of whether or not to start the diet with caloric restriction needs to be made on a case-by-case basis while working with a professional who takes into account your present health and nutrition status. (All the more reason to find an integrative oncologist and keto-savvy nutritionist, if at all possible.) If you are in active treatment, or coping with advanced cancer, you may already be experiencing low body weight, muscle wasting, poor appetite, nausea and vomiting, vitamin and mineral deficiencies, impaired digestion, depressed immune function, and poor absorption of nutrients. This is not the time to add more pressure through caloric restriction!

To sum it up, I believe that caloric restriction can be an incredibly powerful tool, especially at the start of the diet, when properly integrated into a well-formulated ketogenic plan that has weighed risk against benefit in a person who is generally healthy.

## Can You Simply Restrict Calories on a Standard Diet?

Although caloric restriction has great potential to impact cancer-promoting pathways, simply restricting calories does not necessarily eliminate the glucose spikes or the associated rise in insulin. It is also important to remember that severe caloric restriction in a standard diet leaves people reliant on glucose-based metabolism that in turn leaves them hungry, tired, weak, and ultimately non-adherent with their treatment plans. Obviously, these side effects take a toll on quality of life. Also, not all calorie-restricted diets lower protein intake, and for those who have cancer, excess protein may result in higher glucose levels and/or directly fuel tumor growth (through activation of mTOR and the utilization of amino acids as an energy substrate). As noted earlier, extreme calorie restriction with any diet may have a negative impact on the immune system. And the problem is magnified when caloric restriction is combined with standard therapies that also depress immune function.

# The Perks of Intermittent Fasting

There has been a recent surge in research on the effects of fasting in both humans and animal models. The new development that separates most of the current investigations from those of the past is that many of the newer studies are not limited to extended water-only fasting. Instead, they are testing a range of hypotheses that attempt to identify both the benefits and risks of different modified fasting protocols. Of course, this introduces a whole host of variables that warrant further research.

There are some standouts in this research. For one, I was thrilled when I found an interesting review in the journal *PLoS ONE*, looking at research on energy restriction in animal models of cancer.[13] (I encourage you to read this study not only for the interesting information it provides, but also for the list of references that it cites.) The review included studies on caloric restriction, a ketogenic diet, and intermittent fasting and concluded that caloric restriction and a ketogenic diet improved outcomes, whereas intermittent fasting did not appear to have an impact. Nevertheless, it's intriguing to think about the possible role of intermittent fasting as an add-on therapy to either caloric restriction or a ketogenic diet. (Recall that Dr. Seyfried's research showed significantly improved outcomes only in the mice fed restricted amounts of a ketogenic diet). And what might a combination of all three strategies yield? This warrants study in humans, not just animal models, to determine the ideal combination of nutritional strategies that yields the most benefit with the fewest risks.

## The Many Variations of Intermittent Fasting

"Fasting" means many things to many people. Let's take a closer look at the many variations:

- Alternate-day fasting (including variations that allow for 20 percent of normal calorie intake on fasting days alternating with a 20 percent increase in calorie consumption on non-fasting days).
- 48-hour cycles of fasting (water only)
- One day per week of water-only fasting
- 5:2 (5 days of normal eating; 2 days of modified fasting, such as 20 percent of normal caloric intake)
- "Time-restricted feeding," a scientific but awkward name used to describe daily fasting with varying "windows" of eating hours versus fasting hours. I prefer to call this "daily intermittent fasting."

Note: A study by Longo and Panda, published in the journal *Cell Metabolism*, includes an in-depth examination of factors influencing circadian rhythm that leads to a discussion of the potential impact of various fasting protocols.[14] The authors acknowledge that these results are too preliminary to draw any conclusions, but this does open up speculation that some types of fasting may disrupt circadian rhythm and endocrine function while others may actually enhance normal function. They also suggest that age-related changes in circadian rhythm may be addressed through the timing of food intake relative to sleep. More research is needed here to test these new questions.

Given these options, how do you choose which, if any, may work in your favor? Hands down, I prefer to keep it simple, at least early on, with a time-restricted daily intermittent fasting plan. Simply limit your eating window to 8 to 10 hours by allowing at least 3 hours between your last meal and bedtime, then delaying your first meal of the day by an hour or more. If this sounds too challenging, start with a 12-hour window of eating and gradually reduce it as you adapt to your new plan. Over time, this will result in a daily 14- to 16-hour fast. In contrast to water-only or other extended fasts, this pattern has the added benefit of helping nutrition-compromised people retain their current weight.

Energy needs drop and metabolism slows overnight, so there's no need to fuel your body close to bedtime. Overnight fasting also allows your body the needed time to perform its maintenance and repair activities and keeps your glycogen stores low so your body will continue to burn fat for energy. Also, allowing more pre-sleep time for digestion can ease GERD symptoms. A dinner-to-breakfast (or beyond) fast is more tolerable because you're sleeping through most of the fasting hours and because you are consistent from day to day. This makes it easier to adopt the pattern as one of your healthy habits. Commit to giving this plan a two-week trial. If it feels right, commit for the long term. *(Note: If you need to take bedtime medication with food, just keep it light, such as a few teaspoons of nut butter.)*

## The "Bulletproof" Model

In case you haven't yet heard of the Bulletproof plan, here it is in a nutshell: You begin the day with a cup of coffee loaded with fats, pushing your first meal of the day a few hours into the future. Entrepreneur and fitness blogger Dave Asprey initially introduced the concept into the fitness world, where it was an instant hit. Dave's original Bulletproof coffee is a proprietary blend of his organic coffee, ghee, and MCT oil (as XCT or Brain Octane). Although in fact this is a *modified* rather than a true fast, it's caught on like wildfire, with many people concocting their own versions (for example, using tea in place of coffee or substituting other brands of MCT oil, MCT powder, coconut oil, or unsalted butter). The critical takeaway is to keep it free of any carbs or protein that would boost glucose or stimulate a release of insulin.

How far should you take the Bulletproof protocol? In my opinion, unless you are an athlete with the need for a lot of extra fat calories, limit your Bulletproof coffee or tea to a morning cup or two but keep your total intake to a maximum of 3 tablespoons of fats or oils. It is important to note that more is *not* better. Even though it's ketogenic, too much of a good thing may lead to serious gastrointestinal effects, such as bloating, nausea, or diarrhea. Also, be aware that Bulletproof reduces hunger; don't allow it to interfere with your intake of other nutrient-dense foods.

## Consider a Combination of Fasting Options

First, revisit the factors that will help you decide if calorie restriction is a good option at this time. In any case, you will need to track your weight. Is it trending in the direction that you want? If not, where can you add or subtract fat calories? Next, test your blood glucose upon awakening and again at bedtime. Record and/or graph these numbers.

Keep in mind that too few calories overall or too long a fast can backfire, as these are known stressors with the potential to drive up your fasting blood glucose (primarily through the secretion of stress hormones). If you delay eating (with or without Bulletproof coffee), test your blood glucose just prior to your first meal of the day. If it's higher than your fasting level, adjust your schedule so that you're eating that first meal earlier. (Remember that although MCT in Bulletproof drinks can boost your ketones, this is not likely to be as therapeutic if glucose levels remain high.) Another issue: Squeezing all your fat calories into just a few hours per day may not be tolerable, and discomfort or indigestion will interfere with compliance. Experiment with meal timing to find out what's best for you. *Remember to allow three hours or more between your last meal and bedtime if at all possible.*

## Short-Term Fasting as an Adjunct to Chemotherapy

There's been an explosion of published research on the effect of short-term fasting in cancer. You can access this wealth of information easily by going to PubMed.gov and searching for "short term fasting cancer." There's a good chance you'll find a study that relates to your cancer type. I'm excited by what people who try this fasting regimen report back to me, so I want to highlight the potential benefits, some of which you can reap even if you are not yet up to speed with your ketogenic plan.

Nausea and vomiting associated with drug therapies make it difficult to consume *any* food other than drinks, such as Ensure and Boost, which are loaded with easily digestible carbohydrates and added sugars. This is obviously a huge problem if you are following a ketogenic diet! At its most basic, short-term fasting during chemotherapy can reduce both the number and severity of treatment-related side effects.[15] There is also evidence that short-term fasting protects normal cells from damage while sensitizing cancer cells to drug therapies, enhancing the therapy's efficacy. There are now several clinical trials investigating a number of other effects of short-term fasts during chemotherapy. In other words, it's OK to *not* eat if you don't feel like it. Of course, it's best that you remain under the watchful eye of a dedicated caregiver anytime you receive chemotherapy, fasting or not.

Most of my clients who have tried short-term fasting while undergoing chemotherapy are very surprised at how easy it is *not* to eat when in ketosis. This is because keto-adaptation makes the body less reliant on a steady intake of food to meet its energy needs. Worried about losing weight? Those who

## The Basics of Short-Term Fasting during Chemotherapy

- Stop eating 24 to 36 hours before treatment.
- Fast the day of the treatment.
- Resume eating 24 hours post-treatment.
- Stay hydrated! Water protects the kidneys and helps flush out toxins.
- Some people may choose to drink soothing bone broth (modified fasting!).

Note: Short-term fasting is not suitable for everyone. Do not fast if your blood glucose numbers are erratic or if you are taking high-dose steroids that interfere with glucose control. Nor is a full short-term fast an option if you take medications that must be taken with food. (Will a cup of broth work for you?) If you can't completely fast on your treatment day, then perhaps you can still sharply decrease your calorie intake (500 to 800 calories, mostly as fats).

fast during therapy generally do not experience significantly greater weight loss than those who don't, mostly because even those who aren't fasting are usually consuming less food anyway because of the side effects of treatment.

## Therapeutic Weight Loss versus Cancer Cachexia

When making dietary recommendations, doctors rarely draw a distinction between *therapeutic* weight loss associated with a well-planned ketogenic diet, *functional* weight loss from poor tolerance to treatment, and *pathological* weight loss due to cancer cachexia. Cachexia is a wasting syndrome commonly associated with late-stage disease in pancreatic, colon, lung, stomach, and many other cancers. The conventional advice given in response to *any* type of weight loss is the same: Drink Ensure or Boost to add calories. How misguided! In addition to being loaded with carbohydrates, these drinks are overloaded with low-quality synthetic vitamins. Worse, this method of feeding your body feeds your cancer cells!

Cancer cachexia is the polar opposite of beneficial weight loss. It is a complex and often irreversible syndrome characterized by the breakdown of lean body tissue, especially muscle, which liberates amino acids that in turn fuel cancer's

## Ketones and Cachexia

Ketones lower levels of the inflammation that drives cachexia and also help preserve muscle mass. To date there have been few published studies looking at the potential of a ketogenic diet (or ketone supplementation) to prevent or reverse cachexia. That's why it was exciting to read the paper "Metabolic Reprogramming Induced by Ketone Bodies Diminishes Pancreatic Cancer Cachexia," published in 2014 in the journal *Cancer and Metabolism*.[16] In this study it was found that in cultured pancreatic cancer cells, the addition of ketones greatly slowed the flow of glucose and glutamine into the cells. (Pancreatic cancer uses both glucose and glutamine as fuel.) In theory, ketones provide a non-fermentable energy source that spares lean protein, including muscle tissue, from being catabolized.[17] Even more interesting, the researchers implanted tumors in the pancreases of immune-compromised nude mice that were then randomized to receive either their standard food or a ketogenic diet. After three weeks all of the mice were sacrificed. Among other significant findings, the mice fed the ketogenic diet showed a slowing in the rate of muscle wasting, diminished tumor growth and proliferation, and a 20 percent increase in carcass weight when compared to the mice fed a standard diet. These are strong indicators that the ketogenic diet is effective in inhibiting cancer cachexia (at least in this group of mice).

increasing energy needs. Greatly reduced food intake is a hallmark of cachexia, driven in part by inflammation-related anorexia (loss of appetite). The problem is compounded by the curtailment of physical activity.[21] Advanced (refractory) cachexia is very complex and poorly understood, and to date no single treatment has shown broad success. Research is ongoing and is now looking at whether the use of the ketogenic diet and ketone supplements—known to reduce inflammation and spare protein in healthy people—may prove beneficial in those with cachexia from cancer as well.

Recently, the potential for branched-chain amino acid supplementation to maintain and perhaps even rebuild muscle mass has been explored.[22] A supplement called hydroxymethylbutyrate (HMB), a metabolite of the branched-chain amino acid leucine, shows promise in slowing muscle loss.[23,24]

Looking back a bit further, I was surprised to discover a series of studies that looked at a mouse model of colon cancer. In these studies, mice were fed a diet high in MCTs, a dietary source of fat that produces abundant ketone bodies. The first study compared control mice fed standard chow with mice fed diets high in MCTs (with and without exogenous ketones). Tumor-bearing mice that were fed the diet with the highest proportion of MCTs experienced the least amount of weight loss.[18] Another study compared the MCT group with groups fed either a diet high in long-chain fats or a standard diet and found that the MCT group showed reduced weight loss and a reduction in tumor size.[19] In the third study, weight loss and tumor size in mice fed an 80 percent MCT diet were compared with mice that received daily insulin injections. Although both interventions significantly reduced weight loss, only the mice fed the 80 percent MCT diet experienced a reduction in tumor size. In fact, the tumor weight in mice receiving insulin was 50 percent greater than that in saline-infused controls, leading the researcher to suggest that "a ketogenic diet is more effective than insulin administration in reversing the cachectic process and has the advantage of a concomitant reduction in tumour weight."[20] Why hasn't this research received more attention given the dire consequences of cachexia? Instead, patients at risk are advised to simply take in more calories in the form of easy-to-digest insulin-boosting starches.

Supplementation with non-glucogenic amino acids (so far studied in conjunction with an otherwise standard diet) may also help maintain muscle mass.[25] Future research will examine amino acid supplementation in the context of ketogenic rather than standard diets. Dr. Dominic D'Agostino and his team at the University of South Florida are conducting exciting studies that may lead to better ways to prevent or reverse cachexia by targeting inflammation and anti-catabolic pathways using metabolic-based approaches.

Here I want to acknowledge the valuable input I received for this section from Angela Poff, PhD, and cachexia researcher Andrew Koutnik (both at the University of South Florida). Help fund this important lab! (If you are interested, learn how you can do this in the afterword, page 323.)

# CHAPTER 8

# Get Started!

There is already a vast amount of information about the ketogenic diet online, and new sites and blogs pop up almost daily. Without a doubt, you'll find a lot of very useful information there, but currently the majority of it is directed at those focused on maximizing weight loss. That's not your goal. I recommend a few of the best sites in the resources section. These sites provide sound, cancer-specific science without the hype.

There are obvious pitfalls to watch out for online, including those that I call "fountains of misinformation," often well intentioned but misguided. You may read testimonials from those who believe that they've "cured" their cancer with a ketogenic diet. Understand that these personal stories may represent an amazing and wonderful response, but how can they be declaring themselves "cured" in just a few weeks or months? And what about the sites that are intentionally misleading, offering a sliver of science to draw you into buying proprietary, often very expensive "cures"? Although there may be a nugget of truth mixed in with the rubble, my advice is "buyer beware": If a treatment is marketed as a stand-alone cure, it's snake oil. There is no single food, supplement, or other therapy that is a universal cure for cancer. If and when the medical community discovers a cure for this dreadful disease, you will already have benefited from the changes you make now to your diet and lifestyle.

## Put Your Toolkit Together

Are you ready to make the changes that will start you down this path? If so, let me help! There are no hard-and-fast rules here. So much depends on how much time and energy you can devote to this. For example, if you have never read a scientific paper in your life, stick to reading the abstract (a short summary) and scanning the body of the paper for the parts that make sense right now. You can always revisit them later.

## Quick Tips for Getting Started

- Skim this chapter and highlight or bookmark the sections you'll want to revisit. This information is so new to you that I expect you'll need to look it over several times. With each reading, your understanding will deepen and you will begin to incorporate more bits of knowledge into your burgeoning keto framework. You will also formulate new questions by identifying the gaps in your understanding.
- Review the list of recommended books (also listed in the resources section). Order the ones you may need right away and keep a list of those that you may want to read once you are up and running with the diet.
- The resources section contains a list of recommended, vetted websites, interviews, and videos. Prioritize how you will work through them. Can you listen to podcasts while you're performing routine tasks, such as washing the dishes or commuting to work? Can you watch the videos on your TV screen to shorten the amount of time you spend staring at your device? Can you "outsource" some of the research to friends or family who can summarize it for you? Do try to think of creative ways to reduce the amount of time you spend at your computer.

## Basic Keto-for-Cancer Tools

I use a variety of tools in my work and have included here the ones that I see as priorities. I'll describe how to use each of them in detail as we move through the book. For now, I recommend bookmarking these sites on your computer so you can refer back to them easily:

### The USDA Food Composition Database

This is the database used by most online food tracking tools, such as Cronometer and My Fitness Pal. The USDA site provides detailed nutrition data for many of the whole foods that will be an integral part of your keto plan. I'll explain how to use this tool in chapter 12 ("The USDA Food Composition Database," page 200).

## Meal Planner/Tracker

After years of frustration with online food trackers, I've finally found one I can wholeheartedly recommend: Cronometer (www.cronometer.com). And it's free! The Mercola version of the platform allows you to share your data anonymously and also has a few enhancements, including dashboard dials to help you track important ratios, such as your omega-6 to omega-3 ratio. The developer, Aaron Davidson, combined his interest in anti-aging science with his skills as a software developer to design a platform that has, in his words, "dense functionality." That's an understatement! Aaron is constantly upgrading this program, adding new features that enhance and expand the platform's capabilities.

Cronometer uses vetted databases that provide not only macronutrient data but also background information on vitamins, minerals, amino acids, and individual lipids. By sticking to a tracker that uses only high-quality databases, you'll be spared the guesswork and inaccuracies found in other trackers. Cronometer also provides the option of entering your own preferred foods, recipes, and supplements that aren't in the main database. You can even share your recipes with friends. Personalizing your entries in this way requires some time and effort on your part, but there's a huge long-term payoff in knowing exactly what you take in on a daily basis.

Cronometer's "dense functionality" extends way beyond the foods that you eat. As I mentioned, Aaron is an anti-aging advocate. He's also a biohacker (a kind of do-it-yourself biology explorer and inventor), so he's included features that allow you to enter biometrics, such as your blood glucose and ketone measurements, to help you more easily track your personal data, both for your keto plan and for general health improvement. There are many other features that allow you to monitor your progress. See for yourself!

Go to https://cronometer.com (or https://cronometer.com/mercola) to sign up for a free account. For now, when you set up your profile, select the "High Fat/Ketogenic" diet option under "Macronutrient Target" and, under "Strictness," choose "Rigorous." You may end up changing this later, but I want you to become familiar with some of the features before you actually need to use it to create a plan and track your foods. I'll go into more detail in chapter 9.

My effusive praise for this program might lead you to believe that there's some financial gain for me, but let me assure you there isn't. And for the sake of full disclosure, I should tell you that the program does have its quirks. Since the developer is dedicated to constant improvement of the product, however, I expect these minor issues will be ironed out soon. Also, keep in mind that getting started with *any* new computer program can be a bit of a challenge for many of us. If that's the case, don't go it alone. Cronometer offers email support. If the instruction manual and embedded videos aren't enough to get you started, ask a tech-savvy person to help you sort it out. You can also ease in by recording just one meal a day and building up from there.

### The Ankerl KetoCalculator

This tool (https://Keto-Calculator.ankerl.com/) will help you determine the starting point for your personal diet prescription. You will be entering your demographics (age, gender, height, weight, body fat percentage) along with information about your activity level and body-fat percentage. This will be used to determine your "macronutrient prescription," or your beginning requirement for total calories divided between carbohydrates, protein, and fat.

### The Charlie Foundation List of
### Low-Carb Medications and Hygiene Products

Review the lists of low-carb medications and hygiene products (https://www .charliefoundation.org/resources-tools/resources-2/low-carb). What an eye-opener about how often we unwittingly invite carbs into our lives in so many ways!

## Blood Glucose and Ketone Monitoring Products

I've included details on these products in chapter 11 ("Blood Meters," page 186), but I also encourage you to go to my website for information on your options as products and recommendations are likely to change over time. Here's what you'll need:

- blood glucose/ketone monitors and supplies
- urine ketone test strips
- breath-testing devices

## Kitchen Equipment

First and foremost: You need a sturdy and accurate kitchen scale. While not strictly necessary, you can make your life easier with a set of silicone spatulas, wire whisks, and an immersion blender. You may also want to purchase some silicone molds, and a whipped cream canister. Specifics are in chapter 11 ("An Accurate Scale and Other Kitchen Essentials," page 173).

## Supplements

Use caution here! If you're actively undergoing treatment with prooxidative therapies, such as chemotherapy, radiation, hyperbaric oxygen, or intravenous vitamin C, you will need to avoid many antioxidant supplements (not foods), as these can interfere with your treatment. You may still need to include nutritional supplements, however, mostly the vitamins and minerals that are challenging to get from diet alone. (A list is included in chapter 14.) Of course, you may also want to explore some of the better-researched anti-inflammatory and immune-boosting herbals and botanicals (such as curcumin and berberine), but I strongly advise you to find a savvy integrative professional here to guide you, as your protocol must be personalized. Ask your consultant to back up their recommendations with published scientific papers. Be wary of anyone who offers only testimonials, or pushes you toward buying a cartload of expensive, often proprietary supplements. Also, keep in mind that claims of benefits from herbals and botanicals aren't verified since their manufacture is not regulated. Purity and potency can be a huge issue as well, so look for products from suppliers you trust. (The website www.labdoor.com/rankings is a good starting point.)

## Macronutrients

Macronutrients (carbohydrates, proteins, and fats) are a convenient way to group and describe the substances we consume in large amounts to power our bodies and provide the nutrients we need for the development and maintenance of every cell in our bodies. (Some people view ketones as a fourth macronutrient because they also power the body and act as signaling molecules.) We typically think of carbohydrate-containing foods as primarily supplying energy and nutrients; proteins provide amino acids, our body's building blocks; and fats furnish essential nutrients integral to cell membranes as well as aid in the absorption of necessary fat-soluble vitamins.

Although minimum requirements have been established for essential proteins and fats, it is a well-kept secret in the conventional nutrition community that there is no true requirement for carbohydrate. This is somewhat puzzling, given that the government guidelines would have you believe that there is a good reason we need to obtain over half of our calories from carbohydrates, including dense sources of sugars and starches. That said, I firmly believe that it's normal, natural, and healthy for you to eat nutrient-rich foods that contain carbohydrates, such as non-starchy vegetables, nuts and seeds, and some berries. Let's look at the changes you will need to make in your food choices to meet your new macronutrient goals.

## A Different Mix of Familiar Foods

You will be ridding your kitchen space of foods that are no longer part of your plan and restocking your shelves and refrigerator with keto-friendly foods. Remember, to be successful, your shift in metabolism must be accompanied by a shift in your attitude regarding the role of food in your life.

# Redefine Your Relationship with Sugar

We all grew up with sugar. Unfortunately, we have been led to believe that its only drawback is that it can cause cavities or lead to excessive weight. Until very recently, government guidelines allowed up to 25 percent of our daily calories to be in the form of added sugars. (The guideline now stands at 10 percent.) That doesn't even take into consideration foods that are naturally high in sugars, like tropical fruits, and it doesn't include starches, either, even though they are simply chains of glucose molecules that are easily digested and absorbed.

The sugar industry has a massive ongoing campaign to try to sway our thinking here, calling for an end to "demonization" of sugar. It claims that the science against sugar is "inconclusive," the same tactic that the tobacco

## The "Healthy Sugars" Contradiction

A common myth is that some sugars, including honey or maple syrup, are healthy for us because they are closer to the source, unrefined, and assumed to have essential micronutrients in them. But when you actually look for those micronutrients, you'll learn that these exist only in minuscule amounts, generally a few hundredths of a milligram per serving—far too little to offer any benefit, especially when weighed against the health issues associated with sugar in all its forms. There is also misinformation in the blogosphere about agave nectar. Yes, it is low-glycemic, but only because it is so high in fructose!

## Beware of Sneaky Sugars

What we call "sugars" are most often a single molecule of glucose (a "monosaccharide") bound to another monosaccharide. Sucrose ("table sugar") consists of one molecule of glucose and one molecule of fructose. Lactose ("milk sugar") is made up of glucose bound to galactose. It is crucial that you read *all* ingredient as well as nutrition labels. This way you can avoid foods containing sucrose, fructose, lactose, and the other sugars that can easily be identified by their "-ose" endings. (Sucralose is an artificial sweetener and therefore technically OK, but not recommended.)

Beware of sneaky sugars, too, including maltodextrin, corn-based sweeteners, and glycerin/glycerol. Learning the names of all these sugars won't be necessary if you focus on switching over to eating mostly whole foods (which I strongly recommend). Still, this list is a handy reference:

- agave juice, nectar, sap, syrup
- Barbados sugar
- barley malt or barley malt syrup
- beet sugar
- brown rice syrup
- brown sugar
- buttered syrup
- cane sugar, juice, or syrup
- caramel
- carob syrup
- castor sugar
- coconut sugar
- confectioners' or powdered sugar
- corn glucose syrup
- corn sweetener or syrup
- date sugar
- dextrin and dextrose
- dried raisin sweetener
- fructose
- fruit juice
- golden syrup
- granular sweetener or sugar
- grape sugar
- high-fructose corn syrup
- honey
- invert sugar
- isoglucose or isomaltulose
- lactose
- liquid sweetener
- malt sweetener or syrup
- maltose and maltodextrin
- maple sugar or syrup
- molasses
- raw sugar
- refiner's syrup
- rice syrup
- saccharose
- sorghum
- starch sweetener
- sucrose
- sugar
- treacle
- turbinado sugar

industry successfully used for decades to push back against those who blew the whistle on tobacco's dangers. Its mantra is "Just move more!" *Really?* That's great advice, but who seriously believes that movement alone will stem the rising tide of obesity and type 2 diabetes?

The *New York Times* and science writer Gary Taubes, among others, have brought to light decades of shady practices in the sugar industry.[1,2] There are also revelations, unsurprisingly, that several prominent organizations (the Academy of Dietetics and Nutrition, the American Heart Association, and the American Diabetes Association, among others) have accepted large sums of money from Coke and Pepsi.[3] And, as you're now learning, there are other less obvious risks to sugar as well: Diseases such as cancer, type 2 diabetes, and some forms of dementia are also linked to sugar consumption. (I certainly don't say this to make you feel in some way guilty for developing cancer; instead, I want to open your eyes to the underlying cause of so many of our current health woes.)

Thankfully, there has been some movement in the right direction here. Recent changes to food labeling requirements will mandate manufacturers to add a new line for "added sugars." This is an improvement over the old system, but it doesn't go far enough. In fact, it's bound to create some additional confusion if you believe that the "added sugars" line tells you the whole story. You still need to pay careful attention to the "total carbohydrates": That includes a tally of *all* forms of sugar molecules in the product. Under the "carbohydrates" line, you'll see "fiber." Subtract the grams of fiber from the figure for total carbs to arrive at net carbs: This is the real focus of our attention.

## Say Good-bye to Grains and Starches

You may not realize that grains and starches are made up mostly of chains of glucose molecules. Starch is the plant equivalent of our glycogen stores, held in reserve to provide energy to the plant as needed. With few exceptions, the bonds holding these chains are easily broken apart during digestion and the glucose is then absorbed into the bloodstream from the intestines. Plants also use glucose molecules as part of their structure: Cellulose is one example. Humans don't have the enzymes needed to break those bonds, so glucose molecules in these fibers never enter the bloodstream. Instead, they either feed our gut bacteria or are passed out in our feces as fiber residue.

Grains and starches are a dense source of glucose and there is no room for them in a ketogenic diet. Eliminate *all* grains, including wheat, corn, oats, rice,

## Are You Still Feeding
## Grains and Starches to Your Dog?

When our standard poodle, Amos, was 12 years old, he was diagnosed with lymphoma. His prognosis was given as three months with no treatment and three to nine months with treatment. His protocol would include the drugs cyclophosphamide and prednisone; both were drugs that Raffi had received as part of his chemotherapy protocol. We said "no thanks" to the drugs, but immediately switched our dog from a grain-based kibble to a homemade ketogenic diet. Within a few weeks, all signs of lymphoma had disappeared. I'm not suggesting he was "cured" but I can tell you that he lived longer than the projected nine months and died of an unrelated disease.

Cancer has become a scourge for dogs. Think about it: Dogs have absolutely no history of eating grains before modern times. (Ever see a wolf take down an ear of corn?) As you learn the benefits of eliminating grains from your own diet, you'll see plenty of reasons to police what your pets are eating as well.

If you're a dog lover, then you need to know about the exciting work going on at KetoPet Sanctuary in Georgetown, Texas. The owners of Quest Nutrition founded a nonprofit group (Epigenix Foundation) that is carrying out research on dogs with terminal cancers using a combination of conventional and experimental therapies, including the ketogenic diet and hyperbaric oxygen treatments. There is more information about it in the resources section, along with a link to a video presentation in Tampa, Florida.

rye, barley, bulgur, spelt, and triticale, as well as those gray-area grains that you might believe are healthier, such as amaranth and quinoa. Also eliminate breads made from sprouted grains. At least for the first few months, you will need to eliminate most starches, not just potatoes and peas but also starches deemed "healthy," such as sweet potatoes, yams, and root vegetables. Once you are keto-adapted, you can experiment with the effect of adding back small portions (meaning no more than a few tablespoons) of the less concentrated sources of starch—such as acorn squash, rutabaga, raw carrot, or beet—as long as net carbs per serving don't exceed 2 to 4 grams. If you are following a less rigorous keto plan (over 20 net carbs per day), you may want to include these from the start, but only if they don't cause your glucose level to spike. In chapter 16 you will find guidelines for testing this ("Assess Your Response to Foods," page 289).

## Remember, Fruits Are High in Sugars

This reminder often makes my clients very sad. If it wasn't for the high sugar content of most fruits, the nutrients in them would be an excellent addition to your diet. But unfortunately you will never reach ketosis or experience the benefits of keto-adaptation if you keep most types of fruits in your plan. So it's time to eliminate bananas, tropical fruits, pears, grapes, dates, and melons. Most other fruits are also too high in sugar to be a regular part of a keto plan, especially during the transition while your body is adapting to the ketogenic diet. Even the carbs in such low-glycemic varieties as stone fruits (cherries, peaches, plums, apricots) will throw you off. But you'll be happy to hear that nutrient-rich berries can be added back early on if you can keep portions small (around 2 grams of net carbs' worth in a day).

## Eliminate Most Legumes to Start

Here is another entire category of food that we've always heard is healthy for us, primarily because legumes are plant-based proteins that are also high in fiber. As a group, however, legumes—while low glycemic—still contain too many carbs for your starter keto plan. The legume family includes peanuts, soybeans, chickpeas (garbanzo beans), any kind of bean, dried peas, and lentils.

## Cut Dairy Products with More Than a Gram of Lactose

This list includes milk, cottage cheese, ricotta, and even yogurt. High-fat dairy products, like ghee, butter, and heavy whipping cream, are great choices as they are very low in lactose (milk sugar) and contain very little casein, a milk protein that is problematic for many people. Other dairy products, like cream cheese and sour cream, may also be good choices in smaller amounts, but you *must* read the label to screen them for sneaky sugars or starches. Dairy fats and proteins do have a few specific issues, however; you will read more about the "dairy dilemma" shortly!

## Say "No" to Artificial Sweeteners and Most Sugar Alcohols

Although artificial sweeteners do not raise blood glucose, they are used mostly to sweeten poor-quality products. So use this opportunity to remove these from your diet. Artificial sweeteners are marketed under a variety of brand names and include acesulfame potassium, aspartame, neotame, saccharin, and sucralose. Be particularly mindful of the health risks of aspartame, which is added to many low-sugar or sugar-free foods and beverages. (Read more about sugar substitutes later in this chapter.)

Sugar alcohols occur in nature, but that's no guarantee that they are healthy for you, especially given the manner in which most of them are manufactured. In the human body, most are metabolized as carbohydrates, and all but one ferment in the gut to some degree, causing bloating and loose stools. You can identify them by their "-ol" endings: Maltitol, mannitol, and sorbitol are the main culprits. These are found in abundance in sugar-free foods, toothpastes, and even some beauty products. There are two exceptions to this ban: xylitol and erythritol (or stevia/erythritol blends such as in the brand Pyure Organic).

## Embrace "Gluten-Free"

Quite often when I'm reviewing a new client's intake information, I'll notice that they've included "gluten sensitivity" or "gluten intolerance" as one of their food aversions. Most conventional dietitians and nutritionists would attempt to debunk this belief, given that the majority of people who believe that they have gluten "issues" have not tested positive for celiac disease but self-diagnose when they noticed that some of their symptoms eased when gluten was removed from their diets. In truth, most testing for anything

### A Word on Alcohol

You will need to refrain from drinking alcohol until you are keto-adapted. Then you may find that a single shot of straight spirits or a glass of dry wine fits into your plan. But be careful here: Many people report having a much lower tolerance for alcohol once they are keto-adapted.

more subtle than frank celiac disease is usually quite inconclusive, so basing this particular decision on symptom relief is justifiable. No matter whether it's based on an actual diagnosis or not, I'm relieved when I see "gluten-free" on intake forms because it means that my new client has already made an important step on the path to keto: They've eliminated wheat. And as there is significant cross-reactivity between the gluten protein and similar proteins in other grains, eliminating those as well will feel like less of a hardship. (If you wish to read more about the downsides of wheat and other grains, I suggest *Grain Brain* by Dr. David Perlmutter and/or *Wheat Belly* by Dr. William Davis.)

But there's a hazard that has developed surrounding gluten-free products, one that you definitely need to be warned about before you embark on keto: That is, the food industry has seized on our fears and concerns about gluten and responded by creating a whole new category of products. "Gluten-free" is certainly not "carb-free"; in fact, many gluten-free foods are higher in carbs than the foods that they're replacing. Gluten-free breads and baked goods are loaded up with poor-quality, non-grain starchy substitutes, like tapioca, potato, and rice starch.

The industry's marketing strategy is very pervasive and persuasive! I feel sorry for its citizen victims, but I have to say I do find it interesting that

## Misguided Nutritional Advice

Many people are shocked and dismayed when their conventional medical oncology team (doctor, nurse, dietitian) recommends that they, or their loved one with advanced cancer, consume carb-laden liquid shakes and meal replacement drinks, such as Ensure and Boost, to provide the extra calories they are told will help stem weight loss. They ask me, "But doesn't this feed the cancer?" The unfortunate and simple answer is, "Yes, of course it does!" What the team is offering is either a short-term fix for the impact of the cancer therapy on the gastrointestinal tract or misguided advice with regard to treating cachexia, the muscle-wasting syndrome that is often the actual cause of death in someone with advanced disease. How ironic—and sad—that these individuals don't yet acknowledge that there are other options that will actually improve *nutrition*, not just calorie intake.

gluten-free labels have popped up on foods that have nothing to do with gluten, such as butter and eggs. This may be very important information for those with celiac disease, but in the context of this diet, it's not necessary to ensure that even your toilet paper is gluten-free! (Seriously, I've seen that label on a shelf of toilet paper in my local supermarket.) I won't leave you high and dry with regard to what you can do to replace the grains in your diet. That will be thoroughly covered later in this chapter in our discussion of keto-friendly foods.

## Five Steps for Successful Pre-Planning

Pre-planning starts with finding keto foods, recipes, and meals that interest you. If whole-food cooking is new to you, start simply. Select a handful of keto-friendly recipes that call for only a few ingredients and come with basic instructions for preparation. You can build on this foundation over time.

### 1. Consult a good cookbook and build your meal template

Start with *The Ketogenic Kitchen* by Domini Kemp and Patricia Daly (Chelsea Green, 2016). There are several other great cookbooks already in print, and more on the way. A few are standouts. I've listed my current favorites in the resources section and will update my website regularly to include my new finds. (Please feel free to email me with a review of your favorite if it's not on my list.) Many keto cookbooks also include meal plans—some elaborate, some simple. I've also included a Simple Keto Meal Template (page 217) that you can use as the foundation for your own plan. Meal plans can be very helpful even if you only need that degree of support for the first few weeks. The beauty of this approach is that you can't go too far wrong if you follow a specific plan in one of my recommended books. Another plus of referring to cookbooks rather than online sites is that cookbooks often include more keto cooking tips and suggestions for incorporating fat into your diet.

### 2. Go keto food shopping

Take a list and allow extra time for locating new foods and for careful label reading. You don't need to buy everything in one trip; focus on the foods you'll need for a week's worth of meals. You may also need to visit specialty stores or order some hard-to-locate items online.

## 3. Experiment with new recipes

Experiment with your new recipes even before you make the switch to a keto-genic diet. You want to have a set of keto meals that you can rely on in the first few weeks. This is *not* the time to strive for variety. Keeping your menu plan simple and straightforward will go a long way in helping you make a smooth transition. This is especially important if you're planning to start with a fast: Without a plan in place for what comes next, your efforts will be wasted.

## 4. Eat a lot of fat

It's very likely that you will easily catch on to how to lower carbs. It's a bit more of a stretch to truly understand how little protein you need. But the real challenge here is becoming comfortable with the amount of fat needed to maintain ketosis. Initially, you may get away with shorting yourself on fats and still make great ketones (but know that you can only do this while you're carrying extra weight). But if you are of low weight or have other reasons for wanting to avoid an initial weight loss, be absolutely sure that you are meeting your fat intake goal before you remove all the excess pro-tein and carbs.

## 5. Set your house in order

There is no doubt as to the importance of removing foods from your home that are not keto-friendly and restocking your cupboards, refrigerator, and freezer with the new foods you'll be incorporating into your plan. Set your mind to completing this task as quickly as possible.

Before making changes to your diet, take stock of what you have in your home. If you have already made huge changes in the past—for example, if you switched from a standard diet to a Paleo pattern—then you may already have many of the staples that you'll need for keto. But if you're like most people who embark on this plan, you will need to make some changes in what you keep on hand. You can either do it all at once or take it on over a period of days or even weeks. That depends on your personal style, the amount of space you have on hand, and how attached you are to your current pattern. Your finances may also influence how quickly you replace your old foods with keto staples. If you can complete this phase quickly, that's great. But if you truly need time to work through the process (and you're not just using it as an excuse to delay your start date), then take it step by step.

By the way, don't expect your loved ones to be on board with what you're doing, no matter how much you may want them to move with you toward better health. Remember that a large part of your own motivation right now is tied to the health crisis caused by your disease. Still, it's amazing to me just how many people will deny that foods can make an impact on health, choosing instead to defend their old patterns with statements like "I don't eat much sugar" (despite evidence to the contrary). Instead, focus on the changes you need to make in your *own* life and hope your loved ones learn by example. In reviewing this book, Dr. William LaValley stressed this important point for those about to embark on the keto journey:

> Remember, this is *your* diet for *your* health and well-being—and it is not required for your spouse/parent/child/loved one to adopt the same diet. It is often an emotional recipe for distress, pain, and suffering to maintain the expectation that the ketogenic diet "should" be adopted by other family members as a show of support. Don't go down that path because it may backfire and cause unnecessary and undesirable stress on relationships. Instead, it's healthiest if you adopt the perspective that everyone has the right to choose whichever diet they want.

Start with "easy pickings," the foods that clearly don't belong in *anyone's* home. These include anything that lists high-fructose corn syrup, hydrogenated fats or oils, corn or soy oil, and any canola oil that is not organic. These are just plain evil, so you should feel no guilt or remorse whatsoever when you toss these into the garbage, where they belong.

Continuing with the pantry sweep, your next step is to pull out the sugar and flour. There is no need for these pantry staples, as you won't be using them in your meals any longer. Make the commitment, then say good-bye and never revisit that decision. While you're at it, remove any foods made from these staples, such as pasta.

Now take it to the next level and get rid of those snack foods. All of them, including chips, crackers, cookies, breakfast bars, power bars, dried fruit and fruit leathers, and nuts with coatings on them. Even if they don't have added sugars, they are way too high in carbs for your new plan. Your family doesn't need these either, but sometimes that decision is not yours alone to make. If your spouse or adult child objects strongly, then ask them to relocate these items away from the kitchen. And if your younger children are feeling deprived, remember that you are setting a great example for them.

## Hitting Close to Home

My mother is definitely not interested in keto! In fact, it was my repeated lectures to her about cutting back on the grains in her diet that finally brought me to my own edge. For the third time, I was explaining to her the role that grains play in autoimmune disease. With her history, I couldn't understand why she wouldn't go without gluten, even for just a few weeks, to see if any of her debilitating symptoms would improve. I hung up the phone and it hit me: Why did I think that it was OK for *me* to eat grains? Yes, I could reason that the amounts were tiny and the servings few, but the fact remained that I was in danger of traveling down that same road if I didn't change my ways. I went to the cupboard and ferreted out the few remaining offenders: a package of shortbread cookies, a box of whole-wheat crackers, and a bag of corn chips. I thought briefly about who I might give these to, but ultimately put them in the trash. Honestly, when you *truly* commit to a change, it becomes so much easier to see these foods for what they are: land mines along the road to better health.

Besides, they will most definitely find these foods in abundance outside of your home. Kids are especially adept at scoring low-quality foods, so don't feel that you need to hold on to that bag of M&Ms to keep life "normal" for their sake! Just think of all the other "treats" they have easy access to, from chocolates at the register of your local store, to power bars at the gym, items in the vending machines at school, even jelly beans at the pharmacy. Still, some families have compromised by designating cupboard shelves as "keto" or "non-keto."

Then there are the foods that may be decent choices for other members of your family or given away to your local food bank. These include beans, peas, rice, and certain condiments. Over time, phase out the rest of the foods that contain sugar, such as canned tomatoes, or those with other dubious ingredients, such as in most canned soups (notorious for harboring monosodium glutamate, or MSG).

With cupboards cleaned, it's time to attack the fridge and freezer. You'll be amazed at what you'll find there! Unless you are already a very vigilant shopper, you are likely to learn that at least a few of your condiments, jarred

## Raffi's Entry into Keto

How I wish a book like this one had been available when Raffi started the ketogenic diet! We were 2,800 miles from home and living under what I still remember as "combat conditions." Even worse, I had this nagging fear that I didn't fully understand what I was doing. No wonder: At that point and place, I didn't have much of a toolkit.

Somehow, we muddled through those early weeks: weighing and measuring all his foods and hand-calculating the macronutrient content of each meal and snack. I went for simplicity and palatability over food quality, relying on ham roll-ups with cream cheese, sugar-free gelatin parfaits, hot dogs, and commercial ranch dressing with MSG. Along the way I discovered new books and other resources. I promise, we cleaned up our act over time, but for those of you caught in the same cross fire, I say, "Just do it." You are wasting valuable time if you wait until *all* your supplies, *all* your foods, and *all* your recipes and meal plans are in perfect order.

foods, or frozen foods have high-fructose corn syrup or poor-quality oils. Look closely at the ingredient list on that jar of mayonnaise or bottle of dressing labeled "made with olive oil"; you may be shocked to see that soybean and/or canola are among the first ingredients. Toss it.

### SUMMARY OF FOODS TO ELIMINATE

- sugars
- grains
- starchy vegetables
- fruits (to start)
- legumes (to start)
- milk and milk products (except for high-fat dairy and high-fat dairy proteins)
- sweeteners and sugar alcohols (except stevia, luo han guo, and erythritol)

## Stock Up on Keto-Friendly Foods

Ready to go food shopping? In this section I offer a summary of the main points you need to keep in mind as you venture out into the keto world. First, use this list as a quick guide to help you get into the swing of choosing keto-friendly foods. (There's more detail about each of these foods later in this chapter.)

## VEGETABLES

- □ asparagus
- □ broccoli
- □ Brussels sprouts
- □ cabbage
- □ cauliflower
- □ celery
- □ cucumbers
- □ kale
- □ mushrooms
- □ salad greens
- □ sauté greens
  (such as chard,
  beet greens, and
  mustard greens)
- □ spinach
- □ zucchini

*After you are keto-adapted,*
*you can add back limited*
*amounts of these vegetables:*

- □ eggplant
- □ garlic (powder has
  fewer carbs than fresh)
- □ onions (powder has
  fewer carbs than fresh)
- □ peppers
- □ tomatoes
- □ turnips
- □ winter squash
  (keep it to 2 to 3 net
  carbs per meal)

## FRUITS

- □ apple (a few very
  thin slices)
- □ avocados (Hass)
- □ berries (keep it to < 2
  grams of carb per meal)
- □ grapefruit
  (a few sections)
- □ olives (use more like
  a condiment)

## PROTEINS

- □ beef
- □ eggs (preferably from
  free-range hens)
- □ lamb
- □ pork (including limited
  amounts of bacon
  and sausage)
- □ poultry
- □ seafood (wild-caught
  fish and shellfish)
- □ wild game meats

## DAIRY

- □ cheese (hard cheeses,
  such as cheddar or Parmesan;
  or soft, high-fat cheeses,
  such as Brie)
- □ full-fat "original" cream cheese
- □ heavy whipping cream
- □ sour cream (cultured, without
  added starches or fillers)

## NUTS AND SEEDS

- □ almonds (including almond
  butter, almond flour,
  almond milk)
- □ Brazil nuts (rich in selenium!)
- □ chia seeds
- □ coconut (including
  unsweetened meat, milk,
  cream, or flour)
- □ flaxseed (rich in healthy
  omega-3s and fiber; grind and
  store in the refrigerator)
- □ hazelnuts
- □ hemp hearts/seeds
- □ macadamias (good choice:
  high in fat, low in carbs
  and protein)
- □ pecans
- □ walnuts (good choice: fewer
  omega-6s than most nuts)

## FATS AND OILS

- □ almond, macadamia,
  or sesame oils
  (in small amounts to
  add variety to meals)
- □ avocado or extra
  virgin olive oils
  (for dressings or
  homemade
  mayonnaise)
- □ butter or ghee
  (if you include dairy
  fats in your plan)
- □ buttery spreads
  (such as Earth Balance
  or Melt, preferably
  organic; especially
  good if you need a
  substitute for dairy fat)
- □ coconut and MCT oil
- □ lard, tallow, or other
  saturated animal fats
  (such as duck fat)
- □ omega-3 fish oils
  (either as fresh fish—
  e.g., wild-caught
  salmon—or in
  purified supplements)
- □ salad dressings
  and mayonnaise
  (organic or homemade)

## SWEETENERS

- □ Pyure Organic or Truvia
  (blended stevia
  and erythritol)
- □ Splenda (use only
  until you transition
  to stevia)
- □ stevia (liquid drops,
  preferably organic)
- □ xylitol (careful: it's toxic
  to dogs!)

**Figure 8.1.** Keto-friendly food list.

## First, Prepare a Shopping List

You'll likely be visiting new sections of your supermarket or finding entirely new markets that contain more of the foods you'll need. Make a copy of figure 8.1 (or download it from my website) and bring it along with you.

## Choose the Highest-Quality Foods You Can Afford

The top tier in meats includes those from pasture-raised animals on organic farms. The step-down are those that are organically raised. "Natural" is a meaningless, throwaway term—don't pay more for this label! When choosing vegetables, go with organic and local whenever possible. Familiarize yourself with two important lists, both updated yearly by the Environmental Working Group, a nonprofit human and environmental health advocacy organization: the Dirty Dozen (most highly contaminated with pesticides) and the Clean Fifteen (fewest issues). The lists are easy to find if you type their names in your browser's search engine (or go to www.ewg.org).

## Keep Your Foods as "Clean" as Possible

Avoid products that have long lists of additives, including MSG, which may be disguised as "hydrolyzed vegetable protein" or "flavor enhancer." Flavor additives are used in a mind-boggling number of foods, including meat and poultry coming from factory farms. Also be aware that deli meats may contain nitrates that the producer touts as "naturally occurring in celery juice." How deceptive! Wean yourself from overdependence on these.

## Read Labels

Look for hidden sugars and poor-quality fats, as mentioned earlier. Also study the nutrition label to see how many net carbs are contained in one serving (net carbs = total carbohydrates − fiber).

## "What Should I Eat?"

I can't begin to tell you how often I've been asked this question! The answer is really much simpler than you might think: Eat low-carbohydrate whole foods, just enough protein to fill your needs, and lots of healthy fats and oils. Look at figure 8.1 (page 123) for a quick refresher on what foods are keto-friendly. Understand that

## Organic Is the Goal:
## Take Small Steps Here, Not Giant Leaps

There are a multitude of reasons to choose organic as often as you can. Here are just a few.

- Organic farming keeps toxins out of our air, soil, water, and food supply.
- Good farming practices reduce worker exposure to toxins and carcinogens.
- Supporting organic farmers rewards them for their time and effort, as well as for their dedication to improving the quality of what we eat.
- "Organic" is a virtual guarantee that the food is not genetically modified to resist pests.
- Plants have evolved by fighting off their predators naturally; adding herbicides and pesticides disrupts that process.
- Despite its toxicity, Roundup (glyphosate), used with genetically modified crops, is no longer effective against the superweeds that manage to survive, leaving us wondering what plan Monsanto has for us next.
- Roundup is sprayed heavily on genetically modified crops used to make animal feed. This brings us back to my first point: Organic farming practices reduce our toxin load.

there's no requirement for any single item on this list. Instead, choose those that appeal to you. The following list is not complete, but it's a great place to start. Use this information and figure 8.1 to prepare your shopping list, and take this opportunity to try one or two new-to-you foods each week. You're sure to find at least a few new favorites! Now, let's get into the foods in more detail.

## Vegetables

Until you are keto-adapted, stick to greens and non-starchy vegetables, and make an effort to include many from the cruciferous family. When possible, choose organically grown veggies and serve them raw, steamed, roasted, or, less often, sautéed (use medium heat with lard, coconut or avocado oil, or ghee, and keep cooking time short). Use seasonings to add interest. It's best to weigh portions, especially at the start, and to use a reliable database (USDA or Cronometer) to check net carbs to be sure that your choice is within the carbohydrate allowance of your plan. The vegetables listed below are those most commonly included in keto diets in the United States, but there are certainly others:

- arugula*
- asparagus
- bamboo shoots
- broccoli and broccoli sprouts*
- Brussels sprouts*
- cabbage (green, bok choy*)
- cauliflower*
- celery
- cucumbers
- kale*
- leaf vegetables (including endive and chicory)
- leafy greens (including parsley and spinach)
- radishes and daikon
- rutabagas (great replacement for potatoes in slow cookers)
- "sauté greens" (many are also brassicas)
- summer squash and zucchini (referred to as courgette outside the United States)
- turnips

* Indicates a cruciferous vegetable.

The next group of vegetables presents a few more challenges, as they may be too high in carbs for some people—at least at the beginning. After you are keto-adapted, or if you are starting out with a more liberal plan, you can add limited amounts of these, but be careful with portion sizes. Again, I highly recommend that you weigh your portions, keeping net carbs to less than 4 grams so that total carbs in any given meal do not exceed 6 grams:

- artichoke
- beets (also called beetroot; best if eaten raw or lightly steamed)
- bell peppers (red peppers have more carbs than green)
- cabbage, purple (more carbs than green)
- carrot (raw, and only as a condiment; e.g., grated into a salad)
- eggplant
- fennel
- garlic
- green beans
- mushrooms
- onion
- pepper, hot varieties
- tomato (sugar and nutrient content differs widely between varieties)
- winter squash, including acorn and butternut (limited amounts)

If you are on anticoagulant drug therapy, be sure to ask your doctor if there are vegetables that you should avoid. These are the ones that contain higher amounts of vitamin K, such as broccoli. Note, though, that some of the newer anticoagulant drugs do *not* have this dietary restriction. As I said, ask your doctor.

## Berries and Fruits

Including berries and fruits in the first few weeks of your new keto plan may interfere with your transition to ketosis mainly because the portions that you are used to are too high in carbs. Even after you are keto-adapted, tropical fruit (with the exception of a small amount of grapefruit or a squeeze or two of lemon or lime) is so high in sugar that it will never be invited back into your keto plan. Wait until you are keto-adapted before testing limited amounts of other fruits; then keep these to one or two servings per day. When you do eat fruit, always include fat at the same time. (For example, add cream to berries, or almond butter blended with coconut oil to apples.) Check the fruit's effect on your blood glucose by testing the level both before you eat it and an hour afterward. Did your glucose rise more than 20 mg/dL? If so, back down on the portion size.

So what are your options here?

- berries: ¼ cup portions (approximately 30 grams) for strawberries, raspberries, and blackberries; ⅛ cup (15 grams) for blueberries
- apple or pear: a few very thin slices (if you can't control the portion size, don't add this back)
- grapefruit: a few sections at most
- cherries

Portion size is critical! Respect the effect fruit sugars can have on glucose and insulin levels. Weigh each portion of fruit and check its carb content to keep it at or below 4 net carbs.

## Proteins

Let's look at which protein foods can be included in your plan, paying careful attention to prioritizing high-quality sources. Whenever possible, choose meats from pasture-raised animals. These have a healthier fat profile than animals that are fed grains. Poultry should be free-range. Organic is a bonus. Most animal meats contain no carbohydrate, but eggs, shellfish, and liver do contain some carbs that should be counted as part of your daily carbohydrate intake. (Even uncured bacon and sausage usually contain some carbs.)

## Avocados, Olives, and Cacao

It may seem odd that I've put these three keto-friendly foods into their own section, but they do deserve special mention. The flesh of both avocados and olives is unusual in that it's oily and quite rich in mono-unsaturated fats. Avocados are a single-seeded berry, quite an unusual classification. And olives are a fruit, though you may also hear them referred to as drupes. (That designation crosses categories and causes some confusion, however, so I don't use it.) Surprised? Actually, the nomenclature is much less important than the nutrition they offer.

- Choose the smaller Hass avocado instead of the larger Florida variety.
- Half of an average Hass avocado provides 2 teaspoons (approximately 10 grams) of mostly monounsaturated fat packaged with plenty of fiber, just a few carbs, and a little bit of protein.
- Olives are a great snack, and the unrefined oil that's pressed from them is also high in monounsaturated fats. (Eating these types of fats can help keep your LDL low, if that's a concern for you or your doctor.)
- Cacao, the raw material from which chocolate is made, comes from the seeds of the cacao tree. You'll see "high cacao" on many chocolate bars. The higher the percentage of cacao, the fewer carbs it contains. If you enjoy cacao as a satisfying treat, you'll be happy to know that small amounts of high-cacao chocolate (85 percent or higher) are keto-friendly. Bonus: Cacao is high in fiber, minerals, and flavonoids. Cacao can also increase your levels of dopamine, the "feel-good" neurotransmitter.

As you begin your new plan, use familiar cooking methods. This is not the time or the place to overwhelm you or your caregiver with the added burden of sifting through the science before preparing a meal. That said, if you rely heavily on grilling or frying, look into moist cooking with a pressure cooker or a slow cooker (also known as a Crock-Pot). When you're ready, you can develop your knowledge here and explore a multitude of methods to prepare tasty meals, in your own way and at your own pace. Recommended protein foods are as follows:

- beef
- lamb
- pork (including reasonable servings of bacon and sausage)
- poultry (chicken and turkey), preferably free-range and organically fed
- seafood (wild-caught fish and shellfish; be aware of heavy-metal contamination)
- wild game meats
- organ meats
- eggs (farm-raised and organic; or at least choose those that are high in omega-3s)
- dairy (this merits a section of its own; stay tuned)
- protein powders (preferably non-dairy and with fewer than 5 grams of glutamine or glutamic acid per serving)

## Dairy Products

Dairy fats, such as cream, butter, and ghee, are staples in many keto plans. Although some people believe strongly that only raw dairy is acceptable, this presents some challenges. Raw dairy is not available for sale in many states (though workarounds include buying shares of a dairy cow). Even if it's available, the main product that you'll receive is raw milk, not cream or butter. It's also important to understand that there are pathogens in raw dairy, even in the cleanest operations. If contaminants are minimal, most healthy people may not be affected but the same pathogens may be a disaster for you if your immune system is compromised, which it often the case in those with cancer. My advice: Don't stress over this right now. Instead, buy the highest quality available to you (from pasture-raised animals on organic farms).

The next point I want to make is also controversial: It is well documented that dairy fats contain estrogen metabolites (estrogen-like compounds). What is less clear is how this may affect you personally. If you have a hormone-sensitive cancer (such as breast, ovarian, or prostate cancer), you may be weighing whether or not to include dairy in your diet. Understand that all high-fat dairy products—whether from industrial producers or happy cows on organic pastures—contain hormone metabolites, and hormone receptors in humans appear to bind to these. (Note: These hormones are not related to bovine growth hormone—those are hormones that are given to an animal, not ones that they produce on their own.) High-fat goat products contain significantly lower levels of hormones but unfortunately it is nearly impossible to find cream and butter made from goat milk here in the United States.

Here's my take on the estrogen controversy: In theory, estrogen (a protein) should be dismantled during digestion just like other proteins but there are some holes in this argument. First, digestion and absorption are often impaired

## Grass-Fed versus Grain-Fed Meat

This is a hot topic, especially in the Paleo world—and rightly so. The fat from animals that are truly pasture-raised has a different, healthier lipid profile than the fat from grain-fed animals. In 2010, *Nutrition Journal* published a paper, "A Review of Fatty Acid Profiles and Anti-oxidant Content in Grass-Fed and Grain-Fed Beef," that details these differences.[4] Recently the USDA Food Composition Database has started to include nutrient data for meats from grass-fed animals.

Many of the toxins found in our environment are stored in our fat, and this is true for animals as well. Animals that have been raised on organic feed and pasture (grass) should have fewer toxins in their fat. In my opinion, this is even more important in a high-fat diet than it is in a standard diet, as the exposure to these toxins is proportionately greater.

As you can see, choosing well *most* of the time is optimal, but don't let it become an obsession. When you dine out, it's unlikely that the meat will come from happy animals fed on green, toxin-free pastures. The same is true for the butter and half-and-half served in restaurants. Still, the social and emotional benefits gained from a night out will most likely outweigh any downside here. Remember that it's what you do *most* of the time that has the greatest effect on your health.

by leaky gut syndrome or by the drugs commonly used to treat cancer. Second, we know that the consumption of dairy containing these metabolites is associated with higher levels of estrogens in both women and men who consume them.

Is there a way to know for sure if the risks outweigh the harm? Not really, but there are ways to assess relative risk. If you are under the care of a skilled naturopathic doctor, such as my friend and colleague Dr. Nasha Winters, coauthor of *The Metabolic Approach to Cancer*, then you would be monitored for an effect, either positive or negative, with testing for certain biomarkers. I don't list those markers here because I feel strongly that you need to make this decision with the help of someone with Dr. Nasha's skills and experience.

Also, be aware that even though heavy whipping cream contains about 0.4 grams of carbohydrate per tablespoon, the nutrition label will show 0 grams (anything under 0.5 grams is rounded down to zero). This amount, though small, needs to be included in your daily total. If you do decide to include high-fat dairy, choose from these products:

- butter (including ghee and clarified butter)
- heavy whipping cream (preferably without mono- and diglycerides, carrageenan, or polysorbate 80)
- sour cream (cultured, without added starches or fillers)
- full-fat cream cheese (again, look for fillers, including whey protein)
- some types of hard or ripened cheeses (1 ounce or less per serving; count the protein as well)

Milk and cottage cheese are not keto-friendly. Note also that while seemingly thick in consistency, most Greek yogurt is too low in fat and too high in protein for the purposes of this diet.

Dairy proteins have an entirely different set of issues. They are *anabolic*, meaning that they are intended to stimulate growth. This makes perfect sense when you think about why mammals, including humans, produce milk in the first place. Among the many hormones in milk that are associated with growth, the one that concerns me most in cancer is insulin-like growth factor 1 (IGF-1). IGF-1 is crucial in childhood as it works in harmony with other growth factors and hormones important to overall growth and development. But in cancer, it is known to stimulate growth and proliferation in most cancer cells and, unfortunately, these same cells have many more of the receptors for this hormone than normal cells, which helps them to survive and thrive. High intake of dairy proteins is associated with higher blood levels of IGF-1 as well, which is clearly a problem for those with cancer. Looking at the big picture, small portions of cheese, such as a few tablespoons of fresh grated Parmesan, add interest and variety to meals and are not likely to make or break your plan.

There is yet another issue, one that is rarely included in the discussion of dairy proteins in keto. Both whey and casein, the two main proteins found in dairy products, stimulate a release of insulin *independent of a rise in glucose*. What this means is that dairy proteins directly stimulate the pancreas to produce insulin. Again, this is a great evolutionary advantage if you are a young mammal in your growth phase but a poor idea if you have cancer.

In my work with clients, I have occasionally seen issues with even small amounts of protein, such as tiny amounts that may be in cream cheese (read the label—some are fortified with whey protein). I have expressed my concern regarding dairy proteins to multiple sports nutrition companies and hope that

# The Casein Conundrum

Many people, even if they choose not to go totally dairy-free, have opted for a diet that is casein-free. It's clear that for many people, the protein casein is inflammatory and may elicit an unhealthy immune response or exacerbate leaky gut syndrome. Naturally, these issues are problematic for anyone, with or without cancer.

### CASEIN AND DAIRY ALLERGIES

True dairy allergies provoke an immune response. If you have an immune-mediated allergy to casein, you should eliminate all sources of dairy proteins, including the tiny amounts found in butter. If instead you suspect a sensitivity rather than an allergy, you may want to eliminate all casein-containing foods for a two-week trial and note any improvement in your symptoms.

Many keto recipes include dairy but, thankfully, dairy-free recipes are becoming more popular. Just include the words "dairy-free" in your online searches. Some Paleo recipes are dairy-free, but be careful, as Paleo recipes often include sugars.

### CASEIN ALLERGY VERSUS LACTOSE INTOLERANCE

There's a huge difference between casein allergy and lactose intolerance. As I mentioned already, casein *allergy* provokes an immune system response. Lactose *intolerance* is due to insufficient production of the enzyme (lactase) needed to break down the bond in lactose that links glucose to galactose. (That change in enzyme sufficiency often happens as we outgrow our biological need for milk.) Without sufficient production of this enzyme, lactose ferments in the gut and can cause bloating and diarrhea, leading people with lactose intolerance to believe that their bodies are incapable of dealing with *any* dairy products. However, high-fat dairy and keto-friendly cheeses contain very little lactose! Most people retain enough ability to digest these small amounts with no gastrointestinal distress. If in doubt, check it out for yourself.

at least a few will begin to offer a "dairy-free" option. Stay tuned; if that happens, I'll be posting a link to those products on my website.

You must be thinking, "After all this negative press regarding dairy, why in the world would I choose to eat *any* dairy proteins?" Remember, my role is to educate and inform, not to direct your choices. Obviously, you can't check directly for an insulin response but you can check your ketone levels. When insulin levels rise, ketone production is suppressed. So if dairy proteins kill your ketones, then you'll know that you should back off of them, at least for now.

## Nuts and Seeds

Nuts and seeds offer many opportunities to increase your fat intake on a keto plan. There are so many different ways to enjoy nuts: whole, chopped, nut butter, nut flour. . . . They also travel well; take some with you when you're out running errands. This category does come with cautions, though. For one, it's very easy to overeat them! And since they contain carbs and protein as well as fat, "just a handful" can add up quickly. Also, some—such as pumpkin, sesame, and sunflower—are relatively high in pro-inflammatory oils. Choose carefully and use these sparingly, more like a condiment. Others—such as ground flax-seed, chia seed, and hemp hearts—are high in healthy fats and fiber. Add them to salads, puddings, shakes, and baked goods; the fats they contain are very healthy, and they're a great source of fiber as well. Using these will also help keep your omega-6 to omega-3 ratio in a healthier range.

Eating lots of nuts, especially almonds and other varieties that are high in oxalates, may raise your risk of kidney stones. I am not suggesting that you omit these nuts from your plan. Instead, especially in the early days, plan to limit your intake (including all forms) to 4 ounces (112 grams) total per day. (Athletes may need to eat more in order to keep up with their high energy demands. In that case, choose macadamias as they are lower in oxalates and higher in healthy fats than other nuts.)

As you begin your new plan, keep to the following short list of keto-friendly nuts and seeds. You can add to it after you've adapted to keto. Research your favorites and evaluate the pros and cons of each as they relate to you individually. In conducting your search, you are likely to come across a lot of confusing information about oils, oxalate levels, and antinutrients (including oxalates and phytic acid). There is also considerable debate about how they should be eaten: raw versus soaked versus sprouted. After reading this, you may think that it's too hard to incorporate all these recommendations and that maybe you should just stop eating nuts. Don't let that happen. Instead, save the micromanagement for another day when you are comfortably keto-adapted and ready to take on further refinements. One last bit of advice: Rotate your choices to lessen your chance of developing a sensitivity to any one variety. Choose from this list:

- almonds (including almond butter, flour, milk)
- Brazil nuts (rich in selenium but limit these to 2 nuts per day; more is *not* better)
- coconut (including coconut cream, butter, unsweetened meat, flour, and boxed milk)
- macadamias (great choice; high in good fats; low in carbs and protein; low in oxalates)
- pecans (high in fat; low in carbs)
- walnuts (good choice! fewer omega-6s than most nuts)
- chia seeds (rich in healthy omega-3s and fiber; refrigerate)
- hemp hearts/seeds (rich in healthy omega-3s and complete protein)
- flaxseed (rich in healthy omega-3s and fiber; grind it and store in the refrigerator)

I know: Coconut is not a true nut, but I include it on this list to keep life simple. Be especially careful with coconut water; it is relatively high in coconut sugar, so is not part of a keto plan.

## Fats and Oils

Keto diets include a large proportion of fat, so quality, composition, and balance are extremely important. The best practice is to use a combination of the following: animal fats; coconut oil; MCT oil or caprylic acid (C8); monounsaturated oils (olive, avocado); omega-3 oils (from ground flaxseed, chia, hemp hearts, fatty fish, fish oil); and omega-6s (limited amounts, preferably from nuts and seeds, not oils).

When choosing oils, always look for cold-pressed, organic (except avocado, which doesn't need to be organic), and unrefined varieties; although not a guarantee of quality, at least it's a step in the right direction. Read labels and avoid any products made with refined (which means solvent-treated) oils extracted from GMO plants such as soybeans, canola, corn, and safflower. When sautéing or stir-frying, use lard or another animal fat. If you use coconut, olive, or avocado oil, keep the heat below the point at which the oil smokes and minimize cooking times. Also ventilate well to avoid breathing in the airborne by-products of fat combustion: If your airway becomes irritated, the temperature is obviously too high. To learn more about fats, oils, and cooking methods, read Sally Fallon Morell's book *Nourishing Fats*.

It is also good practice to track your intake of fats and oils using a tool such as Cronometer to ensure you are keeping the all-important ratio of omega-6 to omega-3 oils at a healthy 3:1 or lower. Unfortunately, this is still no guarantee that your body metabolizes oils optimally; only blood testing ordered by an integrative practitioner can determine that (yet another reason to add this valued professional to your team).

Choose your fats wisely using the following list:

- Lard, tallow, and other animal fat (such as duck), preferably rendered from organic, pasture-raised animals (Be careful, as the food industry has jumped into this market, and you'll find cheap but unhealthy hydrogenated varieties on supermarket shelves.)
- Butter or ghee (Buy the highest quality you can afford, preferably made from grass-fed animals living on organic and sustainably maintained pastureland.)
- Coconut, MCT, or caprylic (C8) oil
- Omega-3 fish oils, either as fresh fish (e.g., sardines and wild-caught salmon), krill oil, or molecularly distilled supplements high in DHA
- Omega-3 oil from non-animal sources (found in seeds such as flax, chia, and hemp)
- Extra virgin olive oil (cold-pressed and organic) or oil from olives grown, processed, and packaged by California growers (which bypasses the adulteration issues seen in many of the imported brands)
- Avocado and macadamia nut oils (These are high in mono-unsaturated fat.)
- Salad dressings and mayonnaise, organic or homemade, using healthy oils
- Buttery spreads such as Melt or (non-soy) Earth Balance (Both are non-GMO and organic and good to use as a substitute for dairy fat.)
- Other oils used in much smaller amounts, primarily to add flavor (e.g., sesame oil or infusions using garlic or chili)

## Sugar Substitutes

It's impossible to overestimate the importance of lowering your "sweet thermostat," meaning the level at which sweet-tasting foods satisfy you both mentally and physically. A low setting will aid adherence to your new plan as it tempers your brain's hard wiring that triggers cravings for sweets. (Evolutionary biologists suggest that there was a time in our ancient past when sugar-seeking behavior conferred a survival advantage by allowing for more fat storage.)

## Children: Exceptions to the Rule

If you are the parent of a child with cancer, recall or reread what I wrote about sweet treats in chapter 4 ("When the Person with Cancer Is Your Child," page 46). You want your child to feel *special*, not uncomfortably different. This usually means offering them beautiful and tasty treats as "training wheels" to replace their former favorites as they make the transition to the new plan. But you should work at resetting their thermostats as well. Food industry scientists have carefully calculated the amount of sweetness that entices us to select their products. I, for one, choose not to go along with their program. No reason you should, either!

Once you become adapted to the keto diet, almost all commercially available sweetened treats, whether they contain sugars or sugar substitutes, will taste overly sweet to you. Dulling your desire for sweets helps you make better food choices, as you are less likely to turn to the poor-quality, low-nutritive foods marketed as "sugar-free." For all of these reasons, I urge you to cut back on *all* sugar substitutes, allowing the natural flavor of foods to be savored and enjoyed.

The industry that creates sugar substitutes and the food manufacturers that use them in their products would like us to believe that research into the risks of their products is "inconclusive" or "controversial." Doesn't that sound like the same language used by oil companies in the fight over leaded gas, by the tobacco industry leaders as they denied the link to cancer, by the sugar industry to promote its product as safe, and by Monsanto as it continues to defend its abuse of Roundup?

Even if these substitutes are not harmful to *most* people, their use has provoked a lot of controversy. Also, products with these added sweeteners are generally poor quality, and for that reason alone should be excluded from your diet. Start first by weaning yourself from diet drinks, as they are loaded with these sweeteners (not to mention bone-depleting acids and artificial food colorings). Now let's look at the major categories of sugar substitutes.

### Non-caloric artificial sweeteners

These sweeteners are non-caloric and do not raise blood glucose levels; this is why they are commonly found in diet products marketed to people who are either overweight or diabetic. However, there is increasing evidence that this class of artificial sweeteners may have adverse effects on the gut microbiome, with downstream effects that may induce glucose intolerance.[5,6] If you have cancer and are receiving conventional cancer care, your gut is already compromised. Err on the safe side and steer clear of the following sweeteners.

**Aspartame** (marketed as NutraSweet and Equal). This noxious substance is suspected to contribute to numerous health problems. You should be warned that at least some of the reviews that have suggested no harm have been conducted by paid industry consultants. How can we trust this information when there is animal model research suggesting that high doses are toxic to neurons?[7] The neurotoxic effect may even be compounded when aspartame is combined with other food additives, such as dyes.[8] There are also studies that found that the ingestion of aspartame (in amounts nearly equivalent to those consumed by humans) increases the risk of developing leukemias and lymphomas.[9,10] Although it has not been confirmed that aspartame triggers seizures or headaches or any number of other side effects that people have reported, I personally choose not to use it, and strongly urge you to make a similar decision.

**Saccharin** (marketed as Sweet Twin, Sweet'N Low, and Necta Sweet). If you grew up in the 1960s or 1970s, you probably remember the warning label on saccharin that read: "This product contains saccharin, which has been determined to cause cancer in laboratory animals." However, those laboratory studies used extremely high doses—far more than a human would consume—and the mechanism by which saccharin produced cancer in rats doesn't occur in humans. But just because it hasn't been shown to cause cancer in humans doesn't mean you should consume it! It is another artificial sweetener that has been linked to disruptions in the microbiome.

**Acesulfame K** (marketed as Sunett, Sweet One, and Sweet & Safe) has been shown to compromise hippocampal neurons in mice.[11] More research to look at whether it also may precipitate or exacerbate cognitive decline or Alzheimer's disease in humans is needed.

**Sucralose** (marketed as Splenda) may also have a negative impact on the gut microbiome. Although there is not a strong association with cancer in humans, one study that looked at long-term exposure to sucralose in mice did note an increase in their risk of developing certain cancers.[12]

### Erythritol and other sugar alcohols

Sugar alcohols (identified by the "-ol" at the end of their names) are found in nature, although in nowhere near the concentrations found in the products they sweeten. These alcohols are metabolized through the same pathway in the liver that detoxifies more familiar alcohols, like wine and spirits; and, like these other alcohols, they have some caloric value but, with moderate use, not enough to play much of a role in a keto-for-cancer plan. Additionally, there is confusion (and perhaps some obfuscation) regarding a possible glycemic or insulin response. But as you'll soon see, there's no need to look any closer at the options because all but one of the most commonly used sugar alcohols often cause uncomfortable bloating, gas, and diarrhea (due to fermentation in the gut). If you want to avoid these symptoms, there is only one choice: erythritol.

Erythritol is the only sugar alcohol that is completely absorbed from the intestinal tract, leaving nothing behind to ferment in the gut.[13] It is mostly excreted in urine and has an extremely low glycemic effect. It is only 70 percent as sweet as sugar, so it is often combined with stevia to boost the sweetness. Truvia is the most recognizable name, but I don't recommend it because it is made by Cargill, a huge agricultural conglomerate, which extracts it from glyphosate-soaked corn and treats it with chlorine. My personal choice is Pyure Organic, a blend of erythritol and stevia (no GMOs or chlorine used).

## What's the Problem with Xylitol?

Our son, Raffi, loved to chew gum, particularly sugar-free bubble gum sweetened with xylitol. One morning as Raffi got ready for school, our poodle pup, Liam, got into a pack. I'm not sure what attracted him to the gum (then again, I'm equally mystified by why he liked to chew up paper towels and tissues). We caught him in the act as he downed several pieces of Raffi's gum in record time. It probably wasn't enough to harm him, but to be safe we brought him to the vet, where he was given a dose of an emetic.

Xylitol elicits an insulin response that is negligible in humans but significant enough in dogs to cause hypoglycemia, which can be dangerous if left untreated. Worse, the canine liver is unable to process xylitol the way the human liver does. Instead, xylitol overwhelms liver cells with the ROS that are created as the mitochondria unsuccessfully attempt to dispose of this toxic chemical.

As of this writing, no studies I'm aware of have looked at any potential impact of erythritol on the microbiome, and there is no suggestion that it can cause cancer or other diseases. The one unpleasant side effect that I've personally noted is a dry mouth sensation. You may notice this as well, especially if you consume it in large amounts, such as in sodas. Some people also report headaches from its use. (Possibly a consequence of the dehydrating effect.)

Xylitol is another sugar alcohol commonly suggested for those following low-carb or ketogenic diets. It has received a lot of attention as a keto-friendly sweetener, even garnering support in Jeff Volek's and Steve Phinney's books. When added to chewing gum, it protects against cavities. So why isn't it my number one choice? The downsides, for me, are three-fold: (1) It elicits a small but measurable glucose/insulin response; (2) it ferments in the gut to some degree; and, worst of all, (3) it is toxic to pets, especially dogs. Therefore, it has been banned from our dog-friendly home.

Maltitol, mannitol, and sorbitol are the sugar alcohols found in many low-quality sugar-free products. Sorbitol is ubiquitous in non-food products as well: You can find it in everything from toothpaste to sunscreen lotion. None of these three sugar alcohols make it onto my list of keto-friendly foods as they are all too high in carbohydrates and all ferment in the gut.

## Stevia and other natural sweeteners

Stevia is extracted from the leaf of the *Stevia rebaudiana* plant. It is not fermented in vats or concocted in a lab. Instead, dried leaves undergo water extraction followed by crystallization using a solvent, usually either ethanol or methanol. This relatively simple process makes it very appealing to those who want a natural sweetener instead of an artificial sugar substitute. Stevia is non-fermentable and doesn't raise blood glucose levels. It is incredibly sweet, approximately 200 to 300 times the sweetness of sugar. That feature makes it the perfect complement to erythritol (which is less sweet than sugar) as a granulated product, but you can also find it on its own, usually as a liquid. Choose carefully, though, as there are many flavored varieties on the market that contain some carbohydrate. Also, watch that you don't overdo: Stevia drops are highly concentrated.

Many people love stevia and use it in beverages, baking, and treats such as "fat bombs"; others don't care for it at all. My husband is among them, claiming that even a drop or two is too bitter for his palate. (I can pick up on a licorice aftertaste, but I don't find it unpleasant.) Both of our reactions are fairly common, so just give it a try and decide for yourself. Note that stevia has not been well researched by anyone but the companies that produce it, but most of what is known suggests that it is safe when ingested in small amounts, at least in the short term (long-term studies simply don't exist yet). Legal status worldwide varies greatly; in the United States it has been granted "generally regarded as safe" (GRAS) status by the FDA.

Luo han guo, also known as monk fruit, is another natural sweetener. It, too, has GRAS status in the United States, though granted without any investigation into long-term safety. Monk fruit undergoes more processing than stevia: Offending flavors are removed, and enzymatic reactions reduce it to a stable product that can be used as an ingredient in many sugar-free foods, such as bars and ice cream.

Inulin and fructooligosaccharides are technically probiotic fibers that also serve as sweeteners. These are extracted from food sources and added to a variety of products, including protein bars, shakes, and Swerve, another zero-calorie natural sweetener. Because they are fibers, they are fermented by gut bacteria, which may be beneficial to colon health. But if you already know that you are generally not very tolerant of fermentable fibers, you might want to skip this category altogether, as they can cause flatulence and loose stools. Also, some people report a significant rise in glucose levels

## A Word about Glycerin

Glycerol (glycerin) deserves special mention here. It is a sugar alcohol that is often synthesized by food companies and added to all kinds of foods. It's also a common ingredient in many extracts, including stevia drops. Most keto food lists exclude glycerol entirely because it's metabolized as a carbohydrate. In reality, however, the amount you are likely to consume in foods is a *tiny fraction* of the amount your body produces on its own. Glycerol is what forms the backbone of triglycerides, so as your body breaks down fatty acids, the glycerol is freed. Some of it is used to make new triglycerides or phospholipids, and some is also sent to the liver to be recycled into glucose via gluconeogenesis. This is normal and natural, and there's no way around it. The take-home message here is that it is far more important to check the carb content of a food to ensure that it's keto-friendly than to stress over whether or not it may contain a small amount of glycerol.

after consumption of inulin or fructooligosaccharides. My suggestion is to hold off on these until you are totally keto-adapted. If you want to introduce them later on, be sure to test your glucose level both before and after consuming them. If you see a steep rise in glucose levels, then cross them off your list.

Allulose is the new kid on the block. The good news is that it has 90 percent fewer carbs than sugar and it doesn't raise blood glucose. The bad news is that it's made from GMO corn. There are not many products that use this sugar on the market yet. If it catches on, perhaps someone will offer an organic or non-GMO variety, and we won't have to worry about inadvertently contributing to the calamitous impact of GMO products on humans and the environment.

## Spices, Seasonings, and "Those Little Extras"

Spices and seasonings add more than just variety and interest to your meals. Some (turmeric and ginger) have anti-inflammatory and anticancer properties, while others (including cinnamon) are known to lower blood glucose. Look for more information in the resources section.

Feel free to add basil, black pepper, cayenne pepper, chili pepper, chives, cilantro, cinnamon, cloves, coriander seeds, cumin seeds, dill, ginger, mustard seeds and prepared mustard, nutmeg, oregano, paprika, parsley, peppermint, rosemary, sage, and thyme to any dish. (These are suggestions, not a complete list.) Do be careful when using commercial spice mixes, as they often have added sugars or starches (flow agents). Check the ingredients carefully.

Traditional condiments, such as mustard and ketchup, need to be screened, too. Check the labels for sugars and carbs. Standard ketchup is high in added sugars, as either cane sugar or high-fructose corn syrup. Choose gluten-free tamari over soy sauce. Add a good squeeze of lemon juice to your foods! (Don't forget to count the carbs if you use more than a tablespoon a day.) Many vinegars, including apple cider vinegar (with or without "the mother"), slightly dampen the post-meal rise in glucose. Avoid balsamic and malt vinegars; these are too high in sugar.

Experiment with vinegar infusions, such as savory Italian herb, spicy chili, ginger, or turmeric! Be careful, though, as too much vinegar (the amount is hard to define) can etch tooth enamel (best to rinse with water after consuming) and may cause digestive difficulties.

Many people choose to use extracts to flavor treats. We make our own vanilla extract by grinding up 25 vanilla beans (using a blender or food processor),

## Baking Powder and Baking Soda

Both of these commonly used baking ingredients are keto-friendly. Baking *powder* contains some carbohydrate and possibly aluminum as well (check the label). Baking *soda* (sodium bicarbonate) is carb-free and *never* contains aluminum. Some research has suggested the possibility that baking soda added to water and sipped between meals may help reduce metastatic spread in certain cancers that metastasize to the lung, such as breast cancer.[14] (Don't expect this to have an effect in brain cancers.)

A bit of cautionary advice: Don't take baking soda with meals, as it neutralizes stomach acid and interferes with digestion. Also, baking soda is not appropriate for people with sodium sensitivity, as it can affect blood levels of sodium and chloride. And keep an eye on your metabolic panel (blood chemistries); if chloride (but not sodium) appears low, it may be due to overuse of baking soda.

then adding them to a liter bottle of rum (straight up—no sugar, flavorings, or spices). We let it sit for at least a month, then strain it before use.

Finally, you'll want to avoid *any* seasoning that lists MSG or any type of hydrolyzed vegetable / soy protein. These are only found in poor-quality foods and even if you don't have an obvious negative reaction, MSG may still be problematic for people with cancer.

## Salt (Sodium)

Salt is so important that it deserves its own mention. The ketogenic diet changes the way the kidneys handle sodium, resulting in large amounts of it being excreted into the urine. Also, your intake of sodium may be dramatically lowered simply by cutting out sodium-laden processed products as you switch to whole foods. The combination of more excretion and less intake may leave you experiencing what some call "keto flu." One of the best ways to replace sodium losses is to enjoy salted bone broth; it contains other valuable electrolytes as well. The current trend is to move away from conventional iodized salt (which contains ingredients your body doesn't require) and toward specialty versions, like Himalayan or sea salt.

## Do You Love Your Morning Coffee?

If you customarily drink a lot of coffee or tea, plan to cut back to one or two cups a day *before* you start the diet, or else eliminate it entirely—at least for the first month or so. Caffeine may raise blood glucose in susceptible people or contribute slightly to the dehydrating effect of the diet. I would suggest comparing your morning, pre-coffee blood glucose level to one drawn 30 minutes after your first cup. Does the level increase by 15 mg/dL or more? If so, try modifying your drink before deciding that you need to give it up entirely. If you usually drink it black, consider adding cream or turning it into a "Bulletproof" drink (coffee or tea spiked with fats, such as ghee and MCT oil; more detail in chapter 7 ["The 'Bulletproof' Model," page 101]). This makes it keto-friendly and takes care of some of your needed fats for the day.

Why don't I make a blanket suggestion that you stop drinking coffee? Mainly because it may not be an issue in cancer. If you really enjoy it and it's not causing erratic glucose levels, then why not enjoy a cup or two? (Besides, a number of studies now point to the possible health benefits derived from the polyphenols found in coffee—with or without caffeine.[15,16])

## Beverages

The best liquid is water! Keep in mind that the ketogenic diet is slightly dehydrating, so be sure to drink enough to replace what you lose throughout the day. You will also lose electrolytes, especially in the first month or so as your kidneys are keto-adapting. Please don't replace these with sports drinks; use a cup or two of salted bone broth instead.

Beverages other than water add variety. Some options:

- Sparkling water or club soda (Note that club soda contains sodium bicarbonate.)
- Herbal tea (Remember to check the ingredients for "natural flavorings" or other potential sources of carbs.)
- Stevia-sweetened drinks (But read the label carefully to be sure they don't also contain artificial sugars, such as aspartame or sucralose.)

- Unsweetened almond, hemp, and flax milks (These are low in carbs and may be used as a base for high-fat shakes. Watch for added calcium carbonate, which may contribute to constipation.)
- Unsweetened, boxed coconut milk (This is *not* the same as the canned coconut milk used in Asian cooking.)
- Coffee and tea (You'll need to limit caffeine and check for its impact on your blood glucose.)

Review figure 8.1 (page 123) for an easy-to-follow list of these keto-friendly foods. The list can also be downloaded from my website to use as a shopping list as you make the transition to your keto lifestyle.

# CHAPTER 9

# Create Your Personal Plan

There is no one-size-fits-all plan. Each one of us is an individual, and each cancer is idiosyncratic. Our dietary strategies should welcome and reflect these nuances. The best approach to this diet is to create your own personal plan. A ketogenic lifestyle is a journey, not a destination. Where you start isn't as important as having a map that sets you on the right course. Let's look at your options.

## Keto or Low Carb?

There are some scenarios where adopting a low-carb (30 to 40 net grams per day) rather than a full keto plan may be a better fit for your current needs. No matter how motivated you are to get into ketosis, remember that this shift (either from a fast or a ketogenic diet) is usually accompanied by weight loss. If you are already at a low weight or nutritionally compromised, you don't want to lose weight just now. Instead, it may be best to consider such strategies as short-term fasting before and after your chemotherapy infusions.

Understand that I'm not suggesting that you consume sugars, grains, or low-quality starches, such as those found in packaged foods. Instead, obtain most of your carbs from vegetables. Or you may opt instead for a small portion of a legume, such as a couple of tablespoons of peanut butter or a quarter of a cup of cooked lentils or beans. A low-carb diet also allows for slightly more protein, either as part of a meal or as supplemental amino acids (e.g., branched-chain or essential amino acids).

A liberalized low-carb plan may be the best option for you if you are on the other end of the spectrum—you're active or athletic and essentially healthy *despite* your cancer and need to consume more calories. Accomplish this by adding more fats and oils to each meal; in fact, you'll need to add *way* more, since a modest intake of carbs and protein will provide only a small bump in your calorie intake. You may also be a good candidate for a ketogenic supplement, such as MCT oil (or caprylic acid) blended with ghee into coffee. Commercial ketone

## Ketogenic Diet Spin-offs

There is a lot of chatter online about the cyclical ketogenic diet, a spinoff of the more traditional version that is practiced mostly by athletes. Put simply, the cyclical diet is a practice that enhances muscle glycogen stores by cycling between a five-day period of adhering to a ketogenic diet (while simultaneously engaging in intensive training) and a two-day period of carb-loading. Alternating between these eating patterns may have benefits for athletes but I (and many of my colleagues) have questions regarding the use of the technique in the early months of implementing the diet in people with cancer. Cycling in carbs may interfere with the epigenetic changes that slow progression of cancer—plus, cycling may lower resolve and commitment to a keto plan. Hopefully, research will ultimately suggest a best practice in athletes who are managing cancer.

I also field questions about what is known as feast/famine cycling, proposed as an option for those who are dealing with metabolic disorders other than cancer. This plan allows a day or two a week of higher carbohydrate and protein intake followed by a return to a low-carb or ketogenic plan. But remember that cancer is a game-changer! What might have been a good plan before your diagnosis may not serve you well right now. Until there is cancer-specific evidence pointing to benefits that outweigh the potential downside, I will continue to advocate for sustained ketosis. It's also important to stress that any type of feast/famine cycling in people with cancer should be done only under the guidance of someone who can help you determine which foods—and in what amounts—to include on feast days.

supplements are another option to consider, especially for athletes—you could use these in place of a traditional snack or before an event or workout. (Learn more about these in chapter 14, "Boosting Ketosis," page 252.)

## Diet Ratio

Beth Zupec-Kania, consultant nutritionist for The Charlie Foundation, described diet ratio in an email (May 21, 2017): "Ketogenic diets are calculated using either a macronutrient *ratio* or a macronutrient *distribution*. From the

## Raffi's Modified Ketogenic Diet

I messed up badly with Raffi's initial diet calculations, understandably so given my poor grasp of the basics. But despite my amateur efforts, Raffi still had an amazing response to the diet. In only three months, his brain tumor retreated from its relentless advance. Of course we knew we wanted to continue with the diet, but I also knew that I needed professional help. Driven by Raffi's success and my own determination, I was finally able to convince a keto-savvy dietitian to consult with me. What I learned from her was that my son had not been following a 4:1 ratio classic ketogenic diet. I had mistakenly used calories instead of grams to determine the ratio. I've learned since that this is a very common error made by newcomers to keto, so let me emphasize this point: *If you are using diet ratio, calculate using grams instead of calories.* (The next section, "Diet Macros," gives you a different option.)

Fortunately, I had understood the concept of keto well enough to have kept net carbs at 10 to 12 grams. I had set a protein target that met his needs while also cutting total calories by 30 percent (which was appropriate for my son given that his tumor was responsible for what is known as "hypothalamic obesity"). I've long since forgiven myself for this calculation error. Plus, it was instructional in that it gave me an acute awareness of one of the recurring obstacles that complicate diet initiation for many people.

early days of its use as a treatment for children with epilepsy, diet ratio reigned and has been used to describe what is still referred to as a Classic 4:1 Ketogenic Diet (97 percent fat) containing four times the grams of fat as grams of protein and carbohydrate combined. The Classic Ketogenic Diet also uses a 3:1 ratio (87 percent fat). Modern formulations include ratios of 2:1 (82 percent fat) and 1:1 (70 percent) to accommodate more protein."

But the concept of a diet ratio can be confusing, especially because the ratio is based on a system—gram weights of macronutrients—that is foreign to people who are accustomed to thinking of diets in terms of calories, not grams. Where did the idea of a ratio come from in the first place? The short answer: It was developed as a tool for registered dietitians to use in calculating a ketogenic diet prescription for a child with epilepsy, based on that child's protein and energy needs. It was never intended as a user-friendly guide for the general population. Most of the descriptions of "diet ratio" found outside of the clinical setting were in the scientific literature in discussions of the diet's therapeutic use in epilepsy.

That paradigm changed, when the keto team at Johns Hopkins Hospital published a book intended to help medical and nutrition professionals with the details of the diet. Soon their audience had expanded to include parents as well as clinicians, but it was assumed that these families were either working with a keto team or considering the keto option. It was never intended to be a do-it-yourself manual (although of course that's exactly how I used it when I bought my copy of the fourth edition in the spring of 2007!).

Even after studying the book, I still made mistakes in calculating the diet for my son. Remember, at that time I had no knowledge of nutrition science beyond what I'd learned in high school. Essentially, I was on my own except for the book, an Atkins carb counter, a calculator, and the support of a few keto-savvy parents who were willing to answer my many questions. And also remember, I didn't have a moment to spare before embarking on our keto journey.

## Diet Macros

Thankfully, another way of calculating macronutrients became popular as the ketogenic diet began to branch out into uses beyond epilepsy therapy. In the fitness world, use of the term *macronutrients* (or *macros*, as they are more commonly called) quickly gained a foothold, and a *distribution* of macronutrients is now the most common way to describe proportions in low-carb and ketogenic diets. In the distribution model, macronutrients are assigned a percentage based on *calories*, not *grams*. For example, in a 1,600-calorie/day ketogenic diet, carbohydrates typically make up 5 percent of total calories (i.e., 80 calories, or 20 grams). Obesity medicine specialist Eric Westman, along with researchers Jeff Volek and Stephen Phinney, briefly mention this method in their book, *The New Atkins for a New You*.

Without a doubt, macronutrient distribution is more intuitive and user-friendly than the diet ratio. Plus, the conventional nutrition world had been using the term for decades, so it didn't require elaborate explanations to make it understandable to the public. Having a common language also made it much easier to compare the distribution of macronutrients in a standard diet to those in a ketogenic diet (see table 9.1).

As you can see, each macronutrient category is assigned a range that represents its percentage of total calories in an individual's diet. For example,

**Table 9.1.** Macronutrients as a Percentage of Total Daily Calories

|  | Fat (%) | Protein (%) | Carbohydrate (%) |
| --- | --- | --- | --- |
| Standard diet | 20–35 | 10–35 | 45–65 |
| Ketogenic diet | 78–86 | 8–12 | 2–6 |

80 percent fat in a 1,500-calorie plan for a woman amounts to 1,200 calories (approximately 133 grams of fat), while 80 percent fat in a 2,500-calorie plan for a larger man is 2,000 calories (approximately 222 grams of fat). So even though both of these diets contain 80 percent fat, the higher calorie demands in the larger man require an additional 89 grams of fat. That's a difference of over 6 tablespoons of fat per day!

Protein as a percentage of the total calories varies from individual to individual as well, but the absolute amount has much less of a spread as the target is determined not by total energy (calorie) needs but instead by ideal body weight, lean body mass, or some condition that requires a higher intake. Carbs as a percentage of the total also vary depending on total calories. We'll discuss macros in much more detail in the next section as we work through the calculations that will help you determine your personal macro targets.

## Results Trump Ratios (and Macros)

Don't overthink this! Diet efficacy is not tied solely to diet ratios or macronutrient distribution. Keep your eye on the prize: low and steady glucose combined with high ketone levels and a much improved quality of life.

## Determine Your Personal Macros

In this section, we'll look at your needs for each macronutrient. We'll begin with your protein requirement, then set a carb limit, and, finally, calculate how much fat you'll need to meet the balance of your energy needs. Remember that this initial diet prescription is only an estimate of what will work for you. Expect to reassess and refine your prescription over time.

### Calculate Your Protein Target

You already know that your body uses protein to maintain or build muscle mass. But do you also know that protein, broken down into its constituent amino acids, is used in cell cycle activities, such as DNA repair and RNA synthesis? Are

## Important: Read This before Starting Your Child on the Diet

Before embarking on a ketogenic diet, you need to first engage the cooperation of your child's medical team. If the oncologist isn't interested or supportive, seek out a pediatrician who is willing to work with you to provide oversight and to act as a liaison. You also need to connect with an experienced keto dietitian or nutritionist who has access to The Charlie Foundation's KetoDietCalculator.

The dietitian enters the client's demographics and the calculator uses that information to determine your child's protein needs (in grams) and caloric requirements. The dietitian also enters a macronutrient ratio which determines the carb and fat grams needed. All macros are evenly divided between meals. Caregivers are usually granted access to the meal-planning feature, allowing you to choose from a set of precalculated meals or to create new ones from scratch. This tool was originally developed for use in children with epilepsy but can be used by adults as well for any application of the ketogenic diet.

Visit The Charlie Foundation website; you'll find lots of kid-friendly resources there. Also visit the MaxLove Project website and Facebook page. The founders are very supportive of the diet for cancer and offer lots of resources and other support for families.

In no way am I suggesting that the diet itself is dangerous, but there are reasons to seek guidance. First, you are not an expert on the diet—yet. Second, if you run into a problem, such as vomiting or lethargy, you will want immediate access to a professional who can help you troubleshoot the issues. This will be so much easier if your child's team is already aware of the diet and potential side effects.

you aware of protein's role in building hormones and how it participates in the enzymatic reactions that keep you alive? Don't worry if you don't understand the details; it won't keep you from properly implementing this plan. You can catch up on the science later as you become more comfortable with the diet basics.

Determining your individual protein needs is a very important part of your macronutrient calculations. If you are like most people in the United States, you currently eat more protein than you need, and an excessive amount of protein can undermine your efforts at managing cancer through diet. The problem may be compounded if the protein foods you choose are anabolic (as in whey protein).

Most estimates of protein needs are very broad and inclusive. The current RDA stands at 0.8 grams of protein per kilogram of body weight, an amount that the Food and Nutrition Board of the Institute of Medicine views as adequate for over 97 percent of healthy Americans.[1] But there are issues to consider here: (1) This amount was determined by studies of people following a high-carbohydrate standard diet; and (2) This recommendation is based on *actual* body weight instead of *ideal* weight. Let's look at the first issue: Although we could speculate that people following a ketogenic diet need less protein to maintain their muscle mass given the diet's protein-sparing effect, there are simply too many variables to come up with a recommendation that can be generalized to everyone in ketosis. Now let's consider the second issue using this example: Calculate the RDA for protein for an overweight 5'9" individual weighing 220 pounds (100 kilograms):

$$100 \text{ kilograms} \times 0.8 \text{ grams/kilogram} = 80 \text{ grams of protein}$$

Now calculate the RDA for protein for a 5'9" individual weighing an ideal 154 pounds (70 kg):

$$70 \text{ kilograms} \times 0.8 \text{ grams/kilogram} = 56 \text{ grams of protein}$$

Where is the evidence that a heavier person needs an additional 24 grams of protein to maintain what is basically the same lean body mass (weight minus fat)? Some may argue that more protein is needed to maintain the muscle tissue needed to support the extra weight, but, realistically, any additional amount of protein—if needed at all—is likely to be very small, possibly only a few extra grams per day.

Many factors feed into your ideal body weight. I've included a calculator in the resources section to help you sort this out. Note that these estimates are gender-specific and offer a range of weights appropriate for people of varying heights. If you don't know your ideal weight, ask your doctor for advice. If the estimate is in pounds, divide that number by 2.2 to arrive at kilograms, then multiply kilograms by 0.8. That's your estimate of how many grams of protein you need per day. Understand that there are exceptions to this and you may need to set your target higher.

If you want to refine your individualized target, use lean body mass (LBM) instead of ideal body weight and set your protein target at 1.0 gram per

## Protein Intake: Special Cases

Listed here are a few circumstances in which you may need more than the minimum amount of protein.

1. If you are recovering from surgery, are in active treatment, or are losing muscle mass for any reason, ask your team for advice regarding your ideal protein intake (which may include supplemental amino acids).
2. If you are pregnant or lactating, you need to consider the needs of your child first and foremost, even if it means delaying the start of your diet. Again, look to your team for advice.
3. Higher protein intake in people 70 years and older is associated with reduced mortality, even though it may not translate to improved muscle mass. (Factors that affect nutrient intake and digestion may improve your nutrition status, with or without an increase in protein.) Seek advice from your medical team.

kilogram of LBM. To calculate your LBM, you will need to (1) determine your body fat percentage, (2) calculate your body fat in pounds, and (3) subtract fat pounds from total body weight to arrive at your LBM. The quickest and most low-tech way to assess your body fat percentage is to compare your own body to standardized body fat percentage comparison pictures you can easily find online (search for "images body fat comparison pictures").

Similar to ideal body weight, lean body mass estimated in this manner is somewhat subjective, so please ask someone close to you for their assessment as well. Ideally, you will use a more objective assessment tool, such as skinfold calipers. Ask an obesity medicine clinician to take the measurements and perform the calculations for you; or, if you are in more of a "do-it-yourself" mode, you can buy a set of calipers online and learn how to use them.

You can also use a bioelectrical impedance scale. This is similar in appearance to a standard bathroom scale but has a built-in tool that estimates body fat. Under ideal conditions (i.e., proper hydration), it may be an accurate tool to use before you start the diet. However, once you start, it becomes less accurate because it fails to fully account for the change in water content of the lean body tissue.

## Stop Here If You Plan to Use Cronometer

Cronometer, the nutrient tracker that I recommend to all my clients, has tools to help you calculate your protein target without the need to perform all these calculations. You can sign up for a free account at https://cronometer.com and set up your profile right now. The user manual will walk you through all the steps you need in order to set your macronutrient goals, including an estimate of your protein target using a set of body fat comparison pictures (found at https://cronometer.com/help/misc/bodyfat.jsp).

You may ask, what's the harm in eating more protein than you require?

- Amino acids that aren't needed for maintenance and repair are shunted to the liver. There, they may be converted to glucose. (For a refresher on gluconeogenesis, look back to chapter 3, "The Shift to Ketosis," page 21.)
- Cancer cells can use glutamine, one of the amino acids in protein, to fuel their energy needs. (Dr. Seyfried's research is actively homing in on a solution to this, though it is too early to make clinically appropriate recommendations here.)
- Protein increases activity in the mTOR pathway, a problem in cancer as well as in many diseases attributed to aging.
- Protein (especially from dairy and egg) can stimulate an insulin response, which in turn suppresses ketone production.

There is a pervasive myth surrounding protein that pokes its head up frequently. That is the common but flawed belief that physically active people need to double or even triple their intake of protein, especially if they want to build or maintain muscle. The science doesn't support that, even for those keto-adapted people who put some serious effort into resistance training. In an email exchange (April 2017), Dr. Dominic D'Agostino suggested an alternative to adding more protein: Instead, keep macronutrient ratios the same while consuming a surplus of calories (up to 25 percent more than on non-training days) within 24 to 48 hours of intense training. (Please understand that Dr. D'Agostino is not presenting this as an evidence-based protocol, but instead, is simply sharing insights that will hopefully become the subject of formal research.) If you are an athlete and want to continue training, I strongly advise that you work closely with a trainer who is also knowledgeable about the protein-sparing effects of ketogenic diets.

Even if you are not an athlete, it's still important to understand that ketones spare protein. Put another way, if your body is fueled primarily by fat and ketones, you won't *catabolize* (break down) as much muscle during exercise. In fact, it's likely that any extra protein needs you have can be met by supplementing with a few grams of branched-chain amino acids before and during a workout. This will allow for stimulation of muscle protein synthesis without requiring increased protein intake at meals. (The jury is still out on whether or not this will stimulate protein synthesis specific to muscle without activating any of the cancer-promoting pathways. Research is ongoing.)

Putting exceptions aside, let's return to your individual calculations. It is my observation that people have better outcomes if they limit protein intake to 0.8 grams per kilogram of ideal body weight (or 1.0 gram of protein per kilogram of LBM). I have not seen any diet-related problems with low protein or albumin in people who keep to these guidelines (though these numbers may be on the low side because of the adverse effects of some cancer treatments).

## Set Your Carb Limit

Your next step is to set your carbohydrate intake. This is much simpler than determining protein, since there is no requirement for carbs. Go as low as you can, especially in the first few weeks or months of the diet, but keep an eye on your overall nutrient intake. In other words, don't squander your carbs on non-foods like coffee creamers. Instead, use your carb allowance for nutrient-dense, non-starchy vegetables and fat-rich nuts and seeds.

Consider these factors in setting your carb limit:

- If you are healthy enough to jump right in, you can set your net carbs (total carbohydrates minus fiber) at between 12 and 16 grams per day.
- If you have thyroid disease or other hormone imbalances, you will be more successful and feel better during the transition if you set your carb limit between 20 and 25 grams.
- If you are recovering from surgery, or are currently undergoing chemotherapy or radiation, consider a carb intake of 20 to 25 grams.
- If the carbs you crave are found in foods like salad or sautéed greens, it's likely that you can eat all you want and still maintain strong

ketosis, especially if you combine these favorites with oil-based dressings that are also low in carbs.

There are several options in setting up your Cronometer profile. They're described in the Help tutorial. Here are a few tips: (1) Scroll down to Macronutrient Targets and select "High Fat/Ketogenic." If you choose "High Fat/Ketogenic," level "Rigorous," the limit for carbohydrates will default to 20 grams and protein will be at a minimum. (2) If you choose "Moderate," the default will be 40 grams (but note that the default for protein will also be higher). (3) If you want to set an individualized target, you'll need to select "Fixed Targets." I suggest 12 to 25 net grams of carbs as a starting point for almost all of my clients. This virtually guarantees that they will reach and maintain ketosis (as long as protein is kept in check as well). Over time, you can use feedback from monitoring blood glucose and ketones to tweak this amount.

## What If You Have Other Serious Challenges?

If you have bowel disease, poor appetite, or problems with your gastrointestinal tract, or are underweight or malnourished to start, then I strongly recommend that you ease into ketosis over a period of several weeks by first setting your protein target at 1.2 to 1.5 grams per kilogram of LBM while very gradually reducing your intake of carbs. Start by eliminating all added sugars, grains, inflammatory oils, and low-quality starches, such as potatoes and gluten-free breads, while simultaneously increasing your intake of healthy fats and oils, incorporating at least a few extra tablespoons into each of your meals. Identify which high-fat treats appeal to you and use these as snacks (to boost total calories) or desserts (to keep meals from feeling too greasy or oily).

You should also begin to test and record your fasting blood glucose so that you have baseline data for comparison. Don't expect to achieve ketosis until you are able to lower your targets as outlined in the previous section. It must be your priority to troubleshoot any issues that keep you from consuming or tolerating this increase in fat. If you remove carbs before you have accomplished this, you are virtually guaranteed to lose weight or, worse yet, give up on the plan entirely.

## Meet Energy Needs with Fats

Given that fat is so important to a ketogenic diet, you may wonder why I waited so long to get to this section. It's simple: While your protein and carb targets are likely to remain stable over the early weeks and months, the amount of fat you need will increase or decrease depending on your actual (rather than your estimated) energy needs. For example, if you increase your level of physical activity, your calorie needs will naturally rise, and you will want to meet that demand by increasing calories from *fat*, not protein or carbs. You will then need to adjust your Cronometer settings.

Or maybe you'll learn that you overestimated your energy needs to start; if so, you will then adjust your intake by *lowering* the amount of fat calories you take in daily. Again, this only affects the calories you consume from fat, not those from protein or carbs. If you are carrying some extra weight, there is no need to stuff yourself full of fats right now. You will burn your body fat and still make great ketones!

Your fat target includes the fat found in foods. If you are using a food tracker, it will list your intake as grams of fat. As examples, half of an avocado contains about 10 grams of fat, and a 1-ounce serving of macadamia nuts contains 21 grams of fat. When you add fats or oils to meals, it may be easier to think of them in terms of tablespoons, but they also need to be recorded as grams (1 tablespoon of oil = 14 grams). Other foods such as lean protein and vegetables contain almost no fat. We'll cover this in more detail in chapter 12.

## The Question of Calorie Restriction

There's one more question you need to consider: Are you planning to adopt a calorie-restricted ketogenic diet (welcoming a certain amount of weight loss), or do you want to maintain your present weight or even gain a few pounds? Before you decide, please review "Caloric Restriction without Malnutrition" (page 94) in chapter 7. If you are carrying some excess weight but are generally healthy despite your cancer diagnosis, you may want to make a greater "first impression" on your disease by restricting calories for the first few months. To do this in Cronometer, while in your profile scroll down to the "Weight Goal" frame and select one of the weight-loss options, such as "Lose Weight: (–1.0 lb / week)." The program will automatically adjust your calorie target downward by reducing the amount of calories you should consume from fat.

Cronometer will not allow you to set a desired weight loss of more than 2 pounds per week—and that's a good thing! Understand, though, that you are only estimating your energy needs, so you could lose weight at a faster rate, especially in the first few weeks. But please be careful. Even if you've read somewhere that the diet won't be therapeutic unless you severely restrict calories, it's simply not true; so don't go down that road. You can do more damage than good. Too much caloric restriction, practiced daily, may have a negative impact on your immune system that far outweighs any benefit. This is especially true if you are undergoing

## Another Option: The Ankerl KetoCalculator

Cronometer is not the only program capable of helping you calculate your macronutrient targets. You may wish to look at the Ankerl KetoCalculator. You can use this simple program to develop your macronutrient targets, but it does not track your food intake.

1. Go to https://keto-calculator.ankerl.com.
2. Enter your age, gender, height, and weight and select your activity level.
3. Scroll down to enter your estimated body fat percentage, then note your calculated LBM in kilograms.
4. Use this figure to calculate your protein needs (LBM multiplied by 0.8 grams/kilogram, unless you are one of the exceptions discussed in "Protein Intake: Special Cases" on page 152).
5. Then scroll down to the section on protein and enter your target in the middle box. It will be flagged "protein too low." Ignore this warning.
6. Next, enter your limit for net carbohydrates.
7. Finally, enter the degree of calorie restriction as a percentage (no more than 30 percent to start).

Now your complete macro prescription is displayed as "Your Personal Results." This includes an easy-to-read set of macronutrient targets (in grams) as well as their distribution (percent of total calories). Remember, if you follow these guidelines, you'll be counting grams, not calories. You may want to print out the results and bookmark the site on your computer. Revisit this calculation often and make adjustments as needed.

or attempting to recover from cancer treatments that have lowered your blood counts. Also, your body may respond to the perception of starvation by pumping out a lot more stress hormones; this will definitely work against your efforts.

There is another important reason that you don't want to lose weight too quickly: Hormones and fat-soluble toxins are stored in body fat. When weight is lost too quickly, these hormones and toxins can easily overwhelm the body's ability to detoxify. In addition, since vitamin D is stored in fat, I have seen levels jump sharply in people who are losing weight too quickly, and this can also lead to toxicity. And don't think for a minute that coffee enemas or liver flushes are going to save the day. There's a lot of legend but no science to that kind of thinking. Instead, keep your weight loss at or under a few pounds per week and let your liver handle detoxification all on its own.

Keeping all this in mind, how much should you restrict? My recommendation for most people with excess weight is to aim for a 1-pound-per-week

## Trackers and Planners for Nutrition Professionals

Aaron Davidson, the developer of the personal nutrition tracker Cronometer, has developed a "Pro" version intended for use by nutrition consultants and clinic dietitians. As a beta tester for this program, I can assure any "Pros" out there that this tool makes it much easier for you to monitor your clients' entries. As a Pro user, you can move easily from client to client without the need to log in using each individual's credentials. You can also review your clients' profiles and make tweaks to correct the most common set-up errors. Aaron is also working on a way for you to share recipes with your clients so that they don't each individually need to transcribe these into their personal database; this saves time and ensures the accuracy of the nutrition data.

By checking in regularly with your clients, you can offer them targeted feedback. When I review a new client's food diary, I use their own data as a starting point to educate them on how much and what type of foods and supplements they need to cover their nutrition needs. For example, almost everyone following a ketogenic plan falls short of meeting even the lowest threshold for calcium and magnesium. When I call attention to what I see in Cronometer, people are often more open to heeding my suggestion for a high-quality supplement.

weight loss. This rate of loss can help you make the transition to ketosis more quickly and can speed up keto-adaptation as well. If you see that you're losing too much weight too quickly, then adjust your profile setting in Cronometer (see instructions above) or simply add in some fat calories that take you over your target. On the other hand, if you know you have a resistant metabolism, select a weight loss of 2 pounds per week. Remember, you can—and should—make midstream corrections once you're up and running with your new plan. So don't become too fixated on a number right now. You will be adding intermittent fasting (discussed in more detail in chapter 7) to your plan as well, which is yet another tool that can move you into therapeutic ketosis.

What if you don't have an ounce of extra weight to spare? Under "Weight Goal" in your Cronometer profile, select "Maintain Weight." Expect to lose a bit of water weight as you shift to ketosis. Or, if you need to move the needle in the other direction and add a few pounds, choose one of the

Even if your clients are reluctant to start with Cronometer, or don't have the time or energy to fully commit to daily recording, they may eventually get on board, especially if you offer support and encouragement along with some targeted tweaks (there's always room for improvement). Once clients get over the initial steep learning curve, the feedback this program provides often motivates its users to explore deeper layers that optimize nutrition. I routinely check in with people, even those I am no longer actively coaching. If they have been consistent, I can gauge how much they've grown in their understanding of nutrition in general and how over time that information has translated into improvements in their food choices. I find this both personally and professionally rewarding!

Another option for professionals is The Charlie Foundation's Keto-DietCalculator. As I stated earlier in this chapter, this is an essential tool for any professional who plans to work with a child's oncology team. It can also be used as both a planner and a tracker for adults and, like Cronometer, it has a tightly managed database. To gain access, you will need to register your clinic or private practice. There is no fee, but please consider a donation to The Charlie Foundation to help support the wonderful work that it does!

weight-gain options in the profile. The program will add more fat calories to your target.

If all this sounds too confusing, don't despair. It will quickly make more sense once you are up and running with Cronometer.

## Use a Tracker

Over the years I've looked at the practicality, accuracy, and ease of use of many popular online meal planners and food trackers, developed as both desktop versions and phone apps, and I find issues with them all. Most are designed with weight loss as the primary goal, which is not the case for most individuals with cancer; losing weight is a side effect (often an undesirable one) of keeping to a keto plan. Still, I encourage you to use a good tracking tool, even if only occasionally, as this will help take the guesswork out of your food choices. Just as importantly, I have seen for myself how effective trackers are in improving both compliance and personal accountability. After all, if you have to record that bite of cake, then you may decide to skip it. Likewise for that bread that found its way to your table at the restaurant.

One of my frustrations with most trackers is that they allow "serving size" as an entry option. This in itself isn't a flaw, but it does lead to some very inaccurate entries. To avoid error, I encourage *all* of my clients to use a high-quality kitchen scale to weigh all their foods in grams instead of relying on the "serving size" default. My husband and I both use our kitchen scale daily. He finds that periodically spending a week or two weighing and recording all of his foods and tracking his biometrics keeps him focused on his health improvement goals. I no longer track every day, but when we implemented the diet for our son I developed the habit of using a scale. I still use it when developing recipes that I intend to share with clients.

In the first few months of the diet, I highly recommend that you commit to weighing and recording all your foods. Most trackers offer several ways to record quantity (by the cup, tablespoon, and so on), but my recommendation is to select the "gram" option, then enter that food's weight in grams. Soon, it will become a part of your meal prep routine.

# CHAPTER 10

# Plan for Success

As I've said before, there is no need to overthink what is needed to adopt a ketogenic diet. For the most part, keto meals are just a different mix of familiar foods. First, pick a protein. Then prepare a salad or a non-starchy vegetable. Add some fat and a few extras such as nuts, seeds, or berries, and there you have it—the blueprint for every keto meal!

## The Challenge

Most likely, your current diet relies heavily on carb-containing foods. Even if you already "eat clean," grains, legumes, starchy vegetables, fruit, and milk products are most likely providing over half of your daily calories. But if you are like most people who start a keto plan, you will quickly learn how to cut back on carbs. In fact, that part is often easier than reducing protein. And, of course, you'll need to get comfortable with more than doubling your intake of fats and oils. The diet may seem daunting at first, but know that many others have successfully dealt with its challenges!

As a person with cancer, you may also be neck deep in juggling the many changes bombarding you from all sides. Work and family life may now revolve around your treatment schedule and energy level. If you're undergoing conventional therapies, it is also likely that you are dealing with side effects. Managing cancer often depletes your mental and physical reserves, and you want meals to take *less* rather than *more* of your time and energy! The most important thing to remember, however, is that while the ketogenic diet might seem complicated in terms of rethinking your balance of protein and fat and carbohydrates, its actual implementation does not have to be difficult.

If you are the caregiver of a person with cancer, many of these same challenges apply to you as well. In addition to your general caregiving, you are now tasked with a new twist to food shopping and meal planning and preparation, initially perhaps leaving you with less time for activities that are important to your own well-being. My advice is to take advantage of offers of help from family and friends. They can pick up a few items for you while they're doing their own shopping or prepare a keto meal using one of your recipes.

Read through these three options. Which one is the best fit for your set of circumstances?

## Option #1: Jump In with a Fast

Are you thinking of jumping into a fast right now, pushing through the transition quickly so you can enter the therapeutic zone with lightning speed? Or perhaps the idea of a fast appeals to you because you're scared, and taking bold and immediate action may help restore your sense of control over your life? Or are you contemplating a fast because you're overwhelmed by the details of the plan and you want to skip over them for the moment? Take a deep breath. Wherever your motivation lies, there are some things you need to consider first.

Despite your enthusiasm, remember that there are medical reasons why fasting may not be your best option. If you are older, in frail health, recovering from surgery, low weight to start, or need medication that has to be taken with food, then you should not start with a fast. If you have experienced a recent significant weight loss, or if you are taking thyroid medication or are on hormone therapy, I suggest that you ease into ketosis so that your body can adapt comfortably to the changes; you can always opt for a therapeutic fast at a future date. If you have a history of heart arrhythmia or palpitations or if prior drug therapies have caused an elongated QT interval (a heart condition), you need to talk to your medical team before initiating a fast as it can cause some initial disruption in electrolyte balance. And, of course, if you are pregnant or lactating, rule out a fast for now.

Fasting is also not the best option during the workweek; save it for the weekend. And I *strongly* advise against fasting if you live alone or are a single parent with young children. Why? Even though fasting is generally safe and very therapeutic, there are times when you may feel dizzy or light-headed, or your thinking may not be clear. That puts you at a higher risk of a fall or a lapse in judgment. It's best to have someone close by who knows you well enough to step in if needed, either by taking over responsibility for the children or by making sure you drink extra liquids (like salted bone broth or an electrolyte drink) to get you through the transition period. Remember, it takes at least a few days for your body and brain to make the shift to ketosis. These symptoms will ease up as your brain begins to use ketones as its main fuel.

If you are interested in fasting, make sure you have your blood glucose testing supplies on hand and know how to use them. Record several blood glucose measurements in advance to use as a baseline, then take and record your glucose levels throughout the fasting period. At a minimum, test first thing in the morning and again at bedtime. You should also test any time that you experience any minor symptoms, such as light-headedness, or more extreme symptoms, such as vomiting or heart palpitations. Expect your numbers to bounce around quite a bit as you transition to ketosis, but if in these first few days you experience low readings and symptoms, you may need to take action. Also remember that you may not be able to distinguish between mild low blood sugar and acidosis, so always err on the safe side by reversing ketosis or even visiting the emergency department of the hospital if your symptoms persist or worsen.

During the fast you will want to test for ketones as well, using either your meter or Bayer Ketostix. You should see a steady rise in ketones by the second day of your fast. The longer you fast, the higher they may go. Expect them to reach at least 3 mmol/L. They may top out at around 5 mmol/L, though some people, especially children, may reach levels as high as 7 mmol/L. If you're using the urine strips, you will most likely see colors indicating moderate to large ketones.

If you do move ahead with a fast, you'll need to decide whether it will be water-only or modified by the addition of salted broth with added fats or oils. The latter option will still move you into ketosis quickly but with fewer side effects than a water-only fast. For now, leave the length of the fast open-ended. Give yourself permission to break your fast at any time if you feel like it's no longer serving you well. I highly recommend reading about Jimmy Moore's experience with multiple types of fasts, which he recounts in the book *The Complete Guide to Fasting*, coauthored with Dr. Jason Fung. Although it's great to read about others' successes, always remember to focus on what's right for you.

One last word of advice about beginning the diet with a fast: Be sure that you've prepared for the steps that immediately follow the end of your fast. Do this before you begin fasting. Stock up on the foods and other supplies you'll need and "field test" a few recipes beforehand to be sure that they are doable, palatable, and will meet your macro targets. You'll lose valuable ground and experience disappointment in yourself if you complete your fast only to resume your old patterns.

## Option #2: Start with a Rigorous Keto Plan

Although fasting is the quickest way to reach ketosis, starting with a classic ketogenic diet will also get you there. First, consider your net carb intake. If you are facing an aggressive cancer (such as brain cancer) and time is of the essence, paring your carb intake down to the minimum will help you focus on eliminating all nonessential carbohydrates in your diet. In fact, limiting your net carbs to 12 grams a day, the most rigorous option, might also be your best option if you are in good health overall. But there are lots of situations where you may need more wiggle room: for example, if you take thyroid medication or are at risk of too rapid a weight loss. Then I suggest that you start with a more moderate carb intake of 20 net grams.

Another factor in your decision relates to the glycemic index (GI) of the foods you choose most often; that is, how much of an impact on glucose is the food predicted to have—especially when you account for portion size (glycemic load, or GL) and the macro content of the rest of the meal (fat dampens the glycemic response). Variations in metabolism and insulin resistance also factor into this equation so it's no wonder that there is a huge variation in theoretical versus actual response. In fact, I could line up 10 people and feed them each the exact same meal and expect to see 10 different glycemic responses.

Because of the enormous range of variation between individuals, glycemic index and glycemic load, by themselves, are too vague to base your choices on. So if you choose to consider it at all, use GI only as a guide to screen your choices in carbs. For example, if you plan to derive most of your carbs from leafy greens and a few cruciferous vegetables (especially green cabbage, which has a negligible GI impact), then you will most likely see a quick transition to ketosis, even at 20 net carbs a day. Choosing low GI foods will allow for the most variety in non-starchy vegetables, which are also rich in nutrients and fiber. However, if you can't live without blueberries (which are also rich in nutrients but have a GI of 40 to 50), then it's best to limit yourself to 12 net carbs per day at the start. This is usually low enough to prevent spikes in glucose even if you do choose higher GI foods. Once you are keto-adapted, however, you will have more leeway in your choices, but you will need to use a home blood glucose meter to test your actual response to the type and amount of carbs you're eating.

If you are the partner of a person with cancer and want to show solidarity with your loved one, a switch to a low-carb diet may improve your own health as well. The switch to burning fat as your main fuel is associated with lower levels of inflammation, less insulin resistance, and other benefits, such as improved mitochondrial health. You may want to set your initial target at 20 net grams of carbs per day, but my guess is that over time you can raise this number to 40 to 60 grams (as I have done) and still maintain the health benefits of nutritional ketosis.

The transition to keto will be easier for you if you are already familiar with what foods are included in a very-low-carbohydrate diet and which are definitely off-limits. (Refer back to the lists in chapter 8.) Knowing your way around the kitchen and prior experience with whole-food cooking are also definite advantages in the transition to planning and preparing keto meals. You may be pleased to learn that you can modify many of your favorite dishes from the past by substituting keto-friendly ingredients for the more traditional carb-loaded ones. To see what I mean, just conduct an online search for a favorite meal, inserting the keyword "keto" first (e.g., "keto lasagna" or "keto pancakes"). You can also use "low-carb" in your search, but expect those recipes to be too high in either carbs or protein—you'll need to modify them. As I've mentioned, Domini Kemp and Patricia Daly provide many great recipes in their cookbook, *The Ketogenic Kitchen*.

If you are carrying a bit of extra weight, it may now work to your advantage as you move into ketosis. But a long history of obesity is often associated with other metabolic issues, such as insulin resistance or hyperinsulinemia. This generally does not interfere with the initial shift to ketosis, but bear in mind that it can extend the amount of time you will experience transition symptoms. If you have underlying metabolic issues, it may also take longer for you to reverse insulin resistance. Your age may be a factor here as well, since metabolic issues tend to creep up on most people over time. If you already know from past low-carb efforts that you have a resistant metabolism, you may need to eliminate dairy proteins, at least to start, even if you crave these foods. Protein cravings are almost always a sign of a resistant metabolism, and these cravings may intensify temporarily when you adopt a ketogenic plan. Listen to your body and be prepared and proactive when it comes to dealing with the side effects of switching to a primarily fat-based metabolism.

Again, let me emphasize how important it is to test blood glucose and ketones. The feedback is invaluable in helping you determine if you're on the right track. And don't underestimate how empowering it is to see your numbers trending in the right direction! I also highly recommend that you track your food intake in Cronometer. Even if you don't find every food item you consume, the simple act of recording keeps you accountable for what you choose to eat and drink, and that goes a long way toward reinforcing your commitment to the plan. The Food Diary page in Cronometer can also be used to keep track of glucose and ketone measurements, and document physical activity and changes in weight—a powerful set of tools!

## Option #3: Ease Into Ketosis

I've worked with many people who are already quite compromised by their disease or its treatments. Or they may have a number of other complex health issues in addition to cancer. If you fall into this group, I highly recommend that you ease into rather than jump into a ketogenic plan. Easing in is also a great way to shape a child's diet. A slower transition is easier for anyone who is moving to a ketogenic plan directly from a standard diet; there's more time to find keto-friendly substitutes for the foods you now eat and to properly prepare your kitchen and pantry.

To start, eliminate all grains, gluten-free flours, and added sugars of any kind. Cut back on portion sizes and servings of starchy vegetables, legumes, and fruits. As I've suggested before, add a tablespoon or two of fat or oil to each meal; choose olive, avocado, and coconut oil as often as possible. And now is a good time to begin to supplement your diet with MCT oil. If dairy is part of your plan, you'll find it easy to add fats such as butter and ghee. (Heavy whipping cream has moisture as well as fat, so count two tablespoons of cream as one tablespoon of fat, and be sure to count the carbs using information from Cronometer or the USDA website.) Once you are comfortable with one to two tablespoons of added fat, bump it up further by adding one more tablespoon at each meal, while simultaneously cutting out other concentrated sources of carbs in your diet, such as starchy vegetables, legumes, fruits (as well as concentrated sources of dairy sugars, such as milk and cottage cheese). Finally,

### Ask for Help

If you are trying to do this on your own, or if you are the head of a household with others who are dependent on you, then I strongly urge you to reach out to friends and family members for support. Trust me, people want to help, and you will be doing them a favor by guiding them toward what you really need. Be specific: Do you want someone to run a few errands? Shop for keto foods? Help you with the laundry? If someone offers to bring you food, be bold enough to give them some simple keto recipes; that way, you'll have keto-friendly, ready-made meals that you can just pop in the oven or heat in the microwave.

rein in your protein. If you make an effort to stick to these guidelines, you'll get through the transition in good shape and are also more likely to experience fewer cravings and other distractions that can interfere with your adherence to the plan.

Keep a food diary and track your glucose, first thing in the morning and again at bedtime. Test your bedtime urine ketones as well. You can begin to test blood ketones once urine ketone strips start showing some color (pink or purple), but don't waste precious blood ketone strips until the less expensive urine strips show you are in sustained ketosis. Use the same guidelines for tracking food and biometrics that I outlined in Option #2.

## Why Meal Planning Is So Important

Over the years I learned that planning meals for my adult clients is much more challenging than it is for children. I would start with a list of my client's food preferences, then develop some starter meals that fit the macro targets. This was very labor-intensive because it meant ensuring that each meal had the exact amount of protein, carbs, and fat, customized for each individual's targets. Despite my attention to detail, it was the rare individual who followed my plan precisely! And no wonder: From the start, people had no choice but to adapt their personal plans to accommodate life's continually changing circumstances. If they tried to adhere to a rigid and precise meal plan, they would easily be overwhelmed by the inevitable challenges, such as trying to make up for a meal skipped because appointments, nausea, or lack of appetite got in the way. What people needed were tools they could use to help adapt their plan on the fly. That's why I created a meal template that sidesteps the confusion surrounding proper meal planning. If you identify with these challenges, relax a bit. I'll present the plan soon in chapter 13, "Simple Keto Meal Template," page 217.

### Keep It Simple!

Meal planning is easier than you may think if you are willing to forgo complicated gourmet meals and focus instead on putting together simple combinations of protein, carbohydrates, and fat, at least until you feel comfortable with your new way of eating. This usually takes a few weeks, faster if you already feel at home in the kitchen and are used to preparing meals using whole foods. If you have followed a low-carb diet for weight loss sometime in your past, you already know most of what you'll need to get started with a ketogenic diet for cancer. You may have recipes that you liked and these will

## Patricia Daly's Meal Plans

Of course, it's fun to look ahead at some cancer-specific keto meal plans, to motivate you to move from this simple start to a more interesting long-term plan. You may even have enough kitchen experience that you can start at this more advanced point, but be sure you are working with meal plans and recipes designed for cancer: that is, those that are both low carb *and* low protein. That's why Patricia Daly's contributions, which fit this low-carb, low-protein model, make *The Ketogenic Kitchen* such a valuable resource. Instead of the typical weight-loss plans that are too high in protein and too low in quality, Patricia's meal plans were thoughtfully developed for those people following a well-designed keto-for-cancer plan. She's adept at creating family-friendly meals, too, and suggests tasty ways of using leftovers and rotating food choices.

need only slight modifications to lower the amount of protein and raise the proportion of fat.

Cancer is a strong motivator to make these changes, but it's important to keep this motivation from turning into a stressor. Putting too much pressure on yourself at this vulnerable point in time can backfire. There is no need to have every ingredient on hand and all the tools in place before you make your first keto meal. You are more likely to be successful—and less stressed—if you learn to simplify, simplify, simplify! Find a handful of recipes using a few keto-friendly ingredients. (Check the resources section for recommended websites and cookbooks.) Learn from your mistakes as well as your successes. Recycle your favorites, tweaking them slightly by changing the vegetable or the meat. Use leftovers whenever you can, and if you dine out, take half of the protein food back home to eat for lunch or dinner the next day.

## Cronometer Is Your Friend

As I've made clear throughout this book, my favorite nutrient tracker is Cronometer, and I highly recommend that you weigh and record there everything you eat or drink, especially in the first few weeks of the diet and again as a check at any point in the future. You may think that this is not in line with my advice to "keep it simple," but in fact it's easier than winging it because it elimi-nates the guesswork. Plus, it helps with compliance and makes you accountable for your choices. And Cronometer makes it so simple: If you eat more or less the same foods from day to day, as you might choose to do at the start, you can copy an entire day's record, then just make a few minor tweaks that reflect any variations, such as an alternative protein food or different vegetable.

Cronometer can also be used as a meal planner. (First, however, you'll have to upgrade to the Gold version to access the expanded features. This is a minor cost, and I want to reiterate that I don't make a dime from this endorsement.) One of the first things you'll want to do with the Gold version is to edit your Food Diary page so that you can divide your day into segments that fit your new schedule. For example, your meal schedule may not fit a traditional breakfast/lunch/dinner plan, so why not customize your segments with terms such as "Bulletproof" or "First Meal"? (If you need help figuring out how to do this, find Cronometer's user manual and look for information on how to edit the Food Diary.)

Next, enter all the foods in the amounts you plan to use. Is this a good match to your macro targets? If not, adjust your entries and prepare your meal accordingly. If you think that you want a more precise meal planner, then find a keto-savvy nutritionist or dietitian who can grant you access to The Charlie Foundation's KetoDietCalculator. In my experience, though, only about 1 in 10 adults who think they want to go this route actually end up using the planner once they see what it involves. (However, this is the tool that should be used with any child who is on this diet for any reason. A skilled keto nutritionist needs to be part of the team as well if you're implementing this diet for your child.)

Here comes the caveat: Many of my clients who have used Cronometer report back that they are frustrated by the glitches they find when they are entering custom recipes. Specifically, they note the problems they have with putting in the information about serving or portion size. Although there is a tutorial that walks you through adding recipes, there are many nuances that result in a steep learning curve for first-time users. (The developer is constantly upgrading the site, and I'm sure that over time these issues will be resolved and the interface for recipes will be easier to navigate.)

Despite my praise for Cronometer, I do understand that it may not be the best option for you right now. Of course, you are free to choose another app, or even a paper diary if that's all you can manage at the start. The point is to make it a priority to record what you eat, not just for the feedback it provides but also to enhance your commitment to the plan. Cronometer will still be there—if and when you are ready to make that move.

## What Makes a Keto Plan Successful?

Successful keto meal plans share several common characteristics:

- Carb targets are very low and most carbs come mainly from non-starchy vegetables, nuts and seeds, and small amounts of other low-sugar foods, such as high-fat dairy. (Keep berries out of the plan in these first few weeks.)
- Protein intake is kept low but adequate. (Calculate your needs using the tools in chapter 9.) High-quality animal protein is preferred over processed meats or vegetable protein. If you are a vegetarian or vegan, make sure you are meeting your needs for essential amino acids (Cronometer includes these targets).
- Fat intake is high—80 percent or more of total calories—with an emphasis on quality and balance for optimum health. (See chapter 12, "Fat Is Your New Best Friend," page 206.)

# How to Approach Meal Preparation

If you are switching from a standard Western diet, there's definitely a learning curve. But my advice about preparation is the same as for meal planning: Keep your meals as simple as possible during the first few weeks. You may have been led to believe that ketogenic plans are too complex, but when you boil everything down to the essence, you are simply eating a different combination of mostly familiar foods. It will be an easier transition if you stay away from restaurants or cafeterias right now, even if this means taking your lunch to work. Also, you won't find what you need in the low-carb section of your supermarket, as these products are generally poor in quality and too high in protein and/or supplemental fiber. Instead, spend that time and money in the produce aisle, as whole foods are always the better option.

One of the biggest challenges in these first few weeks may involve learning to prepare and cook real foods instead of packaged, processed, and "convenience" versions. Besides *The Ketogenic Kitchen*, there are numerous online resources for this, many with how-to videos. (Check the resources section for some suggestions.) Without a doubt, you'll be spending more time in your kitchen at the beginning, but as you begin to view food in a different light—as fuel instead of as convenience or comfort—your eyes will be opened to a whole new world of higher-quality options, like nuts and seeds (in moderation, of course). By keeping your plan simple, you can forget the sense of being overwhelmed and instead delight in how easy it is to live a keto lifestyle. The bonus: You will soon be free from cravings that have driven your hunger (and food choices) in the past.

## Start by Modifying Familiar Meals

Most likely you already enjoy some meals that are basically keto-friendly, such as eggs and bacon, chicken salad, meat and veggies, or salads with a nice olive oil dressing. Make these more keto-friendly with a few simple modifications:

- Cook your eggs in butter or coconut oil, or add a teaspoon or two of coconut oil to your morning coffee for a bit of added fat.
- Substitute a non-starchy vegetable, such as lightly sautéed spinach, for the traditional toast or fruit at breakfast.
- Enjoy a serving of a keto muffin with coconut butter or cream cheese. (You can find a recipe in the appendix, page 332.)
- Keep a slip of paper at your place at the table that reminds you to "Eat More Fat!" And while you're at it, another that reads "Drink More Water!"
- Weigh your portions. You can then construct a visual cue to help you guesstimate this moving forward. For example, you may find that your protein portion of meat is visually equivalent to two-thirds of a deck of cards. For fish, it may be equivalent to two-thirds of checkbook.
- Use this same technique for the vegetables you choose most often. Again, start by weighing your portions, then creating a visual cue. For example, your portion of broccoli may look close in size to a tennis ball. Or you may find that six medium spears of asparagus are a perfect portion for you.
- Take photographs! You can easily snap a picture of the correct portion size for each of the foods that you choose most often. These pictures can serve as visual cues.
- If you are accustomed to dining out often, consider a short break from this routine until you get up to speed with your guesstimates. (Tips for dining out are coming up in chapter 13.)
- Many foods cannot be classified strictly as either carbohydrate, protein, or fat. For example, a tablespoon of almond butter contains

8.8 grams of fat, 3.4 grams of protein, and approximately 1.4 grams of net carbs. Create cheat sheets of your favorites, either as a written log or as a spreadsheet.

- Learn the macros for the foods you use most often. For example, an egg yields 6 or 7 grams of protein, hard cheese yields about 6 or 7 grams of protein per ounce, and heavy whipping cream contains 0.3 to 0.4 grams of carbohydrate per tablespoon. Again, cheat sheets of the foods you use most often will simplify your efforts.

Feeling better prepared? Then let's move on to putting your new plan into action!

# CHAPTER 11

# Put Your Plan into Action

A s with any new venture, the process of switching to a ketogenic plan will be so much smoother if you have the right tools. Start with what you need for the kitchen. Your initial outlay here may be minimal (under $100)—especially if your kitchen is already set up for cooking with whole foods—or more significant if you are moving from a standard diet and don't even own a vegetable steamer. Consider it a smart investment in your health!

## An Accurate Scale and Other Kitchen Essentials

As I stated in the last chapter, if you do not already possess a sturdy, reliable, and accurate scale, this should be one of your first purchases. Here are the necessary features:

- 0.1 or 0.5 grams accuracy (ensures precise ingredient weights, especially important when preparing batched recipes and baked goods)
- 1,500 to 2,500 grams total capacity (allows you to use your regular plates and bowls when you are weighing foods and simplifies making batched recipes)
- a large, easy-to-read digital display
- easy to clean, such as a removable platform and a protected display
- AC adaptor

I find food preparation easier when the following items are on hand:

- a variety of heat-resistant, flexible silicone spatulas, including some that are small and narrow enough for scraping bowls
- silicone spoons in several sizes; some for baking and others for getting the last drop of oil from your salad bowl

- a small handheld immersion blender, especially helpful if you intend to drink Bulletproof coffee or other hot drinks in which fats need to be blended into the beverage, such as in hot cocoa (The battery-operated ones are lightweight and portable; for travel, I pack mine inside a cardboard paper towel roll.)
- wire whisks in a variety of sizes (mini whisks for sauces, medium whisks for beating eggs, and larger whisks for blending ingredients used in baking)
- a vegetable steamer basket
- a "spiralizer" (a tool that turns zucchini into "noodles"; you can use a veggie peeler for a similar effect)
- Vitamix, Nutribullet, Cuisinart, or other high-end blender/mixer (These are great kitchen accessories, but pricey. If you don't have one already, you may want to wait and see which will suit your purposes best, or pick one up at a thrift store.)
- an electric pressure cooker (such as Instant Pot) or slow cooker (such as Crock-Pot). (There are several excellent recipes in *The Ketogenic Kitchen*; with these cookers, you can "set it and forget it," then come back to a delicious one-pot meal.)
- stylish and visually appealing luncheon plates; 8 to 9 inches, round or square (Because of the calorie density of fats as opposed to starches, keto foods take up less space. Why not feature your meal instead of letting it get lost on a huge dinner plate? This is especially important for kids; take them to a thrift or dollar store and let them pick their own.)
- a whipped cream canister (I prefer those made by iSi Pro.)
- silicone molds for keto treats and muffins (These are readily available online; read the reviews and avoid those made with fillers.)
- silicone cookie sheets (great for baking keto crackers)
- lots of small and medium-sized containers with leak-resistant snap-on lids (Glass doesn't stain or pick up odors, but plastic is more practical for travel.)

## Use a Bathroom Scale

As you will want to monitor your weight, a good bathroom scale is a must. Remember, weight loss is one of the side effects of switching to a keto plan. Initially this is due mostly to a loss of water weight, but it's also because it takes time for most people to wrap their heads around properly implementing a diet consisting of 80 to 85 percent fat! Weigh yourself twice a week at the same time of day, usually just after you wake and urinate. Wear light clothing or no clothing at all, and use the same scale each time. Your scale doesn't have to be doctor's-office accurate. You mainly need to know if your weight is trending in the right direction. Remember that rapid weight loss is not the goal. If you continue with an unintended weight loss beyond the first few weeks, it is usually a sign that you need to pay closer attention to meeting your fat macro. If you record your weights in Cronometer's biometric entry form, you will be able to see your trend in graph form.

## Prepare for the Transition

My goal here is to help you understand some of the common issues that may arise as you make the transition to ketosis from your current diet. Preparation is key. If you are proactive, you are much more likely to sail through the transition with few if any physical symptoms. In fact, many people feel better shortly after eliminating the non-keto foods that were the underlying cause of inflammation. I also strongly advise you to make this shift during downtime from work or family responsibilities. (I recognize that this may be impossible for some of you, especially if you are the head of your household.)

### First, Cook Up a Pot of Broth

It would be wise to make some homemade salted bone broth *before* launching into the diet. (You can also prepare meat/poultry/fish broth, but be sure to count the animal protein in your totals for the day). Make a big batch and freeze it in smaller portions (no more than what you can use in a few days). Or better yet, ask a friend or relative who has offered to help "in any way" to prepare this for you. There are great recipes online at www.whole9life.com or on the Weston A. Price Foundation website.

Why broth? Simple—the electrolytes in bone broth are the perfect replacement for the electrolytes that are lost in urine as you make the metabolic shift to ketosis (covered in greater depth in the next section). Be sure to salt the broth. Your need for sodium will increase greatly, especially in the first few weeks and months of the diet. Increasing your sodium intake may take some conscious effort, since there is an ongoing campaign in conventional nutrition to reduce sodium because of the growing number of sodium-sensitive people. Himalayan and sea salts are good choices; you won't overload on the iodine and anticaking agents found in most conventional salts. Broth is also an excellent place to hide some extra fat, such as butter or duck fat.

## A Word on Ketone Supplements

Ketone supplements (also referred to as exogenous ketones) are relatively new to the keto scene. (An exception is the MCTs derived from coconut oil, which have been a part of keto diets for children for several decades. See chapter 14, "Boosting Ketosis," page 252). I've just begun to explore the use of other types of exogenous ketones to ease the transition to the diet. Data, or even anecdotal reports, about the use of these supplements in cancer is scarce, as most of the emphasis has been on their use in weight loss or athletic performance. That said, several of my clients use the commercially available proprietary blends of βHB salts, and other options, including ketone esters, are expected to be commercially available in the very near future. I will help you keep up with the science and practical implications by posting updates on my website.

There are a few drawbacks, though, in over-relying on bone broth in a keto plan: (1) Broth is naturally high in glucogenic amino acids such as glycine and proline—great for collagen, but bad for cancer because these amino acids are readily converted to glucose by the liver; (2) it's nearly impossible to estimate how much protein is in homemade broth, so it's best to keep your intake to a cup or two per day; and (3) even bones from animals raised on organic pastures may contain heavy metals, including lead, which is another reason to keep portions to reasonable amounts.

## The Importance of Managing Your Medications during the Transition

If you are taking any medications, either prescription drugs or over-the-counter remedies, you need to give this topic some attention right now, before you start the diet. Be smart about this. Never decide on your own to lower dosages or discontinue a drug prescribed to treat a specific condition without first checking in with the doctor who prescribed it. This includes (but is not limited to) medications to treat high blood pressure, thyroid disease, heart conditions, cholesterol, autoimmune disease, or diabetes. The doses should be altered only under medical supervision. As an example, it's not uncommon for blood pressure to drop shortly after starting a keto plan. This is great news if your blood pressure is high and you are currently taking medication to lower it. But if this does happen to you, the dosage of your medication should be titrated only with specific direction from your doctor.

If you are taking steroid medications, such as prednisone or dexamethasone, it is *critical* that you follow your doctor's instructions on dosage carefully, including any weaning schedules.

If you use opioid pain medications, you already know that they cause intractable constipation along with other gastrointestinal side effects. Since constipation is also a common side effect of the ketogenic diet (especially in the first few weeks or months), be sure to enlist your team in staying ahead of this problem before you even start the diet.

On the upside, you may experience an improvement in mood on the diet; but don't let this sway you into thinking that you can stop taking your antidepressants or anti-anxiety drugs without first talking to the prescribing doctor. There can be dire consequences if you abruptly discontinue medication of this kind.

If you take drugs for diabetes, you will need to monitor your blood glucose levels more frequently. It is also essential that you discuss this diet with your medical team, as you will undoubtedly need to adjust dosages (and you may even be able to eliminate some drugs entirely), *but only under medical supervision.* (And don't forget the danger of combining SGLT2 inhibitors, such as canagliflozin, with a low-carb or ketogenic diet.)

The ketogenic diet increases the risk of developing kidney stones. If you have a personal or family history of this, you may want to add a potassium citrate/citric acid supplement, either prescribed by your doctor or bought over-the-counter. Children on the diet for epilepsy are often prescribed this supplement prophylactically. However, be aware that you cannot take potassium supplements concurrent with certain potassium-sparing drugs, such as lisinopril or losartan, as the combination can lead to dangerously high blood levels of potassium. Also, there are certain medical conditions that preclude the use of this supplement. So discuss your medication options and clear any additional supplementation with your doctor before adding anything on your own.

## Transition Side Effects

You may experience some temporary side effects during the transition and knowing what to expect makes it easier for you to take them in stride. The ketogenic diet alters how your body processes nutrients for energy, and this results in several fairly predictable changes in how you feel during the transition. If you've tried a low-carb diet for weight loss before, you'll understand what I'm saying. In fact, the transition symptoms you might have experienced in the past may have led you to abandon your efforts. But realize that your goals and your motivation are quite different this time around. The best advice I can offer you is to welcome this shift by preparing ahead of time for these common transition symptoms.

## Hunger and Cravings

One of the most vexing problems with conventional dieting is dealing with the hunger and cravings that accompany a restriction in calories. Rest assured that the ketogenic diet for cancer is *not* a conventional diet. Let's start by looking at a positive side effect: a steep drop in hunger and cravings. When you're not driven by hunger, you are able to mindfully choose foods that nourish your body instead of simply taking in calories that only temporarily ease your cravings. To understand why a keto diet eases these symptoms, you need to understand what's happening in your current default mode: a diet where half your total energy as calories is coming from carbohydrate-containing foods.

In a conventional diet, hormone signaling cues your system that glucose levels are dropping. You perceive this as hunger, a hard-wired warning that you'd better seek out more food. Opioid receptors in the brain add their signals as well, and that's one reason why you may experience food cravings that are so strong they mimic those of a drug addict. In fact, those people who self-identify as "carb addicts" have hit the nail on the head! And just as in drug addicts who miss a fix, "carb withdrawal" can have some unpleasant side effects. Responding to these signals by continuing with your current pattern would virtually guarantee a vicious cycle. Fortunately, the presence of ketones abruptly interrupts this pattern, and most people get past their hunger and cravings very quickly. So plan to ride it out, knowing that in just a few days you will no longer be "under the influence."

## Keto Flu

In the first few days or weeks, many people experience symptoms associated with what is now commonly referred to as "keto flu." This usually involves some combination of headaches, fatigue, light-headedness, poor concentration, muscle cramps, body aches, and constipation. This is another form of carb withdrawal, and it takes some time to adapt to the metabolic shift that allows your body to use fats more efficiently to meet your energy needs.

At the system level, the drop in insulin changes the way your kidneys handle sodium. As you cut back on carbs, you'll lose water and, with it, sodium and other electrolytes. Replenishing what you lose in urine can go a long way in easing your symptoms. I am not suggesting that you buy costly electrolyte replacement drinks. Instead, drink more water and sip on the salted home-made broth that you should have prepared before diving into the diet.

There are epigenetic changes going on at the cellular level as well. In response to the drop in glucose and insulin, your cells will increase the number of a specific type of transporter embedded in their membranes to allow for a greater influx of ketone bodies into the cytoplasm. The mitochondria also respond to the change in nutrients by increasing the amount of enzyme needed to break down ketones, allowing them to be readily utilized for energy within the mitochondria. Cancer cells are not as metabolically flexible as normal cells.[1,2] They are limited in their ability to produce this enzyme. So even when ketones are present they are not able to use them effectively to meet their huge demand for energy.

How long does it take to get past this? Expect many of these symptoms to ease up quickly, especially if you are paying close attention to replenishing fluids and electrolytes. But you may experience a few lingering symptoms, especially if you have accumulated metabolic challenges, such as insulin resistance. In that case, it could take weeks or even months to become fully keto-adapted, but remember that during that time your new way of eating is still having an impact on cancer.

## Hypoglycemia

Changes in glucose metabolism begin within a few hours of your last carb-heavy meal. When the internal signals for more glucose are not met with more carbs, you will then begin to deplete your liver glycogen stores. Simultaneously, your liver begins to make new glucose as well. It can take a few days for your glucose "thermostat" to reset, and during that time your blood glucose levels may bounce around quite a bit, often dipping into territory known as hypoglycemia, or low blood sugar.

Most people with hypoglycemia have few or no symptoms, while others experience a transient dizziness or light-headed feeling. This is your brain's way of telling you that it's not getting enough energy to meet its needs, but it will self-correct quickly (unless you are taking a drug that interferes with this process; another reason for discussing your medications with your doctor before you begin). Check your blood glucose level with your home blood glucose meter. If you get a low reading (50 to 60 mg/dL) *and* you feel shaky, sweaty, or lethargic, drink two table-spoons of apple or orange juice, and test again in a half hour. If your glucose is still low or symptoms persist, drink another two tablespoons. Keep in mind that

## One Essential Caveat for Those with Diabetes

If you have type 1 diabetes or poorly controlled type 2 diabetes, with or without frequent hypoglycemic episodes, you *must not* adopt a ketogenic diet unless you are under the supervision of a keto-savvy team (HEAL-clinic is one option). "Hypoglycemic unawareness" is a real risk with the diet, as are other potential complications. (If you haven't heard this term before, please discuss what it means with your endocrinologist.)

People with diabetes can practice daily management using Bayer Diastix urine test strips (not the same as Bayer Ketostix) to measure both ketones and glucose. *If both glucose and ketones are detected at the same time, stop the diet and immediately report to your doctor or emergency department.*

readings of 60 mg/dL or even 50 mg/dL will soon be very desirable and virtually symptom-free once you start making and using ketones. Your brain will readily adapt to this new form of energy, usually within just a few days.

## Acidosis versus Diabetic Ketoacidosis

Acidosis that can result from a ketogenic diet typically is limited to a slight and easily reversible disruption in blood pH (not the same thing as the fairly benign swings seen in urine pH). In contrast, diabetic ketoacidosis (DKA) is a severe derangement that manifests as extremely elevated blood glucose (usually well over 200 mg/dL) along with high levels of blood ketones (well over 14 mmol/L). DKA happens only when there's a shortage of insulin in people with type 1 diabetes or poorly controlled type 2 diabetes. (In my decade of experience with this diet, I have never seen a single case of DKA develop in a person with cancer.)

A different sort of metabolic acidosis is associated with the type of diabetes medication called an SGLT2 inhibitor (canagliflozin, for example). *As previously mentioned, a ketogenic diet is incompatible with taking any of this family of drugs.* Discuss other treatment options with your endocrinologist.

Acidosis (which, by the way, is not a common side effect) may pop up during the transition, especially if you are fasting, or during times of illness or unusual metabolic stress that causes a sharp increase in ketones, usually with concurrent dehydration. In acidosis, you typically experience extreme versions of the symptoms you may feel when hypoglycemic: lethargy, more nausea, vomiting, flushing, panting, and a rapid heart rate. If you are experiencing these symptoms and your ketone levels are relatively high for an adult (5 to 6 mmol/L or higher), drink two tablespoons of apple or orange juice as well as ½ teaspoon of baking soda in a glass of water. Repeat in 15 minutes if necessary. You may be reluctant to do this because you believe that it will slow your transition to ketosis, but understand that the negative impact of over-ketosis far outweighs any benefits. Please don't rely on your gut instincts here. *Call your doctor or go to the emergency department if your symptoms don't resolve quickly.* A simple blood test including a check of your $CO_2$ levels will determine if you are acidotic or simply experiencing some transition symptoms.

If you are the parent of a young child who is starting this diet, watch for the symptoms noted previously. Acidosis is more common in children, but also easily reversed. Still, err on the side of caution and call your child's pediatrician for advice if symptoms persist or seem to be worsening.

## Dizziness, Light-headedness, or Shakiness

These symptoms may indicate hypoglycemia. However, these symptoms may also be attributable to a drop in your blood pressure as you eliminate water. Don't put yourself in a risky situation that requires good balance or a sudden increase in effort, such as climbing a ladder or working out with weights, until you are symptom-free. If the feeling persists more than a few days, have your health care practitioner check your blood pressure. If it's normal, then your symptoms may be due to mild hypoglycemia (which will resolve quickly once you are in ketosis) or to the brain needing a bit more time to adapt to using ketones instead of glucose for energy.

## Constipation

Most people have fewer bowel movements on a ketogenic diet than they may have had previously. This decrease is normal and does not qualify as constipation (which is straining to pass hard stool). True constipation, however, is such a common issue that I've devoted a whole section to it in chapter 15. For now, be sure that you're drinking plenty of water and replacing sodium by salting your foods (unless you've been told by your doctor to limit sodium intake). You may also want to carefully monitor your fiber intake and add some supplemental fiber, such as ground psyllium seed husk or ground flaxseed. Certain forms of magnesium can also be a huge help; learn about them in chapter 14 before you start the transition to a ketogenic diet.

## Muscle Aches, Cramping, Weakness, and General Fatigue

Some of these sensations can be attributed to the energy gap as your body adjusts to burning fat instead of glucose as its primary fuel. Or they can be one of many symptoms associated with dehydration and/or loss of electrolytes. Salted homemade broth can replace both. If you don't have broth handy, you can use bouillon (no MSG, please!) or even salted water. (Salted water replaces sodium and chloride but none of the other electrolytes unless you use Morton Lite salt, which contains potassium as well). Also be sure to get enough magnesium.

## Headache

A headache is yet another symptom of dehydration. It may persist for a while, even if you are careful to rehydrate. A cup of salted homemade broth along with ensuring adequate hydration overall will go a long way in resolving this. (Remember, too, that you are not to drink alcohol as you are adapting to the diet.)

## Change in Blood Pressure

If you have a heart condition or high blood pressure, speak with the doctor who manages your condition *before* you begin the diet, especially if you take medication. Your blood pressure is likely to drop soon after you make the shift to ketosis, and while lower blood pressure is a welcome bonus for many people, it may drop too low if the medication is not adjusted appropriately. Track your blood pressure and talk to your doctor about possibly reducing your dosage.

## Heart Rate or Rhythm Changes, Including Palpitations

A change in blood volume brought on by dehydration and loss of electrolytes, including sodium and potassium, may cause your heart to beat faster and/or harder. Salted broth and proper hydration help to replenish these losses. If you have pre-existing heart disease or rhythm issues (such as atrial fibrillation), dehydration and electrolyte imbalance can possibly trigger an episode. Please discuss this with your doctor before starting this diet. Also, if you have ever received any drugs with prolonged QT interval as a possible side effect, you absolutely need to rule out this condition before deciding to start a ketogenic diet.

## Meal Replacement Shakes

Whether you start with a fast or transition more gradually, you need to have a plan in place. If you don't have time for proper planning, you can simplify initiation of the diet by using a homemade meal replacement shake for one meal a day. It's easy to get the macros right, especially if you're using Cronometer or another tracking tool. You can get all the nutrients you need by upgrading a basic protein shake to a green smoothie—simply combine the ingredients in a high-powered blender. Here are some tips:

- Start with full-fat canned coconut milk. (There are several brands; choose one that contains only coconut, water, and guar gum, a soluble fiber that acts as an emulsifier to hold oils in suspension.)
- Add sufficient protein powder to meet your protein target for that meal. (Use vegan powders like Veggie Elite or Sunwarrior Warrior Blend instead of whey proteins, which can provoke insulin and stimulate other anabolic activities.)
- Add enough oil to meet your target for that meal. Include MCT or caprylic (C8) oil (start with just a teaspoon or two until you're sure you can tolerate more) or an MCT powder, such as Quest's (you may find it easier on the gastrointestinal tract). You can also include other mild-tasting oils that are high in monounsaturated fats, such as avocado or macadamia nut oil. You can even add heavy whipping cream.
- Add greens. Stick to very low-carb choices. Kale is an option but not a requirement, especially since the oxalates in it can provoke diarrhea. Choose broccoli sprouts, not raw broccoli. Avocado is a great choice. You can also add cucumber, celery, radishes, and a berry or two.
- If you want, you can flavor the shake with extracts such as vanilla or orange oil. (Avoid overuse of those with glycerin or glycerol.)
- Blend well and sip slowly over 15 to 20 minutes. Store any leftovers in the refrigerator and discard any remaining after 24 hours.

Be sure to test your meal replacement shake before you start your transition. If you don't love it, you may be tempted to scrap it in favor of a less keto-friendly meal. So now is the time to tweak the ingredients until you arrive at a tasty and satisfying drink.

## Change in Exercise Tolerance or Physical Performance

Given the many adjustments your body will need to make as you adapt to the diet, it's best to limit your physical activities until you are mostly keto-adapted (past transition symptoms and maintaining steady ketosis). Instead of intense workouts or training, it's wise to switch to walking, cycling, or lap swimming. Keep it gentle. Still, I've worked with several ultra-athletes who just can't imagine backing off of their current routines, even for a few weeks. For them, the transition is frustrating as it takes some time—from weeks to months—for muscle tissue to adjust to primarily burning fat for fuel. This may seem odd given that muscle tissue prefers fatty acid oxidation over glucose, but the phenomenon is well documented and a reality I urge you to accept. Rest assured that once you are adapted, you will have an edge over your carb-dependent competition, especially in endurance events.

## Keto Rash

Prurigo pigmentosa, often called "keto rash," is an uncommon and poorly understood potential side effect of the diet. It may be due to either acetone in sweat or a change in the skin microbiome. A few online forums and blogs, most notably Diet Doctor, share information about possible treatments (for example, see https://blog.kettleandfire.com/keto-rash). I expect that the science behind this condition will become clearer over time.

## Your First Three Weeks: The "Make-or-Break" Period

I've learned that the first three weeks of the ketogenic diet is often the "make-or-break" period, so it's crucial to make a strong commitment at the start. This will go a long way toward ensuring your success with the transition. Along with commitment, you need the following tools and strategies to enhance both adherence and accountability. If you're working with a coach, she or he can help you tremendously here. If you're on your own, see if you can interest a friend or relative to start the diet with you. Remember, the basic keto plan for cancer has many health benefits for most adults, so you would actually be helping them to clean up their act and move toward better health!

Before you start, please review the following:

- Have you removed non-keto foods from your cupboards, fridge, and freezer?

## Keep It Simple

As you transition, focus your efforts on adapting to your new anticancer lifestyle. This will come more easily if you stick to the basics. For now, skip over the gourmet recipes in favor of those that allow you to put a meal on the table with a minimum amount of time and effort. Also forgo variety for now and recycle the ketogenic meals that you find most palatable and easiest to prepare. You can work on variety and food quality when you are more comfortable with basic meal planning.

- Did you buy your new keto-friendly fresh foods and food staples?
- Do you have your blood glucose meter? If so, have you practiced with it yet?
- How will you test ketones in these first few weeks? Blood ketone strips that work with the Precision Xtra are the most accurate tool, but if the cost is prohibitive, buy Bayer Ketostix (urine strips). These are a good indicator of ketosis in the first few weeks.
- Do you have a kitchen gram scale? If so, are you familiar with how to use it?
- Did you find some good online keto recipe resources? I've listed my current favorites in the resources section at the end of this book. Prepare a few that look interesting so that you have some simple go-to meals. As I've mentioned, don't concern yourself with variety right now. It's smarter and easier to make up a batch that can carry you past several meals. And remember that you can always add a green salad.
- Have you invested in Domini Kemp and Patricia Daly's cookbook, *The Ketogenic Kitchen*? This is a great resource for everyone just starting out, but particularly important if you want meal plans and recipes that spell out exactly what you should eat for a week at a time. Another one of my go-to recipe books is Dana Carpender's *200 Low-Carb High-Fat Recipes*. These are easy and practical recipes that need few if any modifications to make them keto-friendly. (Over time, you can add to your keto cookbook library with other books that you'll find in the resources section.)
- If the idea of meal planning sounds too daunting right now, use the template found in chapter 13 ("Simple Keto Meal Template," page 217).

## Do You Have Concerns about Low Body Weight?

If your current body weight is low or you are nutritionally compromised (from treatments or disease), ease into the diet by adding fats and oils to familiar meals while simultaneously cutting down on grains and sugars. Then start with one fully ketogenic meal a day and build from there. Most people find breakfast the easiest meal to adapt to keto. (Think eggs cooked in lots of butter and perhaps a strip or two of bacon and some grated cheese. Add interest with a steamed or sautéed vegetable, such as spinach or zucchini or asparagus—just remember to add some fats or oils there as well. Be sure to enter this into Cronometer and check to see if you're meeting your macros for that meal.)

- Mark a day on your calendar as the official kick-off date for your transition to the keto plan. If you can, minimize your other responsibilities so you can devote the time and energy you need to your new lifestyle.

## Blood Meters

I often hear "Do I have to?" in objection to blood testing, but honestly, testing your blood for glucose and ketones is almost indispensable right now. To put it in perspective, conventional care usually involves being pricked and prodded, with routine venous blood draws to monitor the side effects of your treatment. The mild discomfort of a finger prick pales in comparison to those procedures. Of course you can proceed without testing, but how will you gauge the impact of your new diet on your blood glucose and ketones? (Children are the exception. If making a game of it with points and rewards still doesn't gain their cooperation, you can make a fair guesstimate based on urine ketones. And what kid doesn't enjoy peeing on a stick?)

Since you are adopting this plan with the hope of achieving a therapeutic effect, it just makes sense that you will need an objective measure not just to assess your progress but also to help you troubleshoot issues and tweak the diet to best meet your personal targets. If you are feeling reluctant or even squeamish about taking that step, just think of the millions of people, including very young children, who are required to test their blood glucose in order to manage type 1 diabetes. They do it or they die. It's that simple.

## Abbott's Precision Xtra Meter

By most accounts, this is currently the most accurate home meter for testing blood ketones. Ask your oncologist for a prescription. If your oncologist won't order it, ask your primary care doctor. If you can't get a prescription, you can buy everything you need at a local pharmacy or online. Just be sure that you have the correct model. It may have a different name outside of the United States.

If you do get a prescription, ask your pharmacist to check your insurance plan to see what part of the kit, if any, is covered. Co-pays may ultimately cost you more than if you were to buy the kit online. Abbott USA has kept the cost of strips quite high. With price gouging becoming increasingly more common, and no real competition in the market at this time, I wouldn't be surprised if the costs continue to climb. Currently, ketone strips purchased in the United States cost $3 to $6 apiece and are sold in boxes of 10. Sometimes I can find reasonably priced boxes on Amazon or eBay, but I also recommend that you check with Universal Drugstore in Canada. They offer them for substantially less, and I've never had an issue except for the occasional delay in cross-border delivery.

Diabetes is so prevalent that you are likely to have a family member or close friend who uses a home glucose meter. Ask them to walk you through the process. If that's not an option, you can ask your primary care team for help. I also suggest that you watch a video on the steps needed to obtain an accurate measurement. My favorite so far is a video of a British gent who neatly guides you through the steps in just under three minutes.[3] I've listed this video in the resources section. You may want to bookmark the website and review the video until you are comfortable with the process.

At the time of this writing there are a zillion options for meters that test blood glucose, but precious few that can test both glucose and ketones. More are in development, but I don't know if and when these will be brought to market. I strongly advise you to also incorporate routine blood ketone testing, as this is the standard used to clinically assess βHB levels. Test strips are pricey, so I keep two meters: the Precision Xtra for ketones and a glucose-only meter for testing glucose. (I'll go into the details of how to incorporate testing into your plan later in this chapter.)

## Precision Xtra Glucose and Ketone Testing Kit

You can order your kit online or through your health care provider. It should include the following: Precision Xtra Glucose and Ketone meter; glucose test strips (usually prescribed as one or two boxes of 50 per month); ketone test strips (usually prescribed as one or two boxes of 10 per month); and lancets to fit the included finger prick device (don't use alternate-site testing).

## Nova Max Glucose and Ketone Testing Kit

The Nova Max meter also tests both glucose and ketones, and the ketone strips cost less. So if finances are limited, you can choose this model. Note, though, that it may not be as accurate as the Precision Xtra.

## Glucose-Only Blood Meters

I use a glucose-only blood meter because of its low cost. You can easily purchase these online. The glucose test strips are less expensive than the glucose strips needed for the Precision Xtra and most models are just as accurate—if not more so! Keep in mind that all glucose meters are intended only as screening devices. They have a high tolerance for error (up to 20 percent on either side of actual blood glucose levels).

## Continuous Glucose Monitors (CGMs)

These monitors were developed for people with type 1 diabetes. Rather than relying on finger pricks, CGM sensors are inserted below the skin and left in place for about a week before needing to be replaced. They take readings every

### Tips on Using a Blood Glucose Meter

Ask a friend or family member with diabetes to walk you through this, as it's close to impossible to describe adequately in text. As I mentioned before, you can also follow along with this great You-Tube video demonstrating the proper procedure for testing glucose: https://www.youtube.com/watch?v=rMMpeLLgdgY.

few minutes, offering crucial feedback on changes in blood glucose levels that diabetics use to regulate the amount of insulin they inject. Recently, biohackers have co-opted use of these meters, and the newest models can now send blood glucose data to a smartphone. These are expensive units to rent or purchase, but I mention them here because you are likely to come across online keto or low-carb forums that serve as data-sharing platforms for users of these devices.

There are new high-tech continuous monitoring systems in development that will hopefully provide good data but be less costly and not as invasive as the current CGMs. I'll keep you posted about new products on my website.

## Track Your Blood Glucose and Ketones

Testing your blood glucose and ketone levels is the only way to properly assess the impact of the dietary changes you're making. Understand, though, that home devices can provide only approximations, not exact measurements. Home glucose testing is designed to help people with diabetes track their glucose levels as a way to provide feedback on their blood glucose control or to ensure that their prescribed medications are working as intended. The ketone strips were initially developed for people at high risk of developing diabetic ketoacidosis.

Dr. Seyfried and his colleagues have developed a very useful calculation called the glucose ketone index (GKI) to help with tracking your progress. To see if you're meeting Dr. Seyfried's targets, take your blood glucose and ketone measurements at the same time, then divide your glucose reading by 18 (to convert it from mg/dL to mmol/L). Next, divide that number by your blood ketone reading (already expressed as mmol/L). According to the developers of the GKI, a therapeutic target is a GKI of 1.0 to 2.0. (Note that you can't use the reading from urine strips for this calculation.) For more information on how to calculate and interpret the GKI, refer to Dr. Seyfried's paper, "The Glucose Ketone Index Calculator: A Simple Tool to Monitor Therapeutic Efficacy for Metabolic Management of Brain Cancer."[4] In my experience, the GKI for cancers other than brain cancer may be higher than 2.0, especially in older adults, but even with these higher numbers, I have still seen what I believe to be a therapeutic effect. I've included information on how to calculate this index in chapter 16 ("Monitoring Your Glucose Ketone Index [GKI]," page 306).

## Alternate Ketone Testing Tools

As a reminder, there are three types of ketone bodies: beta-hydroxybutyrate, or βHB (detected in blood), acetoacetate (detected in urine), and acetone

## Your First Three Weeks of Blood Monitoring

Testing is the only way to know for certain if the changes you are making are lowering your blood glucose and raising ketones. Your results provide you with information that will help you to shape your plan as you move beyond the first few weeks.

- Begin by testing your fasting blood glucose (FBG) first thing in the morning, before eating or drinking anything. Record that measurement.
- If you have chosen to delay your first meal of the day (this would be considered daily intermittent fasting), test first thing in the morning and then again just before you eat. Most likely your measurement will be lower just before the meal. If it's higher, you may be waiting too long before you eat. Don't rely on a single day's numbers: Test this on several days before making changes to meal timing.
- Test your blood glucose just before bedtime.
- Also test your blood glucose in the middle of the afternoon, either before a meal or at least two hours after.
- Once you are comfortable with glucose testing, move to testing your blood ketones. (This may take a week or two.) Do not use the same drop of blood for both glucose and ketone tests. You will need a larger drop of blood for the ketone strip. Optimally, you will be testing your blood ketones several times a week.
- Vary your test times to get more feedback on your trends. For example, test at bedtime one day and just before a meal on a different day.
- If you get an unusual reading and it concerns you, then immediately retest using a new drop of blood from the same finger. If the two readings are close, take the average. If the second one is more believable, go with that one.
- Eventually, you will want to test your response to specific foods, meals, exercise, and even stress. See chapter 16 for more monitoring suggestions.

## Factors That Can Impact Blood Glucose Readings

There are a myriad of factors influencing your blood glucose measurements. This list will help you identify a few of the more common causes:

- the dawn effect (This is due to the normal circadian rhythm of cortisol, which causes morning glucose to be higher and ketones lower than at other times of the day.)
- circulation (Cold hands can interfere with test accuracy.)
- dirt, grease, or soap on your hands
- squeezing your finger too hard to get a large enough drop of blood
- hormones and other stressors (A poor night's sleep, headache, argument, or other stressful event can raise blood glucose.)
- low hematocrit (A low proportion of red blood cells in the blood can throw off the measurement because the test strips are calibrated only for normal blood counts. More information on this in the resources section.)

You may wish to bring your glucose meter to your blood draw at a lab. The measurements are not likely to be the same because home glucose meters test capillary blood and lab assays test venous blood, but at least you'll have a rough idea of a correlation between the two.

(detected in breath). Blood testing is the standard used in research, but testing urine and breath can also provide you with valuable feedback, so let's look at those testing options as well.

## Urine Testing

Urine test strips use a chemical called nitroprusside to detect the presence of acetoacetate in the urine. Nitroprusside changes to a pink tone ranging from just a blush of color to deep purple. The darker the shade of purple, the more ketones are present. You may have heard or read that urine testing is not accurate. This is true after keto-adaptation for many reasons: (1) After a period of adjustment, the kidneys do a better job of returning ketones to the bloodstream; (2) there is a higher rate of conversion of acetoacetate to $\beta$HB;

(3) an increase in ketolytic enzymes and membrane transporters catches up with the supply of ketones. But these changes don't tell the whole story: That is, most low-carb (compared to ketogenic) diets contain a greater proportion of protein, resulting in lower (and sometimes undetectable) urine ketone levels.

While there's no question that measuring urine ketones is not as accurate as measuring blood ketones, it is still a decent tool in these first few weeks to assure you that you are staying ketogenic, which can help with both compliance and accountability. Urine ketones are usually affected by something you ate or drank a few hours prior to the test, and this retrospective view is helpful in determining if a meal (or even a specific food) was not in keeping with keto.

A major benefit of testing urine ketones is that the test strips are inexpensive, non-invasive, and easy to use. Buy the best: Bayer Ketostix. These strips were developed for people with diabetes, so the quality and reliability are better than the strips that have come to market exclusively for dieters who aren't using them for therapeutic purposes. You can order these online or ask for them at most pharmacy desks. Toss the insert; it doesn't apply to you. Also, disregard the unit of measurement (either as mg/dL or mmol/L) displayed on the container and just go by the color. Any color at all indicates that you are in ketosis (assuming you are achieving natural ketosis, without the addition of ketone supplements) and that's what provides the feedback on food choices.

Ketone readings should be taken 15 seconds after passing the test strip through the urine stream. During the first three weeks, plan to test for urine ketones at least three times a day: first thing in the morning, mid-afternoon, and at bedtime. Write down the results using the color scale (negative, trace, small, moderate, large). Although most biometrics can be recorded in Cronometer, there isn't a good option there (yet) for urine ketones. A notepad kept in the bathroom is good enough, since this is mostly for screening and for viewing trends. Ideally, most ketone readings taken in the first few weeks will be "moderate" or "large."

Tracking urine ketones can help you identify patterns and trends. If you experience a sudden drop in urine ketones, look back at your food choices over the past few hours. You may find hidden carbs, such as wheat in soy sauce. A drop in ketones may also indicate too high an intake of protein. Expect ketones to be lighter in the morning (due to the "dawn effect") and darker in the evening. Your level of hydration will also affect the color. The strips may be lighter if you're well hydrated (due to dilution) or darker if you're dehydrated (more concentrated). Avoid testing for a few hours after vigorous exercise or when your hydration levels are either higher or lower than your norm.

If the test strips immediately turn the deepest shade of purple, then your ketone levels are higher than what the strip is designed to measure. High levels of urine ketones usually do not indicate a problem unless they are accompanied by symptoms of acidosis.

High levels of urine ketones after adaptation may also indicate that you are not getting the full benefit of the ketones that your body is producing. This may be due to high consumption of MCT oil. MCT is very ketogenic, but if you make more ketones than your body needs, large numbers of them will be excreted in your urine. You are essentially peeing out some of the energy value of the MCT. This is not an issue in the short term unless you are experiencing unintended weight loss. If that's the case, stop including the MCT when you calculate your fat intake for the day. Instead, consider it a "bonus."

The major drawback in relying on urine test strips is that they don't strongly correlate with blood levels of βHB, the standard used both clinically and in research. For that reason, you cannot use urine ketone levels to calculate your GKI.

## Ketone Breath Analysis

Using Ketonix, a specialized breath analyzer (the only breath analyzer available to the public at this time), you can detect the presence of acetone, another of the ketone bodies. This technology uses a small handheld device that connects to your computer or other USB-supported device. Although it is convenient, inexpensive, and reusable, it has the same limitations as the urine test strips: It can be used as a screening device to detect ketosis but not as a tool to assess your GKI. Some people, notably athletes, prefer this type of testing as part of their routine because it is a reliable and somewhat measurable marker of ketosis that can keep and correlate with blood levels of βHB. However, it is not the best tool to use if your lung capacity is impaired by asthma, age, or disease. Check my website to learn about developments or improvements in breath analyzers.

# CHAPTER 12

# Get to Know Your Macros

I n chapter 8, you were introduced to macronutrients, those foods (fats, proteins, carbohydrates) that are the primary sources of both energy and nutrients for the human body. In this chapter, you'll get to know each macronutrient, often abbreviated "macro," on a first-name basis. Only then can you truly understand why you can let go of the thinking and habits of a lifetime and move forward with a new plan that will serve you better.

## Embrace a "Carb Famine"

You don't have to look too far back into human history to see that we did not evolve alongside full cupboards and well-stocked fridges. In fact, our history has always been rocked by periods of devastating famine, sometimes by our own doing, as when Paleolithic man overhunted animals to extinction, or at other times due to acts of nature, such as cyclical droughts. I often tell my clients that they are about to embark on a famine of sorts, but only with regard to one macronutrient: carbohydrate.

Our dentition and digestion define us as omnivores; we are able to access nutrients from a wide variety of plants and animals. As gatherers, we were undoubtedly drawn to berries and fruits, as "sweet" was usually associated with "safe." And seasonally gorging on these foods helped to create the fat stores we needed to survive during food-restricted times of the year. (This is similar to what bears do in the fall, just before they hibernate.)

Modern man is now up against an evolutionary hurdle: We have opiate-like receptors in the brain that respond to powerful signals that drive cravings for "sweet and safe" foods. Thankfully, one of the wonderful side effects of switching to a low-carb ketogenic plan is that these receptors—at this juncture having zero survival purpose and no dietary reason to be triggered—no longer drive the urge to gorge, and that quells the cravings. Another beneficial side effect of a low-carb diet is the production of ketones, which are known to have a direct impact on hunger signaling. So many clients have told me, after the fact, that they simply didn't believe that this could be true until they experienced the loss of hunger signaling for themselves. You may have even tried low-carb diets in the past but hadn't seen this drastic reduction in cravings. This is not surprising given that you were replacing carbs with protein, and the excess amino acids were converted to glucose via gluconeogenesis. This source of blood glucose in turn stimulated the release of insulin, which dampened the conversion of fats to ketones, effectively keeping you out of deep ketosis.

To layer on even more challenges, remember that the conventional nutritional paradigm (drilled into us by our current dietary guidelines) strongly advises us to consume up to two-thirds of the calories in our diets in the form of carbohydrate-containing foods: "healthy whole grains," fruits, starchy vegetables, legumes, and dairy. We've also been reassured that added sugars, such as sweetened yogurts and sugary treats, are still healthy "in moderation."

Essentially, these flawed guidelines gave you and everyone else the green light to eat in a way that has led our nation to the crisis in health that now threatens to bankrupt us on many levels. This is certainly not meant to be an indictment of how you've lived your life. Instead, it's a statement about the poor state of our country's nutrition guidelines and unhealthy food environment. Even worse, the US Dietary Guidelines have exerted considerable influence on what happens in the rest of the world; sadly, we are witnessing a global explosion of those chronic diseases that used to be confined to the Western world. Today it's equal opportunity for all with a long list of diet-driven diseases that include obesity, type 2 diabetes, polycystic ovary syndrome, heart disease, autoimmune diseases, neurodegenerative diseases, and, of course, cancer. This crisis, however, is preventable, as most of these dire diseases have the same underlying cause: insulin resistance and chronic inflammation.

## Deciphering Carbs on Nutrition Labels

So how do you take the available nutrition information and shape it to develop your personal keto plan? For starters, you will need to become familiar with nutrition labels, starting with the carbohydrate and sugar information. The newest regulations now mandate that nutrition labels point out any sugar (including sucrose and high-fructose corn syrup) that is *added* to a product. That's how you can distinguish the sugar that is added to tomato sauce from the sugar that is naturally occurring in the tomato itself. But this change in labeling does nothing to help the consumer understand that *all* carbohydrates are sugars in one form or another, an awareness that you will need to be diligent about when following a ketogenic diet.

Let's look at the glucose content of a starchy food, such as rice crackers. Typically, these don't contain any added sugar, but they are nonetheless a very dense source of carbohydrates because they are comprised entirely of glucose molecules lightly bonded together. In fact, these bonds are so weak that enzymes in your saliva begin the job of breaking them down into individual glucose molecules while you're still chewing. This is true for all grains, as well as for grain-free, gluten-free products such as tapioca starch and bean flours. Despite their high glucose content, the longer chains of glucose found in starches are not listed as sugars. Instead, you'll find them under the heading of "total carbohydrates." When you look at a nutrition label, pay close attention to total carbohydrates, as that figure contains all the sugars found in the product.

Next, look at the amount of fiber per serving. These are carbohydrates that are not readily broken down by human digestion. Subtract that amount from the total carbohydrates figure to arrive at net carbs. For example, if a label says that the total carbohydrates per serving is 34 grams (yikes!) and total fiber is 4 grams, then that serving portion has 30 net carbs (still a huge problem). While you may have heard that you should count total carbs rather than net carbs in a ketogenic diet, that is only because many low-carb diets adopted for purposes other than cancer therapy allow for a much more liberal intake of carb-containing foods—sometimes as much as 100 grams a day.

In calculating net carbs, there are rounding issues that skew the nutrient information. Labels on foods that contain fewer than 0.5 grams of carbohydrate per serving are allowed to list "0 grams" under total carbs. These hidden carbs can add up fast! Also be sure to carefully read the ingredient list and look for any of the sugars listed in chapter 8 ("Redefine Your Relationship with Sugar," page 111). If a single serving contains 2 grams of sugar per serving and sugar is listed far down on the list of ingredients, chances are good that it won't have much of an impact on your glucose levels. However, if you see a sugar, even a supposedly "healthy" one, such as honey or organic cane juice (or a "low-glycemic" cheater like agave nectar), listed as the first or second ingredient, you are definitely looking at a non-keto food!

Heads up on sugar alcohols: The rules governing how and where they are included on the nutrition label are quite convoluted. Manufacturers of products labeled as "sugar-free" need to list sugar alcohols separately, as do producers of products that contain more than one type of sugar alcohol. However, on other labels, they are simply included under total carbohydrates. (If you're interested in learning more, I've included a link to a fact sheet in the resources section.)

It's simplest and best to learn to avoid almost all processed foods and focus instead on whole foods, where, by and large, what you see is what you get.

## Understanding Digestion of Carb-Containing Foods

Carbohydrates are often introduced into the body as disaccharides, a molecule of glucose bound to another sugar. In sucrose (what we think of as "table sugar"), a molecule of glucose is bound to a molecule of fructose, and this bond is easily broken by an enzyme, sucrase, which is almost universally present in humans. A similar ratio of glucose to fructose exists in maple syrup and honey as well. In high-fructose corn syrup, the ratio of fructose to glucose is often much higher; plus, the glucose and fructose molecules are not bound together. This increases the sweetness (and the profitability) of the foods and beverages sweetened with this industrial poison.

Lactose is another disaccharide: A molecule of glucose is bound to a molecule of galactose. Lactose is also known as "milk sugar," and it's what gives milk its slightly sweet taste. Lactose is found not only in milk, but also in cottage cheese, ice milks, and many other low-fat dairy products that have been fortified with non-fat milk solids. It's also found in cheeses and butter, but only in tiny amounts. Interestingly, the ability to make enough lactase, the enzyme needed to break this bond, often declines with age—rightfully so, given that milk consumption was historically confined to breastfeeding of infants and young children. Poor digestion of lactose is referred to as "lactose intolerance" or, more scientifically, as "lactose malabsorption."

Maltose is yet another disaccharide: a glucose molecule loosely bound to another glucose molecule. Glucose molecules can also be bound together as polysaccharides, either as long chains of glucose molecules or as glucose bound in a branched configuration that we know as "starch." Again, the digestion of foods containing maltose or starches is dependent on the presence of particular enzymes.

All disaccharides and most polysaccharides are broken down into monosaccharides during digestion before entering the bloodstream. Glucose is quickly distributed throughout the body and is readily available to every single cell, but most fructose and galactose must first be sent to the liver for processing. (Ancestral diets contained very little fructose, so our modern bodies are not well adapted to processing large amounts of this sugar. That is a major reason why it wreaks havoc in our bodies, such as a serious liver disease called non-alcoholic fatty liver disease.)

## Choosing Carbs Wisely

In the human diet, glucose is the most common monosaccharide. In most cells and tissues, glucose is transported from the blood into cells, often with the help of insulin. Once inside the cell, it is quickly converted to energy molecules, mostly within the cell's mitochondria, but also in the cell's cytoplasm. In cancer, as in many other diseases, mitochondria can accumulate defects that interfere with mitochondrial energy production.

The amount of glucose contained in foods varies from "very little" to "almost exclusively." For example, salad greens have very little sugar in any form, while bread is made up almost entirely of glucose molecules. Therefore, carb density becomes a huge factor in what foods you choose and how you put them together to make up a meal. Obviously, the most carb-dense foods are not keto-friendly, so be sure to review the lists in chapter 8 that specify which foods to eliminate and which to include.

Remember that the goal of a keto diet plan is to remove almost all sources of dietary carbohydrates (a "carb famine"). However, this will not stop your body from using the process of gluconeogenesis to make the glucose it needs to support red blood cells and a few other cells and tissues that are dependent on glucose. (In essence, you can now think of carbohydrates as the only macro that doesn't need to be included in your diet.) For the first several weeks, most of your carbs should come from greens, non-starchy vegetables, nuts, and seeds. Be sure to include servings of anticancer cruciferous vegetables, such as lightly steamed broccoli, cauliflower, and Brussels sprouts, as well as kale and cabbage.

## The Power of Balanced Glucose Levels

Think of your liver as a furnace with a thermostat that regulates the amount of glucose in your blood. If your level drops too low, the furnace kicks in to restore the set level. If the level is too high, the furnace has no reason to make new glucose (except when recycling metabolic waste, such as glycerol and lactate). People on standard diets live in bodies that have the thermostat set too high. This makes them highly reactive to signals that glucose has dropped below its current set point. Hormones respond to fluctuations in glucose levels by increasing hunger signals, stimulating the release of stored glycogen, or increasing the production of glucose via gluconeogenesis. Once you have settled into a ketogenic diet, you'll notice that the "normal" setting has dropped to a lower level than before, and your liver can seamlessly restore glucose homeostasis. Our bodies are well-tuned machines as long as we provide them with the right fuel and pay attention to maintenance!

Other non-starchy vegetables I recommend are asparagus, celery, cucumber, zucchini, and summer squash. Sprouts and shoots are also great choices, and of course, don't forget avocados, which are nutrient dense and high in good fat! If you are including high-fat dairy, some carbs will trickle in from small amounts of lactose found in butter, heavy whipping cream, sour cream, and cheeses.

In these early weeks, it is crucial to stick closely to your well-formulated plan and keep to a limited list of foods. Once you're keto-adapted, however, you can begin to experiment with larger portions of veggies and small amounts of berries or other fruit.

## Maintaining Vigilance with Carbs

It is critical to be wary of all sources of carbs that can sneak into a meal. These include anti-caking agents (such as those found in packages of shredded or grated cheese), maltodextrin used as a filler, wheat in soy sauce (opt for the wheat-free tamari), and even small amounts of carbs from keto-friendly foods like eggs, mayo, and salad dressings. (Remember what I said about "rounding" of carbs on nutrition labels.)

Today you can access a number of easy-to-use online tools, such as Cronometer, that can help you track your intake of carbs. Use the feedback from these tools to shape your food choices. The more comfortable you become with using a precision tool to track carbs, the fewer mistakes you'll make. Even with the best tools, though, don't expect to be perfect on Day One. And if you're not ready for online tracking, you can always use a carb counter plus a notepad as your diary until you are accustomed to entering what you eat and drink into Cronometer.

## Rein in Your Protein

When you think of protein, what comes to mind? A big steak? A nice salmon fillet? Eggs and bacon? Any chance you thought of peanuts or almonds or even broccoli? In fact, most foods, with the exception of fats, contain some protein.

All dietary protein is made up of amino acids. During digestion, protein is broken down by stomach acid and enzymes into its constituent amino acids, which are then used as the raw materials (building blocks) to increase muscle mass, construct enzymes and hormones, build DNA and RNA, and perform specific functions within cells (e.g., as receptors, transporters, and signaling molecules). These are normal processes that occur in all human beings, regardless of diet.

## The USDA Food Composition Database

The USDA Food Composition Database (https://ndb.nal.usda.gov /ndb/) is an important tool.[1] It contains precise macronutrient content item-by-item (branded and generic) that can be used to guide you in tracking macros and in estimating your serving sizes. It offers information by the gram, cup, measuring spoon, or portion size, such as "1 large spear." Total carbohydrates are listed as "Carbohydrate, by difference," and fiber as "Fiber, total dietary." Subtract fiber from the total to arrive at net carbs.

Since Cronometer interfaces with the USDA database, most of the basic information about macros, vitamins, and minerals can be accessed through your Food Diary. However, there may be times when you are curious about a food's extended nutrient profile (including flavonoids, phenols, and so on) and want to see *all* of the available data from the USDA. This is easy to do using the food search page on the USDA site: Enter the item into the search bar, then click on the name of the item you want to view to see the nutrient breakdown. Some items have a "full report" option with an even more detailed listing of nutrients; if available, this option is located under the item name.

The human body requires a core group of 20 amino acids. The 11 that can be made endogenously are designated as "non-essential" amino acids, and the 9 that must come from the diet are referred to as "essential" amino acids. Several fall into a special category called "conditionally essential," meaning that most of the time we can make enough of them on our own, but if this synthesis is slowed down, or the need for repair and maintenance is exceptionally high (as is often the case during conventional cancer treatment), then more of these will need to be obtained from the diet. Foods that provide the 9 essential amino acids in one package are called "complete proteins." Those that don't are called "incomplete." (These are descriptive terms, by the way, not value judgments!)

Omnivores (like humans) can easily obtain what they need from relatively small amounts of animal protein. However, if you are a vegan or vegetarian, you need to pay close attention to meeting your needs, because even if you meet your overall protein target, you may still fall short of the essential amino

## A Warning about Lowered Protein Intake

If you have recently undergone surgery or are nutritionally compromised (your albumin levels are low), you are likely to need more protein than someone who is otherwise healthy. If this is the case, I urge you to discuss your actual needs with your team before you set your protein target. If you make guesses here, you may over- or underestimate your needs.

acids that are more readily obtained from animal sources. (Cronometer tracks amino acid content for you so you can tell at a glance where you stand.)

There's another way to categorize amino acids, and that is by describing what happens to them in the liver. If they can be converted to glucose, they're referred to as *glucogenic*, and if they can be converted to ketones, they're called *ketogenic*. Most amino acids can follow either route, depending on the needs of your body at the time. But a few, including glycine and proline, are exclusively glucogenic and are easily converted to glucose in the liver in just a few steps. In contrast, leucine and lysine are exclusively ketogenic. These two are readily broken down into either acetoacetate, a ketone body, or acetyl CoA, a precursor of ketone production as well as a direct participant in the Krebs cycle.

## Protein and Gluconeogenesis

Gluconeogenesis is a normal and very important process. In fact, we would have never developed as a species if we didn't have this backup system that enables us to survive without consuming carbohydrate-containing foods. So it concerns me that some individuals, even a few in the keto world, paint gluconeogenesis in a bad light, as though it is something we need to stamp out. I wholly agree, however, that *excessive* production of glucose certainly does not work in our favor in cancer and therefore advise you to take in only enough protein to meet your needs, but not so much that you are unintentionally feeding your cancer by providing an excess amount of those glucogenic amino acids.

## Keep an Eye on Glutamine

Glutamine is the most abundant amino acid in the body. It plays an essential role in many biochemical processes and is incredibly important to immune

## What about Red Meat?

There have been a few pretty alarming studies that might have led you to believe that consumption of red meat causes cancer—or, at the very least, raises your risk. On closer reading, though, you can begin to pick out the flaws in the research. For example, these studies have lumped together all red meat without regard to source or quality. Can't we safely assume that meat from animals raised on confined animal feedlot operations, fed grain, and pumped full of antibiotics are not a healthy source of meat? Also, the manner in which meat is prepared, preserved, cooked, and stored also matters. Smoked, processed, or grilled meats are likely contributors to increased cancer incidence; it's best to avoid them.

Another issue with much of the research is that it often refers to "servings," but rarely defines the actual size of the servings under study. If you look at the broader picture, there is no reason to believe that a few small, properly prepared portions a week of good-quality, pasture-raised beef or other red meat are likely to move the needle in the wrong direction.

system function. The dire downside of glutamine is that it can produce cellular energy: In other words, it can feed your cancer. Even if you're conscientiously tracking your intake, it's challenging to know how much is too much, given that in times of greater need your body will increase its biosynthesis of glutamine or mobilize it from liver or muscle tissue, far outpacing the amount that is obtained through diet.

The need for glutamine increases with stress, tissue breakdown, severe illness, and surgery; and the level required can vary greatly from day to day. And cancer has other workarounds for obtaining glutamine: It takes advantage of glutamine that is released when cells die, including those cells that are killed by cancer treatments or acidity in the microenvironment. Cancer cachexia (a wasting syndrome discussed in chapter 7) also provides cancer cells with this fuel through the breakdown of glutamine-rich muscle tissue.

If you consume large portions of animal protein, you may easily take in more glutamine than you currently need. But dietary intake through consumption of keto-friendly portions of protein-rich foods may play a relatively minor role when compared to the intake of glutamine found in supplements often taken by people with cancer. Read your supplement labels carefully to see if they have any added glutamine. Check your protein powder as well (if you're using one) to be sure that it isn't fortified with extra glutamine. (A quick aside: If you're currently using whey protein, consider switching to one of the newer, higher-quality plant protein isolates [e.g., MRM Veggie Elite]. Whey's anabolic effects may be problematic in cancer. Also, it is not unusual for people to show some degree of sensitivity to whey, which is a bovine milk protein.)

I'm often asked, "How much glutamine is safe?" Unfortunately, there is no single right answer. To quote Dr. Seyfried (from personal communication, September 2016):

> The glutamine issue is very important. We need glutamine for many physiological processes. Most importantly, glutamine is a major metabolite for cells of our immune system, including macrophages. But macrophages are the origin of metastatic cancer cells regardless of tissue origin. Metastatic cancer cells produce cachexia through glutamine sequestration from muscle. Glutamine supplementation is often used to reduce cachexia. This is a type of catch-22. Glutamine can suppress cachexia, but glutamine is a major metabolite of those cells that produce cachexia.

So what can be done to limit the negative impact of glutamine in cancer and cancer cachexia? Rein in the total amount of protein. This is the simplest and possibly the best path to take right now. While pharmaceutical companies are choosing to tackle this problem by developing new drugs that block this pathway, Dr. Seyfried's lab is working on nontoxic metabolic therapies using repurposed FDA-approved drugs that will have the same effect, minus the unintended consequences. He describes this research in an important paper entitled "Press-Pulse: A Novel Therapeutic Strategy for the Metabolic Management of Cancer," published in the journal *Nutrition and Metabolism*.[2] Here Dr. Seyfried acknowledges the critical role of glutamine as a major metabolite needed for cells of the immune system, including macrophages and lymphocytes. His "press" therapies included a ketogenic diet, while the "pulse" targeted glutamine-avid cancer cells for destruction.

## Other Negative Impacts of Too Much Protein

I've made several mentions of the fact that keeping protein low but adequate inhibits two of the major cancer-progression pathways: mTOR and IGF-1. But it's also important to know that certain cancers are very dependent on methionine, another one of the amino acids that we get from protein foods.

## Digging Deeper: Glutaminolysis

Glutamine is one of the amino acids found in all animal proteins as well as many plant-based proteins. It can be utilized directly by cancer cells in a process known as *glutaminolysis*. Some types of cancer (i.e., pancreatic, lymphoma, melanoma) are more glutamine-avid than others, meaning the cancer cells consume it at a higher rate. Ironically, our bodies need glutamine most when we are recovering from the effects of surgery or from injury to the digestive tract, such as that caused by many chemotherapy drugs. (Dr. Kara Fitzgerald suggests a "swish and spit" protocol using glutamine to treat stomatitis, the inflammation of the mucous membrane of the mouth, commonly caused by treatment with chemotherapy drugs.)

Should you avoid all foods containing glutamine? Absolutely not! Not only would that be impossible, but even if you tried, you'd be cutting out many beneficial foods. And as I mentioned earlier, if you don't get enough glutamine from your diet, your body will make what it needs.

A word to the wise: A number of integrative and naturopathic doctors believe that even their patients with glutamine-avid cancers will benefit from the immune-boosting effects of supplemental glutamine. Obviously, we need to do more research to determine if this will indeed help the host without feeding the tumor. If supplementation is indicated, we need to understand how best to dose and time the pulsing of glutamine supplementation, and undoubtedly this will need to be individualized further on a case-by-case basis.

Methionine metabolism may contribute to cancer cell metabolism, so it would be wise to avoid any methionine supplementation (i.e., SAMe). In fact, specially formulated methionine-restricted diets have been studied as possible adjuncts during active treatment with chemotherapy drugs, as restriction can sensitize cancer cells, making them more vulnerable to treatment.

Unfortunately, I can't provide you with a list of cancers that are negatively impacted by methionine, and I'm not suggesting you restrict methionine completely—it's one of the essential amino acids we need to get from the foods we eat because our bodies can't synthesize it. It's also important because it combines with lysine to make carnitine, so we don't want to impair that process.

That said, I often see intake at 500 percent of what's needed. (How do I know that? It's simple: I look at my client's Cronometer Food Diary. It displays the amount of methionine both in grams and as a percentage of the daily requirement. This excellent function helps you control your intake so you can meet but not exceed a reasonable amount.)

## Be Precise with Protein

Whenever I work with new clients, I work very hard to educate them about the cancer-specific benefits of keeping their protein intake low. If they're using Cronometer, I can see how much protein they're eating with a quick peek at their Food Diary. Often I see that they are doing a stellar job at keeping carbs low, but protein intake may be twice what they need. Time for more education!

If you are concerned that you will lose muscle mass if you don't eat a lot of protein, understand that this is yet another example of an urban legend that doesn't apply to those who live in the keto universe. In fact, *ketones spare protein*. In other words, if your muscle tissue is fueled by fatty acids and ketones, then there's less need for your body to break down muscle in order to convert those amino acids to glucose.

There are some people, however, who may benefit from some extra protein. If you are an athlete or if you have a heavy workout routine, refer back to chapter 9 ("Calculate Your Protein Target," page 149) before you decide to boost your protein intake postexercise. If you still believe that this is important to your training, you may decide to lightly supplement with the specific branched-chain amino acids (BCAAs) needed to stimulate protein synthesis. Be careful here: Powdered BCAAs have an odd taste, so most are sweetened with sugars and/or artificial flavors. Make sure to read the label very carefully to be sure that they are not supplemented with glutamine.

If you do decide to supplement, time your intake to coincide with your activity. For example, add some BCAA powder (consider 4 or 5 grams) to one of your water bottles and sip on this just before as well as during your workout. This will direct those amino acids toward active working muscle tissue, but there's still no guarantee that this effect won't extend to stimulating pro-cancer molecular signaling. (Remember, we're navigating uncharted waters here.)

You may also have heard about amino acid supplements. The most widely known is Master Amino Acid Pattern (MAP). My physiologist colleagues tell me that this is more hype than science, but I know that some naturopathic doctors do suggest them as a supplement. Since the science is lacking here, I'll leave it up to you to decide if you want to invest in these.

## Estimating the Protein Yield of Foods

There is a difference between the *weight* of a protein food in grams and its protein *yield*, which is also measured in grams. Most likely, you've never given much thought to this before, so let's look at the basics.

Except for isolated protein, such as that found in powders or supplements, protein foods always contain moisture and fat, and this is reflected in their protein yield. For example, most fish has less fat and more moisture than chicken, so a larger portion raw may yield similar protein amounts when it's cooked. Skinless chicken is a more concentrated source of protein as it contains less fat than ground beef or lamb, so you need less of it to derive the same yield. And as I already described, raw foods contain more moisture than cooked ones, so that needs to be factored in as well. Here are some examples of the variation in weight of cooked animal foods (with no fats used in cooking), all yielding the same amount of protein:

**Table 12.1.** Variation in Weight of Cooked Foods

| Cooked Food | Weight (grams) | Protein Yield (grams) |
|---|---|---|
| Chicken breast, no skin | 58 | 18 |
| Ground beef (85% lean) | 65 | 18 |
| Lamb, trimmed | 75 | 18 |
| Coho Salmon, moist cooked | 65 | 18 |
| Eggs, 3 large, poached | 150 | 18 |

# Fat Is Your New Best Friend

More than 80 percent of the calories in a rigorous ketogenic diet come from fats. This presents a huge problem in the conventional nutrition world: Suggesting that a high-fat diet is superior to the current norm is akin to blasphemy. The fear of fat, particularly saturated fat, has been drummed into us from the time we were children, but the beliefs we have come to accept are no more grounded in fact than the tales you once believed about the Tooth Fairy. To better understand the origins of fat phobia, first read Nina Teicholz's eye-opening book *The Big Fat Surprise*, then dive into the denser science in *Good Calories, Bad Calories* by Gary Taubes. Both of these books pull back the curtain to expose how the flawed science surrounding fats in our diet became integrated into our nutritional consciousness.

If you're following a standard diet, carbohydrate-containing foods currently make up over half of your daily calories. In switching to a diet very low in carbs, you will need to make up the calorie shortage by *more than doubling* the percentage of calories that come from fats, from your current intake of 30 to 40 percent of total calories to 80 percent or more. At the start, it can be very challenging to think of ways to incorporate this much more fat into the diet. That is actually one of the many reasons that I suggest you start with a calorie-restricted version of the ketogenic diet (if this is appropriate for you). Lower overall calories mean you don't need to take in as much fat from your diet; instead, your body will rely on its fat stores and you will easily enter deep ketosis. In the meantime, experiment with the best ways to gradually add in the fats and oils so that you can sustain ketosis once you begin to take in more calories. You may even find that you can obtain most of your fat from whole foods, such as nuts, seeds, avocados, and fatty fish.

Even if you rely mostly on whole foods for your fats, you should still become familiar with how best to incorporate fats and oils into your meals and snacks. And, of course, understand how the type and quality of the fats you choose can either support health or contribute to disease. Let's look at some of the general guidelines and key points regarding the best fats, then focus on what you can do to get up to speed quickly using these recommendations. Remember, you have a lifetime to devote to improving food quality, one step at a time.

To describe fats and oils in simple terms, they are actually chains of fatty acids made up of carbon, hydrogen, and oxygen. If every carbon is bonded to hydrogen, you have what we call a *saturated fat*. However, if any of the carbon molecules lacks a hydrogen, then that carbon will instead bond to the next carbon in the chain, forming what's called a double bond. Fatty acids with a double bond are referred to as *unsaturated fats*. Those with a single double bond are classified as *mono*unsaturated, while those with more than one bond are *poly*unsaturated. The structure of polyunsaturated fats makes them inherently more subject to oxidation (a bad thing), but as you will soon see, some of these fats play a vital role in human health.

Fatty acids fall under the umbrella of a more general category: *lipids*. While fatty acids are important to cellular metabolism, lipids form the core of our existence. The membranes so crucial to every cell in your body are made up of lipids, and the myelin sheath that insulates nerves in your central nervous system is primarily lipid-based. Lipids are also crucial to the structure of fat-soluble vitamins. Our bodies synthesize lipids, but most of this process still relies on the dietary intake of fats that can be used as building blocks; so what you choose to eat and how it is handled by your body ultimately affect your health on many levels.

## Get Up to Half Your Fat from Saturated Fats

. . . And preferably from organic sources! Remember, saturated fats have no double bonds. That makes them the most stable of all the fats, and in their purest state they are the most resistant to oxidation and rancidity. When we think of saturated fats, what comes to mind are animal fats, such as butter, ghee, lard, tallow, duck fat, and bacon grease. This is also the type of fat we usually associate with fatty animal meats, such as beef and lamb. But what you may not know is that most of these fats also contain a substantial amount of mono- and polyunsaturated fats, and the quality and balance of these fats depend in part on what that animal ate. For example, cream from a grass-fed cow will contain less of those inflammatory polyunsaturated fats than cream from a grain-fed cow.

Coconut and red palm oil are vegetable sources of saturated fat and are very stable and resistant to oxidation, especially if they are kept at or below room temperature and out of light. Coconut and palm oil are complex blends of saturated fatty acids of differing lengths, and these longer, stiffer chains are why these oils remain mostly solid at normal room temperatures. The MCT oil derived from coconut, however, remains a liquid even at low temperatures (including refrigeration) because it is comprised solely of fatty acid chains only 8 to 10 carbons long, which are too short to stiffen up when chilled. (This difference is just descriptive and doesn't have anything to do with the quality of one over the other.) I have a whole section covering the benefits of coconut and MCT oils in chapter 14 ("Boosting Ketosis," page 252). Be sure you read and incorporate what I've included there into your plan.

## Choose High-Quality Monounsaturated Fats

Monounsaturated fats (MUFAs) should make up another substantial portion of the fats in your diet. As I mentioned, MUFAs have a single double bond in their carbon chains. Good monounsaturated fats include (unadulterated) extra virgin olive oil, as well as avocado and macadamia oils. Canola and high-oleic sunflower are among the other oils that are high in monounsaturated fats. If you want to include these oils, be meticulous about your source and choose only those that are organic, cold expeller pressed, and unrefined.

## Use Caution When Choosing Polyunsaturated Fats

Polyunsaturated fats (PUFAs) have more than one double bond in their carbon chains. This makes them highly subject to oxidation, and oxidized oils can

## A Question about Oleic Acid

There is research suggesting that oleic acid, such as that found in olive and sunflower oils, can both promote and inhibit cancer. Conflicting studies like these can cause a great deal of confusion for people with cancer. Perhaps the best advice I can offer is to vary your sources of oils. You may also want to look at the literature for your specific cancer. For example, limited research suggests that a high intake of oleic acid may promote progression in aggressive, metastatic breast cancer but may suppress progression in less aggressive cancers.[3,4] Unfortunately, not everything is black or white. The best we can do is be as properly informed as possible and update our thinking based on findings from new research.

spark inflammation in the body. This is a bad situation for anyone, but is especially problematic in cancer, as inflammation is one of the prime drivers. That said, you can't (and shouldn't) shun these fats entirely, because a select few of them play a crucial role in maintaining your health. However, in a ketogenic diet, you don't have to go out of your way to find polyunsaturated fats because they are in many of the foods that you will be eating, including most nuts and seeds. In fact, it is way too easy to take in too much oil from these sources. Focus instead on ensuring that you get enough of the following fats.

## Omega-3 Fatty Acids

### Alpha-linolenic acid (ALA)

ALA is found in plant oils that should definitely be included in your plan. Examples include flaxseed, hemp, and chia. Choose the seeds themselves rather than the isolated oil as the seeds contain other valuable vitamins and minerals as well as a healthy dose of fiber. Store them in the refrigerator.

### Docosahexaenoic acid (DHA) and eicosapentaenoic acid (EPA)

Although our bodies have the ability to convert plant-based ALA to DHA and EPA, there is increasing awareness that these two long-chain fats have a profound anti-inflammatory effect, and relying solely on conversion falls far short of the amounts needed for optimal health. DHA in particular is a critical component of neuronal cell membranes, another important reason to ensure that you're getting enough through diet and/or supplements.

The highest amounts of DHA are found in marine animals that are part of the food chain that starts with algae. Sardines are a good food source (unless you have food-based histamine issues), but be careful with other fish sources higher up on the food chain, as they can carry a heavy load of contaminants, including mercury. If natural marine sources don't appeal to you, opt for a supplement, such as krill oil or molecularly distilled fish oil (such as Nordic Naturals Ultimate Omega). Choose one that is independently lab tested and high in DHA and EPA. Keep to the recommended dosage, as this oil has an anticoagulant effect. (Salmon is often touted as a great source of omega-3s, but be certain that you are not buying farmed fish. False advertising here is rampant and challenging to detect.)

## Omega-6 Fatty Acids

### Gamma-linolenic acid (GLA)

If our bodies are working optimally, we can make GLA from linoleic acid (LA), but there's no harm in bumping up your intake of GLA by including borage oil, black currant oil, and evening primrose oil. GLA has benefits that extend well beyond its anti-inflammatory effect in cancer and is often included in supplements that are known to relieve premenstrual and menopausal symptoms.

### Linoleic acid (LA)

Chances are good that you more than meet your requirement for LA, as it is found in many keto-friendly foods, such as chicken, pecans, Brazil nuts, walnuts, and cheese.

### Conjugated linoleic acid (CLA)

CLA is found mostly in dairy products and meats from ruminants, such as beef and sheep. Sheep that are allowed to forage year-round maintain high levels of CLA, and cattle that are truly grass-fed also have extremely high levels. Eggs from chickens that are pasture-raised are another good source. Some research indicates a general health benefit to CLA, and there are even studies that suggest an immune-boosting anticancer effect.

## Fats to Avoid

So now let's look at the fats and oils that you should totally eliminate from your diet. Make this a priority and be sure to share this information with those you love, even if they haven't jumped on the keto wagon.

## Track Your Omega-6 to Omega-3 Ratio

You can use either the Gold or Mercola versions of Cronometer to track your omega-6 to omega-3 ratio. This eliminates the guesswork and provides immediate feedback through the dashboard dials. Be sure to enter any supplements that include these oils, such as fish or krill oil supplements.

## *Trans* Fats as Hydrogenated Vegetable Oils

If *trans* fat is listed among the ingredients, it's obviously in the food even if the nutrition label says 0 grams (which legally means any amount up to 0.5 grams). There's not enough time or space to go into all the reasons why it is so bad for you, but chances are excellent you're already well aware of its dire effects. The exception is this: Dairy products have some naturally occurring *trans* fats, and there is no evidence to suggest that these have a negative impact on your health.

## Low-Quality Fats and Oils

I put all oils that are heat extracted and/or refined with solvents into this category, including most mayonnaise and store-bought salad dressings. Heat extraction and refinement go hand-in-hand, but it may take some label-reading work on your part to get up to speed with how to distinguish between good and poor sources. Unfortunately, low-quality products never sport a label that reads "genetically modified" (hopefully that's changing), "damaged by high heat," "refined with solvents," or "sprayed with toxins that are detrimental to your health and the environment." That's simply implied if you don't see "organic," "non-GMO," "cold-pressed," and "unrefined" on the better-quality choices. (If it's organic, it's not GMO and hasn't been sprayed with Roundup or another dangerous herbicide.) Olive trees are never sprayed with Roundup, but there are other potential problems with olive oil imports: Many packagers adulterate their product using low-quality oils or allowing contaminants. Also, there's a substantial difference between extra *light* olive oil and extra *virgin* olive oil: The former has been chemically refined, so definitely choose the latter.

## Meat from Confined Animal Feeding Operations (CAFOs)

Fat from these animals has a less healthy lipid composition than meat from grass-fed animals. There are also ethical issues with the treatment of the animals. Another huge problem: These factory farms pump toxins into the environment, creating unhealthy conditions for farm workers and people in general.

## Anything That Smells Rancid or Moldy

Even if you just opened a bottle of good oil or just recently bought a bag of organic nuts, return or toss them if they smell rancid or moldy.

# Incorporating Fats and Oils into Your Keto Meals

You may need some time to adjust physically and mentally to this substantial increase in fats and oils in your diet. Even before you initiate the diet, be sure that every meal includes at least one or two tablespoons of some combination of fats or oils. (Of course, your individual needs may be higher or lower than this amount.) Snacks should contain at least one tablespoon. Experiment with new sources, such as ghee or duck fat. By the end of your first few weeks on the diet, you should be able to prepare tasty meals and snacks that include the full amount of fats that you need to meet your needs.

Quality and balance are important and should be a high priority for you over your lifetime. However, understand that it is more important to do what it takes

### Measuring Oils

When adding fats and oils to your meals, you may find it more convenient to use measuring spoons, but in doing so you run the risk of shorting yourself on this important fuel. One tablespoon of mayonnaise is likely to weigh the full 14 grams listed on the label, but when you are measuring a liquid oil, you may be tempted to stop short of a full spoon, simply because you don't want to overfill it. If you're going to use spoons because they're convenient, check the actual weight with your kitchen scale. You may find that your tablespoon only holds 10 or 11 grams instead of the 14 grams you thought you were getting.

*right now* to make the shift to ketosis as quickly as possible. Use fats and oils that you are familiar with, and upgrade your selections as you find time and energy to do so. Some of the better choices may be challenging to locate in supermarkets or even at whole-food specialty stores. Do your homework online.

Even oils marketed as having a high smoke point should not be used with high heat, as they will oxidize during the cooking process—and you will also be breathing those toxins into your airway. Also, these are mostly GMO oils that are heat extracted and refined with solvents. Experiment with using duck fat or lard instead.

Learn how to add fats and oils without using high heat. For example, you can lightly steam veggies or moist cook the meat before adding them to a sauté over medium heat. Or you can forgo heating fats entirely: Spaghetti squash is great with olive oil drizzled on it, coconut oil blended with almond butter has a very pleasant taste, and adding butter to steamed and mashed cauliflower adds flavor and interest.

## The Scoop on Fiber

It's true that most ketogenic diets are "low residue," as fat and protein do not contain fiber. You can choose foods—such as nuts, seeds, and fibrous vegetables—that contain a mix of both soluble and insoluble fiber. You want enough fiber to help with regularity and to serve as a fuel for healthy colonic bacteria. If you fall short, you can supplement with organic ground psyllium seed or ground flaxseed.

### Soluble Fiber

As its name implies, soluble fiber soaks up water. It then forms a gel that slows digestion. This can dampen blood glucose spikes, but don't rely on fiber to rescue you from a high-carb meal! Because of its water-soluble properties, this type of fiber can also help to keep stool soft, making it easier to pass. Soluble fiber also speeds up the secretion of bile and binds to cholesterol, removing it from the body, but the evidence is just not there to support the theory that lowering cholesterol will lower your risk of cardiovascular disease.

Another known benefit of soluble fiber relates to the production of short-chain fatty acids (SCFAs), a by-product of fermentation by gut bacteria. One of these SCFAs, butyrate, is the metabolic fuel of choice for colonocytes, the cells that line and protect your colon. But soluble fiber by itself can't correct a problem with your microbiome (the bacteria—both good and bad—that populate your gastrointestinal tract): First the healthy bacteria must be restored, preferably through dietary intake of fermented foods, such as sauerkraut, or by taking a probiotic supplement. (If you have dietary histamine issues, the latter is a better choice but do your homework as to which strains are best for this purpose.) Simply adding fiber will not correct any pre-existing problems, so address this issue early on.

Despite its benefits, there are also some drawbacks to soluble fiber. Some fibers ferment excessively, causing gas and bloating, and some people are simply not tolerant of certain fibers, such as inulin, the major fiber component in chicory root and Jerusalem artichoke. Inulin is inexpensive to produce, so it's common to see it listed among the ingredients on food labels, including processed products labeled as high fiber or low carb, but people who are allergic to ragweed pollen may have cross-reactivity to inulin.[5] Soluble fiber can also bind to certain minerals and medications, interfering with their absorption. This is not usually an issue with the soluble fiber found in whole foods, but if you are using supplemental fiber, timing can be tricky. Talk to your health care provider if you have specific concerns regarding this.

If you are considering a fiber supplement, I personally prefer food choices, such as chia puddings or ground flaxseed added to salads, shakes, or baked goods. However, many people choose to use psyllium. If that's your choice as well, look for organic ground psyllium *seed* (not husk). You can buy it in bulk online. Stay away from GMO commercial products found on supermarket shelves, as these usually contain unwanted ingredients, such as sugars or artificial sweeteners. Expect some initial issues with gas and bloating as your gut bacteria adjust to this abundance of fuel. Start slow and build your tolerance. Also be sure to drink plenty of water to enhance the effect. Read and heed any warnings you see on labels for these products, as they are not recommended for people with problems swallowing. They can also cause a bowel blockage if you have hard-to-pass or impacted stool, abdominal adhesions, or obstructions (including tumors). Soluble fiber can also decrease absorption of certain drugs and minerals.

## Insoluble Fiber

Insoluble fiber is not broken down during digestion and does not provide any fuel for your microbiome. It remains intact, adding bulk to your stool and speeding "transit time" (the time between ingestion and elimination). Some people still think of fiber as a cure for constipation because it speeds up digestion; it's true that it may aid in "regularity," and many people value that

## Keto-Friendly Foods High in Healthy Fiber

Below is a short list of keto-friendly foods that are high in both soluble and insoluble fiber:

- artichoke hearts
- asparagus
- avocado
- berries (such as keto-friendly blackberries, strawberries, and raspberries)
- broccoli
- Brussels sprouts
- certain varieties of lettuce and leafy greens
- chia seeds
- collard greens
- flaxseed (preferably ground fresh so you can also benefit from the omega-3 oil)
- nuts and nut flours
- unsweetened shredded coconut

highly. Again, whole foods are the best source of fiber, but if you do use fiber supplements, keep doses reasonable. But also keep in mind that you have a protective mucosal barrier in your colon, and too much insoluble fiber can act like sandpaper, scrubbing the barrier away. Ideally, you want enough fiber to nudge toxins along, but not so much that you remove this evolutionarily important protection. The right balance may be found in whole foods such as fibrous non-starchy vegetables, nuts, and seeds. In fact, there are so many contraindications to using supplemental insoluble fiber that you should really discuss this with your health care practitioner before deciding to add it.

## Proper Hydration Is Central to Good Health

Every organ, tissue, and cell in your body needs water. Water keeps your joints, spine, and brain bathed in fluid. Water flushes toxins from your body and helps to keep your kidneys and bowels healthy. Therefore, water lost through urine, sweat, and respiration needs to be replaced throughout the day.

Because it changes the way that the kidneys handle electrolytes, including sodium, the ketogenic diet has a diuretic effect. Most electrolytes will be replaced by the foods you eat. (As a reminder, salted bone broth, which is rich in electrolytes, is a common cure for what some people call "keto flu.") Most people following the diet should make a conscious effort to replace sodium.

Opt for salt that is *not* iodized, as upping your intake of iodine may push you into the toxic zone, especially if you are already struggling with thyroid issues.

Our bodies normally send a thirst signal when we need fluids. However, thirst signaling and your response to it are far from perfect! Don't rely on thirst to keep you well hydrated. You can use a visual reminder, such as a water pitcher left on the table, or develop routines that center on fluid intake, such as drinking a cup of herbal tea after breakfast. For most people, six to eight glasses a day are enough. More may not be better: Overhydration dilutes blood levels of electrolytes, and there is a dire downside to that.

Vomiting and diarrhea can also deplete fluids and electrolytes. Replace the lost fluids and if the problem persists, talk to your medical team about how best to replace lost electrolytes. Also remember that illness and fever increase your need for water. (There is a disorder of diuretic hormone, common in people undergoing cancer treatment, that depletes sodium independent of fluid intake, but this is a special situation that you should discuss with your oncology team.)

Hot weather and vigorous activity increase your need for fluids. You are more likely to notice this while exercising in heat and humidity, but you also perspire at cooler temperatures. Water not only replaces what you've lost, it also helps regulate your body temperature (by increasing the surface area of your blood vessels). You can obtain fluids from a variety of sources: unsweetened beverages or decaffeinated teas, salted broth (which can also replace lost electrolytes), and the foods you eat.

# CHAPTER 13

# Meal Templates

Finally, here's your simple ketogenic meal template! This may be all you need for the first few weeks—for many people, the most challenging period. Also included here is a more detailed meal plan for that demanding first week that you can easily adapt to fit your own needs and preferences. What I emphasize throughout is keeping it simple. Remember, you have a lifetime to work on the tweaks that will improve your plan over time!

## Simple Keto Meal Template

It's as easy as 1-2-3!

## Breakfast

At breakfast, do each of the following:
1. Choose your favorite protein (e.g., eggs, bacon, cheese, protein shake).
2. Select a veggie (e.g., spinach, zucchini) or a keto muffin.
3. Decide which fats and oils work best for you (butter? coconut oil? cream? duck fat?).

*Sample Breakfast*

Start with two eggs cooked in one or two tablespoons of butter, ghee, or coconut oil. (Or melt these and add them to the beaten raw eggs before cooking.) Garnish with freshly grated cheese or serve with a couple of strips of bacon. Add a serving of vegetables that have been steamed and then lightly sautéed and drizzled with avocado or olive oil. You may also want to include a serving of a keto muffin or chia pudding for an omega-3 fat and fiber boost. Need even more fat? Spread cream cheese on the muffin or top the pudding with whipped cream.

## Bulletproof Coffee

As you may recall from chapter 7 ("The 'Bulletproof' Model," page 101), Dave Asprey introduced Bulletproof coffee to the world. His is a proprietary blend of coffee, ghee, and MCT oil, an early morning elixir used by many in the keto world to provide a carb-free source of energy while pushing back the timing of that first meal of the day. Though not part of a true fast, it turns that early morning coffee into a potent ketone booster. But please don't indulge in too much of a good thing. Enjoy a cup or two, but keep these early morning fats to three tablespoons total, especially if it causes gastrointestinal distress or interferes with appetite, thus preventing you from eating other nutrient-dense foods. And feel free to experiment with your own version using coconut oil, MCT powder, or unsalted butter added to coffee (regular or decaf) or tea.

## Tired of Eggs?

Since you are dividing your macros fairly evenly over the day, you may also opt to have a first meal that more closely resembles lunch or dinner.

## Lunch

At lunch, do each of the following:
1. Start with two to four cups of salad greens and half of an avocado. Add keto condiments of your choosing.
2. Add a protein food (e.g., chicken, tuna, sardines).
3. Serve with olive oil and/or salad dressing and/or mayo.

### Sample Lunch

Half an avocado provides two teaspoons (10 grams) of fat so far for this meal, along with a small amount of protein and carbs and a healthy amount of fiber. If you choose, add a few tablespoons of shredded carrot, diced beets, or bell pepper. Add a portion of cooked chicken that falls just shy of your protein macro—even less if you are adding nuts or seeds to the salad (for most people, that amount of animal protein is close to half of the size of a deck of cards). Check your estimate by weighing your portion and entering the amount of grams into Cronometer. Adjust your portion as needed.

Keep in mind that you can combine different protein foods. For example, you may want to reduce the amount of chicken and add two tablespoons of grated Parmesan or a boiled egg. Serve your salad with homemade olive or avocado oil dressing, using the vinegar of your choice. Vary your vinegar: There are some savory choices out there that can change the "mood" of your salad from savory to spicy. Or, you can make your own infusions. (Stay away from balsamic and malt vinegars, though, as they are too high in sugar. And some vinegars may be too high in histamines as well, so do your homework if histamines are an issue for you!)

Weigh out your oil and make sure to consume every drop, using a small silicone spoon to scoop up what settles to the bottom of your bowl—you don't want to short yourself on calories from fat. Vary this as you see fit. For example, you may want tuna or egg salad made with avocado mayo in place of some of the salad dressing. Again, weigh and record your ingredients so you know you're meeting your macros for the meal.

Now, take a picture of your lovely creation and share it with someone who cares about you and your nutrition. It will reassure them (and you) that this is indeed a healthy way to eat! Finally . . . enjoy! Take the time to savor every bite in pleasant surroundings.

## Dinner

To begin, do each of the following:
1. Pick your protein first (e.g., salmon, beef, lamb).
2. Select complementary veggies (e.g., broccoli, cauliflower, asparagus, or cucumbers).
3. Choose complementary fats (e.g., butter, oil, mayonnaise).

### Sample Dinner

One option is baked or poached fish. Again, track your portion on Cronometer to be sure that you're meeting but not exceeding your protein target. Snip some fresh herbs into one or two tablespoons of avocado mayonnaise and use it as a dressing for the fish, or use melted butter with a squeeze of lemon. (Of course, you can also choose to have meat or poultry instead with some combination of

## Be Sure You're Using Quality Oils

Avoid cooking oils labeled as "high heat." Most are heat-extracted from GMO crops and then refined with solvents. Typically, they also contain high levels of inflammatory omega-6 fats. Also avoid refined "extra light olive oil"; this oil is processed the same way. Instead, use extra virgin olive oil, avocado oil, or coconut oil, but keep the heat level low and use the shortest cooking time possible. You may also want to experiment with using duck fat or lard.

butter and oils in place of the mayonnaise.) For the vegetable, steam cauliflower and mash with one or two tablespoons of butter, or lightly sauté a vegetable in coconut or avocado oil using medium heat. If you insist on stir-fry, use lard, as it can handle higher heat than oils. (Remember my rule: If high-heat cooking irritates your airway, listen to what your body is telling you and back off on the heat.)

## Snacks

Use these high-fat snacks only if you really need them—for example, if you are at a low weight, hungry, or experience a dip in energy between meals. Also use them to get over the hump of learning how best to incorporate the fat you need into your meals. Snacks should fall between two meals, not between dinner and bedtime. Snacks should be very high in fat (one or two tablespoons) and very low in carbs and protein.

*Sample Snacks:*
Here are some 200-calorie snack suggestions:

Fat bombs are high-fat savory or sweet treats that can help boost your fat intake. They can also go with you to work or even to restaurants (which never provide a meal high enough in fat). Look online for recipes; these are very common in the keto world, and people love to share their creations. Dana Carpender has included a few in her book *200 Low-Carb High-Fat Recipes*, and KetoDietApp posts "60 Amazing Fat Bombs" online (https://KetoDietApp.com).

Mix 1 tablespoon of almond butter with 2 teaspoons of coconut oil. Spread on celery sticks. How simple is that!

Enjoy a keto muffin (use mini muffin cups or a silicone muffin mold).
For a special treat, top with 1 tablespoon of keto buttercream
frosting (use Swerve Confectioner's Blend or Pyure Organic Blend
that you've powdered in a spice grinder).

Blend 2 tablespoons of sour cream with ½ of an avocado. Season with
garlic powder and serve with a few pork rinds.

And, of course, there's always that handful of macadamia nuts or some
other nut mix that suits you. If you tend to overeat nuts, then weigh
out your portion at the beginning of the day and place it in a small
container or bag. Commit to "that's it for the day"!

## Detailed Meal Plan for the First Week

I'm providing you with the details of an easy meal plan for the first week.
If you need more suggestions regarding the "how-tos" of meal planning or
preparation—or want a more structured meal plan on hand as insurance that
you're starting off on the right foot—I urge you to obtain a copy of *The Ketogenic Kitchen*. In fact, even if you don't need more direction in this first week,
you should still purchase this book for its plans, recipes, and inspiration. You
should also set up your Cronometer Profile page so you can enter your portion sizes prior to preparing the meal. That way, you have time to adjust the
amounts if you need to before you actually prepare the meal.

## Day One

Checklist for the first day:

☐ Modify these meal suggestions to fit your food preferences.
☐ Use your macronutrient prescription to determine your protein portion.
☐ Ease into the recommended amount of fat, and keep carbs very low.
☐ Keep this day "clean." No treats or snacks on the first day, not even keto-
friendly ones, as they may undermine your efforts to deplete glycogen stores.
☐ Drink lots of water throughout the day and a cup or two of salted broth!

*Breakfast: Eggs and Bacon*

**Protein:** Eggs, bacon
**Fat:** Butter, coconut oil, ghee, heavy whipping cream, bacon grease
**Carbohydrate:** Spinach
**Prep:** Cook eggs in butter, ghee, or coconut oil. (You can also add melted butter,
ghee, or coconut oil to beaten raw eggs.) Cook the bacon, then lightly sauté

## Tips for the First Week

Set yourself up for success! You don't need to have all of your supplies, all of your food, all of your supplements, and a 30-day plan in hand, but you do need to be prepared. Note that timing is important, too. The day before a family vacation or business trip is *not* the right time to make these changes. Here are some tips to get you started:

- Review chapter 8. What do you need to ensure that this week goes smoothly?
- Look through the entire week's plan. What meals seem appealing? What ingredients do you have on hand already? Which do you still need to purchase?
- Note that many of the same foods are incorporated into meals on two consecutive days. Leftovers make it simpler to plan and prepare meals.
- Cook up a pot of chicken stock or bone broth. Salt it. You can use this to replace fluids as well as sodium and other electrolytes lost in urine.
- This meal plan is only a suggestion. If you don't like a particular food—beef, for instance—then pick a different protein. If you don't like (or can't find) spaghetti squash, feel free to "spiralize" a zucchini.
- Many of these meals contain cream or butter. If you choose to go dairy-free, what will you use in its place? (One possibility is Melt Organic Spread.)
- Plan to keep physical activity light and mostly recreational (e.g., a gentle walk in nature rather than an extreme workout at the gym).
- Use seasonings as desired to spice up your meal. For example, curry for a stir-fry, or Italian seasonings for veggies. And remember to use that saltshaker!

the spinach in the bacon fat. Add heavy whipping cream to coffee or tea. (Count 2 tablespoons of cream as 1 tablespoon of fat and 1 gram of carb.)

*Lunch: Caesar Salad*
**Protein:** Chicken (optional: grated Parmesan)
**Fat:** Caesar dressing, ½ avocado (contains 2 teaspoons of fat)

**Carbohydrate:** Salad greens. Also count the net carbs from the avocado.

**Prep:** Serve salad greens with grilled, sliced chicken and ½ of an avocado. (Optional: Reduce chicken portion and add 2 tablespoons of grated Parmesan.) Serve with Caesar dressing and boost the fat content with extra virgin olive oil.

### Dinner: Poached Fish with Asparagus

**Protein:** Fish fillet

**Fat:** Butter, mayonnaise, olive oil

**Carbohydrate:** Asparagus

**Prep:** Bake or poach fish. Serve with herbed butter or avocado mayonnaise with snipped fresh herbs. Steam the asparagus and drizzle with melted butter and/or olive oil. (Optional: Add a green salad with olive oil and vinegar dressing.)

## Day Two

Checklist for the second day:

☐ Start measuring and recording your fasting blood glucose level.

☐ Prepare one or two high-fat snacks; you may not need them, but at least you'll have them on hand.

☐ Remember to drink some salted broth to ease mental fog and tired muscles.

☐ Test urine ketones after lunch and at bedtime. The presence of ketones indicates that you've depleted your liver's glycogen stores and have made the shift to ketosis.

### Breakfast: Protein Shake

This can be used as an occasional—but not daily—meal replacement.

**Protein:** Non-dairy protein powder (such as MRM Veggie Elite)

**Fat:** Heavy whipping cream, MCT oil (or, better yet, Brain Octane or another caprylic [C8] oil), and one other oil (e.g., avocado, macadamia)

**Carbohydrate:** Unsweetened almond/coconut milk and a serving of a keto muffin

**Prep:** Blend almond milk, protein powder, C8 oil, other oil, and optional flavorings (extract, stevia). If you're using Brain Octane, start with a small amount and increase this slowly over time. Sip this drink slowly over 15 to 20 minutes. (If this is too much oil to comfortably digest, you can have 1 ounce of macadamia nuts in place of 4 teaspoons of oil.) Enjoy a serving of keto muffin.

## *Lunch: Tuna Salad*

**Protein:** Canned tuna, such as Wild Planet, or sardines packed in water

**Fat:** Non-soy mayonnaise, olive oil

**Carbohydrate:** Salad greens, celery (optional: cucumber)

**Prep:** Mix tuna (or sardines) with mayonnaise. Add diced celery. Serve on a bed of greens with sliced cucumbers (optional). Drizzle extra virgin olive oil over the salad greens.

## *Dinner: Burger with Tomato Slices*

**Protein:** Ground beef

**Fat:** Butter, olive oil, canola oil, olive oil mayonnaise

**Carbohydrate:** 2 tomato slices, zucchini

**Prep:** Shape ground beef into a patty and broil or panfry. Serve with mayonnaise, a slice of tomato, and steamed or spiraled zucchini (with butter). (Other prep options: You can also sauté or microwave the tomato and zucchini and add olive oil.)

## *200-Calorie Snacks*

1 tablespoon (16 grams) almond butter with 2 teaspoons (10 grams) coconut oil

1 ounce macadamia nuts (= 28 grams = 10–12 kernels)

# Day Three

Checklist for the third day:

☐ Test your fasting blood glucose. How does it compare to yesterday's?

☐ Test your urine ketones. Are you consistently seeing a shade of pink or purple? If not, can you connect the dots between your food choices and any "negative" ketone readings?

☐ Are you tracking your macros yet? If not, consider starting. If you are already tracking, how close did you come to your targets yesterday, and what can you improve on today?

☐ Remember to drink some salted broth as it can keep many of the "keto flu" symptoms at bay.

## *Breakfast: French Toast*

**Protein:** Egg(s), sausage (Use Cronometer to balance protein in this meal.)

**Fat:** Butter, coconut oil, cream cheese, cream, Melt Organic Spread

**Carbohydrate:** "Mug muffin" (see resources section), strawberry

**Prep:** Beat egg with melted butter or coconut oil. (Optional: Add vanilla, cream, spices, and stevia to taste.) Slice the keto muffin in half. Soak each piece in the egg mixture and fry in coconut oil using medium heat. (Use a spatula to keep slices from sticking and crumbling.) Spread with butter, cream cheese, or Melt Spread. Top with a finely sliced strawberry and serve with a second egg or 2 small sausage links to keep within your macro targets.

### Lunch: Chicken Salad

**Protein:** Chicken (cooked)
**Fat:** Mayonnaise, olive oil, walnuts or pecans
**Carbohydrate:** Salad greens, celery (optional: cucumber)
**Prep:** Mix diced chicken with mayonnaise. Add diced celery and chopped nuts. Serve on a bed of greens with sliced cucumbers (optional). Drizzle extra virgin olive oil and vinegar (optional) onto the greens.

### Dinner: Lamb Chop with Mashed Cauliflower

**Protein:** Lamb chop(s)
**Fat:** Butter, olive oil, mayonnaise
**Carbohydrate:** Cauliflower
**Prep:** Grill or broil the lamb. Steam the cauliflower, then mash your portion for this meal. Add your choice of fats and oils. Season to taste. Keep leftovers for tomorrow's breakfast. (Yes, you can eat any keto meal you want for breakfast!) You can also "rice" the cauliflower; find instructions on how to do this in *The Ketogenic Kitchen* or other recipe sources online.

### 200-Calorie Snacks

1 tablespoon almond butter mixed with 2 teaspoons coconut oil spread on celery sticks

2 tablespoons sour cream with ½ of an avocado seasoned with garlic powder and served with a few pork rinds

## Day Four

Checklist for the fourth day:

☐ Did you steer clear of food for at least three hours before bedtime? If not, make an effort to move in that direction.

☐ Continue to test blood glucose: fasting and at bedtime. Be sure to keep a record of your numbers, either by logging them into Cronometer, entering them on a spreadsheet, or keeping a logbook.

☐ You should definitely be in ketosis by now, and urine testing should reflect this. Check urine ketones first thing in the morning, in the mid-afternoon, and at bedtime. Are you noticing a pattern where ketones are lighter first thing in the morning and stronger as the day progresses? This is perfectly normal and part of your body's circadian rhythm. Cortisol rises before you wake, stimulating your liver to make glucose. This temporarily suppresses ketones. If at any time your urine stick immediately turns purple, most likely you are burning a lot of body fat. If you are carrying excess weight, this is not usually an issue during the first few days or weeks as long as you don't have any symptoms of acidosis (such as extreme fatigue or lethargy, rapid breathing, or profuse sweating). If you are at a low weight or have other conditions that compromise your health, you need to slow down weight loss by ensuring that you are taking in enough fat in your meals and snacks.

☐ Have you been keeping a good food diary? Even if it seems like more work than you want to commit to right now, I strongly urge you to track what you eat, even if it's only for a single meal or a single day. Add your blood glucose and ketone measurements to your diary. Later, you will begin to use these readings as feedback on your choices. Add notes about how you are feeling as well.

### Breakfast: Eggs with Cauliflower and Cheese Sauce

**Protein:** Eggs, cheese
**Fat:** Butter, coconut oil, cream, Melt Organic Spread
**Carbohydrate:** Leftover mashed or riced cauliflower
**Prep:** Grate a condiment-sized portion of cheese (up to 14 grams) into a pan and add cream or oils. (Optional: Season with onion powder.) Heat briefly. Stir with a wire whisk, then continue heating just until smooth. Ladle cheese sauce over the cauliflower. Serve with eggs, cooked any style.

### Lunch: Chicken Soup with Spinach or Kale

**Protein:** Chicken, chicken broth
**Fat:** Duck fat, olive oil, butter, other oil choice
**Carbohydrate:** Celery, onion, spinach, or kale
**Prep:** Make a new pot of chicken broth. Separate the meat from the bone and remove any vegetables that were used for flavor. Ladle out a bowl of broth and add your portion of chicken along with fresh spinach or kale. Serve when the greens are wilted. Add fats and oils to the soup. Add a small

dressed salad. If you need more fat, eat a handful (28 grams) of macadamia nuts or have a fat bomb for dessert.

### Dinner: Shrimp Scampi with Spinach

**Protein:** Shrimp (frozen and peeled are simplest to prepare), Parmesan
**Fat:** Butter, ghee, Melt Organic Spread, olive oil, heavy cream
**Carbohydrate:** Spinach, garlic, onion
**Prep:** Ready to try a low-carb recipe? You can search online for "keto shrimp scampi" or use the one at www.tasteaholics.com. This recipe's quick and easy, and you'll have leftovers for tomorrow's salad. Careful with portion size, as the recipe as written yields 36 grams of protein. Plan to limit your serving to 5 large shrimp.

### 200-Calorie Snacks

Experiment with some fat bomb recipes. You can press these into silicone candy molds or simply drop them onto wax paper or parchment. (Or, repeat snacks that you liked from the previous two days.)

## Day Five

Checklist for the fifth day:
☐ Use the same glucose and ketone testing schedule as yesterday's.
☐ Did you weigh all of your foods? Did you update your food diary?
☐ Use Cronometer as your health journal. You can use Notes to add times for your meals or tests, or to record how you are feeling. Are you noticing less inflammation? Fewer cravings? More energy? Better mood? What, if any, side effects are you still experiencing?

### Breakfast: Eggs and Bacon

Repeat the breakfast from Day One. Can you incorporate more fat this time? For example, use more butter or coconut oil to prepare your eggs or drizzle some extra olive oil on your veggies.

### Lunch: Shrimp Salad

**Protein:** Shrimp (prepared last night)
**Fat:** Avocado, olive oil, or avocado oil
**Carbohydrate:** Mixed greens, select veggies
**Prep:** Prepare a bed of greens and other veggies. Cube ½ of an avocado. Arrange shrimp and avocado on the greens and dress with olive or avocado oil. Add your favorite seasonings, including salt. How easy was that!

*Dinner: "Noodled" Zucchini with Meat Sauce*

(You can use a vegetable peeler to create long, thin strips of zucchini—or you can buy a spiralizer that does this—which you then steam and use as a noodle substitute.)

**Protein:** Ground beef
**Fat:** Butter, Melt Organic Spread, olive oil
**Carbohydrate:** Red bell pepper or tomato, zucchini
**Prep:** Brown the beef with Italian herbs and fresh onion or garlic (you can also use granules or powder). Simmer with a few tablespoons of red bell pepper or diced tomato. Serve over zucchini noodles with added butter, Melt Spread, or olive oil. Season with salt and pepper.

*200-Calorie Snacks*

1 ounce (28 grams) of mixed nuts (macadamias, pecans, almonds, walnuts)
1 fat bomb

## Day Six

Checklist for the sixth day:

☐ Test your glucose response to one meal. Check glucose just before the meal, then again at one hour and two hours afterward. At one hour did your glucose level rise more than 20 mg/dL above the pre-meal level? If so, can you identify a likely cause, like food choice or portion size? By two hours, did glucose drop back down to pre-meal levels? If not, wait another hour and test again. This type of intensive testing can provide you with great feedback that you can then use to tweak your plan.

☐ Are you testing blood ketones yet? Remember that you need a larger drop of blood for ketone strips. Test either before a meal or at bedtime. Do this at a time when you're also testing glucose so that you can calculate your GKI. (Learn about this in chapter 16, "Monitoring Your Glucose Ketone Index [GKI]," page 306.)

☐ Did you stop eating at least three hours before bedtime? If not, why not? Make this a priority unless you have a medical need (such as taking medication with food) or are low weight and need an extra handful of macadamia nuts or some other snack late in the day to boost your calorie and fat intake.

*Breakfast: Crunchy Nut "Cereal" (as a side dish)*

Today's breakfast invites you to begin to test your skills at putting together a meal using Cronometer. The cereal is low in both protein and fat, so you'll need to find

## How to Determine Your Portion Size with One-Pan Meals

Easy. Plan your serving sizes, in grams, using Cronometer or the USDA site. Include each ingredient, then adjust the amounts to meet your macros. After you've prepared the meal, place your empty plate or bowl on the scale and use the tare feature to reset the scale to zero. Place your serving of "noodles" on the scale, record the weight, and, once again, use the tare feature. Now, add the beef. Continue adding ingredients, recording the weight of each and resetting to zero each time. Use a silicone spoon to scoop up some flavorful liquid from the pan. Add salt, and pepper if desired. Add your oils. (If you are following a rigorous keto plan, leave the garlic and onion in the pan and just enjoy the flavor in the liquid. If your plan is more moderate, you can add these extras to your plate. Just be sure to keep to your macros for the meal.)

other foods to boost those two macros. Let me help you with this first attempt. If this seems too involved for now, recycle a breakfast from earlier this week.

**Protein:** There is some protein in nuts but you'll need to double or triple that amount. Add a boiled egg and/or a slice of ham or a small protein shake.

**Fat:** There is some fat in the cream, coconut, and nuts but it's likely that you'll need more. Some options: Add coconut oil or caprylic (C8) oil or ghee to your hot beverage. Or spread some cream cheese on that slice of ham and roll it up. None of these options take more than a minute or two of your time.

**Carbohydrate:** The cereal substitute has all the carb and fiber you need for this meal.

**Prep:** Weigh out individual amounts of unsweetened shredded coconut and sliced, chopped, or slivered nuts. Enter the weights into Cronometer, keeping net carbs low. Decide on your other proteins and fats, entering those into Cronometer as well. Make sure to include the cream or almond/coconut milk that you plan to use with the cereal. Does this now meet your meal macros? If not, adjust portion sizes. To make the cereal, toast the coconut and nut mixture in a dry pan over medium heat, stirring constantly till golden brown (approximately 3 minutes). Allow to cool slightly. Add cream and some sweetener to taste.

*Lunch: Grilled Hot Dog*

**Protein:** Applegate Organics beef hot dog with a 1-ounce slice of cheese
**Fat:** Add mayonnaise to your wrap or olive oil to your salad dressing.
**Carbohydrate:** Green salad or a lettuce wrap.
**Prep:** No prep instructions needed for this one!

*Dinner: Quick and Easy Curry*

**Protein:** Your choice—beef, lamb, or chicken
**Fat:** Coconut oil and butter or ghee
**Carbohydrate:** Cauliflower
**Prep:** Sauté thinly sliced beef, lamb, or chicken in coconut oil in a pan over
medium heat. Add onion granules, garlic granules, and curry powder (red or
yellow). Steam cauliflower, then chop in food processor until about the consistency of steamed rice. Add butter and serve with beef, lamb, or chicken on top.

*200-Calorie Snacks*

Are 200-calorie snacks still meeting your needs? If not, you can adjust the calorie content up or down as needed. Just be sure that they are high in fat and
low in protein and carbs.

## Day Seven

You made it! Hopefully, you are gaining confidence and can now see that you
don't need to overthink this new way of eating. Here's your checklist for the
seventh day:

☐ If you haven't started using Cronometer or another similar tool, I once
again urge you to set up a profile and begin tracking. This will serve as a
durable record of your efforts moving forward.

☐ Hopefully, you are comfortable with your kitchen scale and are using it to
ensure that your food choices and portion sizes are meeting your target macros.

☐ Continue testing glucose and ketones. In chapter 16 you will learn ways
to gather even more feedback on your individualized response to foods,
exercise, and stressors.

*Breakfast*

At this point, you may no longer be hungry for breakfast, especially if you're
starting your day with a Bulletproof-style hot beverage (coffee or tea with added
ghee, butter, coconut oil, and/or MCT oil). No problem. In fact, there may be
an advantage to delaying breakfast (refer back to "The Perks of Intermittent

Fasting," page 99, in chapter 7). Also, as breakfast creeps closer to the traditional lunch hour, you may find that you no longer need to think in terms of
traditional breakfast foods. Leftovers from last night may serve you just as well.

### Lunch

Look back at the lunches that you enjoyed the most this week. Were they also
easy to prepare? If not, can you think of a way to simplify meal prep?

### Dinner

Protein, fat, and carbs. You've got this!

## Moving Forward: Beyond the First Week

Now it's time to look back on this first week to see how you might improve on
your efforts. Ask yourself these questions:

**Are you meeting your macronutrient needs?** The only way to know for sure
is to either plan your meals or track what you eat and compare your intake
to your macro targets.

**Are you hungry?** If so, you may be going too long between meals or shorting
yourself on fat. For now, you may need to fill in with an extra high-fat
snack or two.

**Have your carb cravings subsided?** If you have kept carbs low, you should be
experiencing fewer (or no) cravings by now. That said, understand that it can
take several weeks for your body to adjust to burning fat instead of sugar.

**Have you gotten into the habit of testing blood glucose and ketones?** Even
if you're hesitant to do this, keep in mind that only testing will provide you
with the information you need to determine if you're on the right track.

**Are you bouncing in and out of ketosis?** If your urine test strips are not
consistently showing some shade of pink or purple, or your blood test strips
indicate that you are just barely into nutritional ketosis (0.5 mmol/L), look
for hidden carbs in the foods you're choosing.

**Do fats and oils make you feel overly full or even slightly nauseous?** Fat slows
digestion, so you may want to move some of the fat from meals into one or
two high-fat snacks, such as fat bombs. Experiment with different combos of
fats and oils; you'll find that some are more digestible than others. If tolerance
continues to be an issue, consider adding Pure Encapsulations Pancreatic
Enzymes to help with fat digestion. You can also add a few grams of sunflower
lecithin to your oils; this can help to emulsify fats, also aiding fat digestion.

**Are you missing your former favorite foods or treats?** You can find substitutes for many of your former favorites, but there's a fine line between keto-friendly and non-compliant. If you substitute sugar-free sweets that look and taste like your favorite sugary candy bar, you run the risk of slipping back into old habits. Instead, keep lowering your sweet thermostat until it's so low that those types of foods are no longer appealing. Children do need foods that replace the treats given to siblings or peers, however. The Charlie Foundation website contains lots of kid and keto-friendly recipes on their "Recipe Resources" page, as does MaxLove Project's website and Facebook page.

**Are you experiencing what you believe to be diet side effects?** Side effects resolve with time. Lingering symptoms may reflect non-diet-related changes to your health or may be associated with your cancer treatment.

**Are you monitoring your weight?** Almost everyone sheds a few pounds as they deplete stored glycogen. If weight loss is excessive or sustained, consult with a keto nutritionist (check the resources section for some guidance here).

**Are you limiting variety by relying too much on just a few foods, such as kale or avocado?** In general, it's preferable to eat from a wide variety of foods, especially seasonal favorites, to ensure that nutrients are derived from a variety of sources. Variety also helps to increase the diversity and health of your microbiome. If you find yourself relying too heavily on one specific food, look for alternatives so that you don't develop sensitivities or get tired of that food. All things in moderation!

As you enter into your second week of the diet, why not simply repeat the meal plan from your first week, adding your own tweaks now that you have a better idea of what you are doing? If you want more variety or are feeling ready to invest more time and energy, start paging through a few keto cookbooks. Hopefully, by this time you'll feel a lot less intimidated and these concepts will have become more intuitive, making them easier to riff on. In time, you'll even come up with your own brilliant keto recipes!

## Update Your Diet Prescription

Be flexible, as your ideal plan will undergo changes over time! If it's reasonable to do so, keep to your initial calculations for the first two to four weeks. Then it's time to reassess. Every few weeks, take note of the following, then look for ways to use this information to keep you moving in the right direction:

- glucose/ketone readings (explained in chapter 16, "Monitoring Your Glucose Ketone Index [GKI]," page 306)
- changes in weight
- changes in health status
- bloodwork and scan results (discuss high/low values with your team)
- changes in your standard protocol (chemotherapy, radiation, surgery)
- changes in your medications or dosages
- changes in alternative or complementary therapies
- changes in dietary or herbal supplements
- satisfaction with food options
- satisfaction with the input you get from your team
- level of support you're receiving from family and friends

## Tips for Dining Out

It's best if you eat most of your meals at home or work until you're feeling comfortable with your new plan. That said, I encourage you to dine out on occasion, especially if it involves good times with family or friends. Just follow these guidelines to make sure you remain on your keto plan:

- In the early weeks and months, choose familiar venues whenever possible so you already have an idea of what keto-friendly foods they offer.
- When dining out with a group of friends, remember that socializing is more important than the meal itself. Keep it simple, especially if there aren't many keto-friendly choices.
- If the restaurant is new to you, go online to look at the menu and start thinking about which meals might work best for you.
- Call ahead and ask if they are willing to accommodate special requests.
- Ask how protein foods are prepared; broiled, poached, or grilled foods are generally better options as most fried foods are breaded, and these will skyrocket your carb intake.
- Hold the bread, but ask for *lots* of butter and then find ways to use it!
- Hold the starches. Ask for double non-starchy veggies instead.
- Avoid sauces and dressings unless you are positive that they don't contain sugar or starch.
- You will almost always be served more protein than you need; take half of it home to eat at another meal.

- You will never be served enough fat! Consider bringing your own salad dressing and fat bombs with you in leakproof containers.
- What will you say to that friend or relative who—for whatever misguided reason—encourages you to have "just one piece" of bread or "just one bite" of dessert? (Hint: Keep the conversation focused on your commitment to your plan.)
- What about alcohol? If that's part of socializing, make that one glass of wine or one shot of straight spirits last for the evening.

## Tips for Smoother Business Travel

Airports, malls, conferences, and the neighborhoods surrounding conference hotels are often food deserts (not to be confused with "desserts"). Scope out your options pre-trip or shortly after you arrive.

### Before Your Trip

When you make your room reservation, ask for a mini fridge and a microwave. You won't be preparing gourmet meals, but a fridge and microwave come in handy for storing and reheating take-home and carry-out foods. Also scope out the setting, looking for what can aid you as well as what can trip you up:

- Does the hotel have a restaurant? If so, what does it serve? What are the hours?
- Do you have time to shop at a nearby grocery store? If so, check to see what's nearby and plan to pick up a few items that will make your stay easier.
- If food shopping isn't an option, bring your own cheese, cream cheese, nut butters, coconut oil, nut mixes, pork rinds, even boiled eggs, and sealed packages of deli meat. Celery sticks, thin slices of carrots, and a few cherry tomatoes are good to have with you as well. Pack some avocados, too, along with a knife (in your checked bag, of course). Store your foods in plastic containers with lockable lids. Tuck a freezer pack in with them if you're flying or use a cooler if traveling by car.
- Do you have a favorite keto muffin or cracker recipe? Make some up ahead of your trip and take them with you. These generally travel well.
- I now travel with packages of powdered βHB supplements. These are much easier and less messy than traveling with MCT oil. If

you do want to take your MCT oil, pour it into a metal container with a leak-resistant cap, triple bag it, and include a label for TSA identifying it as "coconut oil." (I bought a camper's fuel bottle that I used solely for this purpose, but even this was not leakproof, so bring some extra bags for the return trip.)

- Low-carb and keto food companies are popping up, offering you more travel choices, such as bars and snacks. There are even packaged powders you can use to make Bulletproof-style coffee. So bring along your travel mug!
- Fat bombs are also an option, but only if you can keep them chilled.
- Bring some salt! And your favorite seasonings. (I've been known to salt and season chilled butter pats just to get the fats I need. Tastes like herbed cheese!)
- Tinned sardines travel well.
- Always pack some extra ziplock bags. They come in handy for repackaging your bulk foods into briefcase- or purse-sized portions.

Of course, toting all this food means that I will have to check a bag, but I find it's well worth it, especially when the choices at my destination are limited and costly. And it sure saves time as well. The biggest bonus: I get to eat better-quality food than what I'm likely to find on-site.

## At the Airport

I used to stress over not having enough food to get through a long day of air travel. Now, I tend to travel light or sometimes even fast for the day. It's easy to do when you're ketogenic. It also makes travel simpler, less messy, and certainly less costly. Be sure to stay well hydrated, though, even if it means more frequent trips to the restroom. If you do plan to eat, here are some tips:

- Carry individually wrapped packages of foods or ziplock bags of nuts, cheese, even pork rinds. Carry small plastic bags or containers with keto-friendly snacks, such as deli meat rolled up with cream cheese (you're going for convenience here, not quality). For longer trips, keep these in a small insulated bag with a refreezable pack. I like to bring fresh food, such as celery and carrot sticks, or a few thin slices of apple.
- Note that you won't be allowed to carry oils on board unless they are in small, leakproof containers that can be placed in the "liquids" ziplock bag that's allowed in your carry-on baggage. Some exceptions

are made for families traveling with children on the diet who have a
signed note, on letterhead, from a doctor.

- Most airports sell salads. Add olive oil or low-carb salad dressing. If possible, choose a salad that includes a protein food (chicken, boiled egg, deli ham, sliced cheese). It's not ideal, but it will get you through the day.

- If you have a longer layover, you can usually find a burger or grilled chicken. Order yours in a lettuce wrap. Add mayo. Order a small salad with it so you can load up on olive oil and low-carb salad dressing. And, yes, you can expect low quality, but that's the trade-off with most convenience venues of this type.

- Pick up a few mayonnaise packets. You can use them as a dip for your protein food or save them for the hotel room. (This mayonnaise will be made from soybean oil, but a serving or two is not likely to create any issues.) Same with cream cheese: Many breakfast buffets have small packages. Pick up a few.

- As noted earlier, sardines travel well, but they can be messy during travel. Bag these in ziplock bags and eat them at the gate, not at your seat!

- If you enjoy keto muffins or crackers, pack a few in your carry-on bag.

- Ensure that you have enough food with you (or available to you) to get you to your destination. Allow extra for travel delays and as a buffer for the first few hours after your arrival. If this is a business trip, you may want to take a holiday from blood monitoring. Continue to check your urine ketones.

## Navigating Conference Food

Conference fare is a minefield! You may be trapped for an entire day in a room with nothing other than the dreaded luncheon buffet: rolls and whipped butter, finger sandwiches, raw veggie platters with questionable dips, pasta salads, chips, cookies, and desserts. Plan for this! Of course, you can opt to fast till dinner, or you can bring some of the lockable lid containers you carried with you, filled with the real foods you enjoy. Carry these in your insulated bag. (You can refreeze the ice pack in your hotel room's mini fridge.)

## Celebrating Special Occasions

You can either face holidays and other special occasions (such as birthdays and anniversaries) with dread or "defuse" them with some pre-planning.

## A Passable Sample Menu for a Conference Attendee

Start your day with Bulletproof coffee.

### BREAKFAST

At the hotel buffet, stick to eggs with bacon, sausage, or cheese. You can also make an egg salad with hard-boiled eggs and mayonnaise packets. Eat chilled butter pats for extra fat. Pick up extra packets of cream cheese and mayonnaise and take them with you. If you're at a restaurant, order an omelet. That plus your snacks should be enough to hold you until lunchtime.

### LUNCH

If you can't bring your own meal, choose deli meats, tuna, or chicken salad. Toss the bread and double the salad veggies. Look for butter pats and mayonnaise packets and, if available, choose olive oil and vinegar (no balsamic). If you have cream cheese with you, spread some on deli meat, roll it up, and eat it as a finger food.

### DINNER

It's usually easy to find grilled meat, fish, or poultry. When ordering, ask them to replace the bread and starch with an extra serving of vegetables (no sauces). There may be a slight surcharge for this. Add olive oil, butter, or mayonnaise wherever possible. Find a way to gracefully consume all the oils from the bottom of the plate or bowl. Take any leftovers back to your room. If you find yourself at a restaurant not known for low-carb choices, ask your waitperson for help. Chances are good that you are not the first person to request a low-carb meal!

Put some thought into how you will handle the day before the time arrives. Own your decisions. If you choose to have a traditional Thanksgiving, understand that one day of relaxing your diet won't make or break your efforts; just don't make it a habit or allow it to chip away at your commitment. Also consider fasting for a full day after a day off from the diet. That's the fastest way to get back on track. (Again, beware of letting this become a "binge and purge" cycle.)

Also, recall the advice I gave earlier about creating new traditions that don't revolve around food. Of course, this is easier to do on a small scale—like what we did by swapping Raffi's birthday cake for a trip to the hot springs. This won't work for an event such as a wedding, but honestly, it's not likely that anyone is micromanaging your food intake, so chances are good that you can leave that piece of cake on the table and it will be your little secret. (Understand that my suggestions for how to handle these events reflect my strong bias against sugars and starches; if we let them into our lives, they often take up too much of the landscape, like weeds in a hay field.)

# CHAPTER 14

# Nutritional Supplements

**M**ost people consuming standard diets do not take in enough of the right kinds of nutrients on a daily basis. Some of this is obviously related to food choices, but another significant factor is due to soil depletion in large-scale farming, which results in unbalanced trace minerals in the soil and subsequently the food grown in it. That's one compelling reason to buy your produce from small local farms and, whenever possible, from small organic farms that are responsibly managed. But even if you are diligent about purchasing only organic foods, this may not solve the problem. Large-scale organic operations may yield crops that are just as depleted, or even more so, than non-organic varieties. We spent one winter camping in Mexico with Raffi, soaking up the sun. During that time, we observed some growing practices that I'm sure hold true for large-scale farming anywhere in the world. For one, many of the big farms were growing their produce in sandy soil. I can't imagine that these foods contained all the vitamins and minerals that would be found if they had been grown in nutrient-rich soil. (Have you noticed how much of the produce available in the United States comes from Mexico?)

If you're using Cronometer, your Food Diary page will display all the nutrients along with how well you are meeting the minimum daily requirements. Cronometer is linked to vetted databases, so the information is as accurate as it can be given the issues with soil depletion. If you want even more information about the nutrients in a wide variety of brand-name products, visit the searchable USDA Food Composition Database (https://ndb.nal.usda.gov) and click on the food you are interested in to view the nutrient report. This provides you with detailed data, not only for vitamins and minerals, but also for individual fatty acids and amino acids.

## Vitamins and Minerals: Key Considerations

Ideally, you should receive all of the vitamins and minerals you need from the foods that you eat. But the sad reality is that even if you're eating organic or locally grown food, you may still fall short, especially if you are restricting total calories or if your food intake is low for other reasons. You need to either ensure your average nutrient intake is adequate by faithfully tracking everything you consume (with a tool like Cronometer) or take supplements—at least in the beginning as you are adjusting to so many other changes in your life.

Most vitamins serve critical roles in a variety of biological functions and activities. For example, B vitamins are cofactors in enzymatic reactions that support healthy metabolism and brain function; others, such as C and E, act as antioxidants. Vitamin D has an unusual structure that is similar to steroid hormones like estrogen, and in many ways it acts more like a hormone than a vitamin in the body.

If you find you are not getting all the nutrients you need from food, consider adding a good vitamin supplement, along with a few key minerals, to cover your bases. Thankfully, there are many good options available.

## Choosing Multivitamins and Minerals

When I work directly with clients, I dig into the specifics of their health history and food preferences to help me to individualize their plan and suggest supplements where needed. Here, however, I'm simply providing a broad overview. Do your homework and be sure to discuss your choices with your medical team. They may have reasons why they don't want you to take a certain supplement right now. I should also note that there are cancer researchers who believe that defective mitochondria in tumor cells benefit from supplemental vitamins. This is definitely something that needs research!

### Vitamin A

Vitamin A is recognized as an antioxidant. It is fat soluble, so there is a danger of toxicity if you consume too much preformed vitamin A, such as that found in liver and some fish oils, including cod liver oil. However, plant-based provitamin A is a precursor that does not carry this risk. Most multivitamins contain either provitamin A itself or provitamin A along with a low level of preformed vitamin. (There are many different vitamin A precursors, and to complicate matters further, dosages can be given in either micrograms [mcg] or international units [IU].)

### B Vitamins

You'll need to be careful here, as there are a lot of low-quality B vitamins in the marketplace. Pass over those and look for one that provides most of the B vitamins

## Niacin (Vitamin B$_3$): A Special Case

I am particularly interested in this vitamin because of its relationship to the coenzyme NAD$^+$, a molecule that is essential to the signaling and energy-production functions of every cell in your body. In fact, there is ongoing research looking at the role of NAD$^+$ in extending both healthspan and lifespan. Humans cannot benefit from directly ingesting NAD$^+$ but are reliant on sufficient intake of its precursors (of which niacin is one). Once consumed, these then undergo reactions that convert them to NAD$^+$. All multivitamins contain niacin, the *least* active of the B group and the furthest removed in the conversion process to NAD$^+$. Nicotinamide riboside, marketed as Niagen, is a more active form of the vitamin, but it is not yet known if this supplement has a downside in people with cancer.

in more bioavailable forms (for example, B$_{12}$ [cobalamin] as methylcobalamin or hydroxycobalamin instead of cyanocobalamin, and B$_9$ [folate] as methylfolate instead of folic acid). These forms may provide more benefit because they have already undergone some of the reactions that move them closer to their "active" forms. Caution: People with active cancer need to be mindful about the potential downside of hypermethylation. Consult with an integrative doctor before you decide to supplement with methylated forms of these vitamins.

### Vitamin C

It doesn't take much effort to meet the minimum requirement for vitamin C. In the past, I've recommended against taking oral vitamin C supplements because I believed they could interfere with ketosis. However, in my conversations with Dr. Jeanne Drisko at the University of Kansas Integrative Medical Center, I have learned that vitamin C (taken orally as ascorbic acid) will not raise blood glucose levels. But the controversy regarding the impact of vitamin C on glucose levels also reflects confusion between the effect of vitamin C taken orally and its effect when delivered intravenously, at a much higher concentration that can be consumed. Because the chemical structures of glucose and vitamin C are very similar, a home blood glucose meter will erroneously indicate a very high glucose level following an intravenous infusion of the vitamin. (Imagine your surprise at seeing glucose at 260 ml/dL or higher,

## A Word about Vitamin D

I've singled this vitamin out because almost everyone who doesn't supplement is deficient to some degree. Vitamin D is essential not only for bone health but also for immune modulation, which is so critical in cancer and most other chronic diseases. Unfortunately, most conventional health care practitioners don't yet understand how important it is to assess blood levels of this vitamin, and those that do may accept 30 ng/mL as an acceptable threshold. But this is far from optimal!

The RDA for vitamin D is quite low (600 to 800 IU, depending on age) and is met by almost all multivitamins, but this amount does not provide any real health benefit apart from preventing rickets in children. Food sources don't cover our needs either, and people routinely overestimate the amount of vitamin D synthesis from sun exposure (most of the United States is at too high a latitude to activate synthesis for a good part of the year). Other factors, such as darker skin color and advancing age, also lower the amount of vitamin D synthesis. Add to that the fact that most Americans block the sun's rays with sunscreen or UV-resistant clothing and it's no wonder that blood levels of vitamin D throughout this and most other developed countries are dismal.

A February 2016 fact sheet from the government Office of Dietary Supplements suggests that oral supplementation with 4,000 to 5,000 IU of vitamin $D_3$ (cholecalciferol) should be safe for most adults.[1] I suggest that you ask your provider to test your blood level of 25-hydroxyvitamin D (calcidiol, the prehormone form the vitamin takes following metabolism by the liver), then supplement accordingly. In my world, optimal calcidiol levels are thought to be in the range of 50 to 70 ng/mL, though government guidelines suggest keeping levels at or below 60 ng/mL. Depending on your age, skin color, and degree of sun exposure, maintaining those blood levels of calcidiol may require supplementation of anywhere from 2,000 to 5,000 IU of oral vitamin $D_3$ daily (taken at the same time as calcium- and magnesium-containing foods or supplements). Since vitamin D is fat-soluble, take it as a capsule suspended in oil (such as coconut oil). If your baseline levels are deficient (less than 20 ng/dL) or insufficient (less than 30 ng/dL), consider working with a doctor who can prescribe and monitor a therapeutic loading dose.

despite tight adherence to your plan!) This is simply an artifact of testing. In fact, home meters are routinely used as a quick check of vitamin C saturation following an intravenous treatment.

Intravenous infusions of vitamin C are sometimes recommended as a pro-oxidant cancer treatment, usually as an adjunct to conventional prooxidant therapies, such as radiation and some chemotherapy drugs. Prooxidative therapies exert their effect by creating intense oxidative stress that overwhelms dysfunctional cancer cells. If you are supplementing with high-dose *oral* vitamin C, it's likely because you've read that it has a powerful antioxidant effect. But despite extensive research, oral vitamin C supplementation has not been shown to improve outcomes in cancer. In fact, it could work against you. (This is the subject of much controversy and confusion, so it's good to understand the difference in action between oral and intravenous vitamin C.)

But that still leaves us with an unresolved issue: Is there a "safe" amount of oral vitamin C supplementation? I've posed that question to my colleagues, and the answer ranges from "no supplementation beyond food sources" to "it's likely safe to supplement up to bowel tolerance" (in other words, up to the dose that induces diarrhea). Ultimately, we may learn that, as is the case with most other therapies, the safe amount is likely to be situation-specific and vary greatly between individuals.

## Vitamin E

Vitamin E is actually made up of several plant-derived vitamins, some of which are potent antioxidants that help to protect the lipid component of cell membranes from oxidation. Only one form, alpha-tocopherol, is known to be necessary for human health, while others show good evidence of benefit even if they are not considered "essential." (Your oncologist may not want you taking this as an antioxidant supplement while you are receiving chemotherapy, so do check before adding this to your regimen.)

## Vitamin $K_2$

Vitamin $K_2$ is needed to move calcium from blood into bone. It can be derived either directly from the diet or by being converted in the body from vitamin $K_1$. As a supplement, it should be taken as menaquinone-7. Even if you are taking in enough $K_1$ through diet, that's no guarantee that you will convert it efficiently to $K_2$, and low levels of $K_2$ can negatively impact bone health. Fermented vegetables are a source of $K_2$ but you can't assess the dosage accurately. If you are on certain types of anticoagulant therapy (e.g., warfarin), you should adhere to any food or supplement advice from your medical team, as $K_2$ affects blood-clotting factors.

## What I Look for in a Multivitamin

When my clients ask me for a multivitamin recommendation, I do not recommend for or against supplementation as the research here does not conclusively show a benefit. However, if my client wants a general recommendation, I will share the following:

- I prefer multivitamins that only require a single capsule per day. Also, I don't want them to be loaded up with antioxidants that may be contraindicated for those in active treatment.
- No iron or copper—two minerals that can be problematic in cancer—unless of course your doctor prescribes iron for anemia.
- Also, there's no need for a multivitamin that includes the minerals calcium, magnesium, or potassium as these are rarely in the form or the amount that I would personally use.

What it *should* include, and which I find beneficial, are the following:

- microminerals (iodine, zinc, selenium, manganese, chromium, and molybdenum)
- reasonable amounts of good-quality B vitamins (including methylated $B_{12}$ and folate, unless those are contraindicated for your cancer)
- Vitamin $D_3$—most likely you will need to supplement with more than you will find in most multivitamins.
- $K_2$ as menaquinone-7, but this is rare in a multivitamin so you may need to supplement this separately.
- CoQ10 is not a vitamin but many multivitamin supplements include it—it is a powerful mitochondrial oxidant so check with your oncologist to be sure there are no contraindications for use.
- small amounts of other nutrients that are included to support eye or bone health

## Minerals

The supplementation of minerals deserves special attention. Some minerals function within the body as ions; that is, they carry an electrical charge, either positive or negative. These are known as electrolytes (chiefly calcium, chloride, magnesium, phosphate, potassium, and sodium). As ions, they are unstable, which gives their flux within the body a very powerful influence on many of our basic biochemical functions, such as transmitting nerve impulses throughout the body and brain. Our bodies generally do a great job in keeping electrolytes in the proper biochemical balance, but there are many possible disrupters. Any excessive loss of body fluids—whether from urination, sweating, vomiting, or diarrhea—can upset the balance, resulting in a host of issues. Dilution of their concentration, such as happens with overhydration, has its own special set of problems. Disruption in potassium levels, for instance, can cause heart palpitations or arrhythmias. Loss of magnesium may result in severe muscle cramping. Calcium balance is needed for neurotransmitters to function properly. Sodium imbalances cause fluid shifts that can either swell or dehydrate cells, undesirable in either case.

Each mineral can exist in many forms. For example, magnesium can be ionic or combined with other minerals, such as chloride, to form a more stable compound. It can also be chelated with amino acids, such as glycine or threonine, to form magnesium glycinate or threonate. The form that you consume as a supplement or in food makes a difference in how it's absorbed and what effect it has on your body. Again using magnesium as an example, magnesium oxide and hydroxide (and, to a lesser extent, magnesium citrate) draw water into the colon and can loosen stool to the point of causing diarrhea. In fact, I see this effect so often that I mention it to every new client. If you suffer from chronic constipation, however, you can use this to your advantage by adding one of these forms of magnesium (but don't count magnesium oxide / hydroxide as a supplement as this form is poorly absorbed).

The degree of absorption of a mineral into the body is widely variable among individuals. This is partly due to gut health, but also is a function of what else is being consumed at the same time. For example, soluble fiber supplements form a gel that can bind minerals and interfere with their absorption. This effect can be reduced by drinking extra water or by taking the fiber supplement at least an hour away from ingestion of the mineral supplement.

All of these factors, and more that I won't overwhelm you with here, are good reasons to choose the type and dosage of minerals carefully. Although I can offer a general guide, I certainly can't make specific recommendations as to what you should do. This is especially true if you have other conditions that affect mineral balance (such as high blood pressure being treated with potassium-sparing drugs). I strongly urge you to do your own research and then consult with your medical team or pharmacist.

## Calcium and Magnesium

Let me start by commenting on the RDA of these two critical minerals: In my opinion, the RDA for calcium is overstated and the RDA for magnesium is understated. Postmenopausal women, particularly those at risk for osteoporosis, are often told that they need to increase calcium intake through supplementation, without factoring in how much calcium they may already get from their diet. If you fit in this group and choose calcium-rich foods as well as act to enhance calcium's absorption from your intestine, then you may not need to supplement up to the recommended 1,000 to 1,200 mg a day. You also need to consider the source of your calcium supplement. Some elemental forms, like carbonate, may have high levels of lead. They can also neutralize stomach acid and contribute to constipation. I prefer using calcium citrate or gluconate. Absorption of calcium from supplements is not ideal, but even when there are sufficient blood levels, it is important to your health to move calcium from the bloodstream into cells and bone. (As noted earlier, that's vitamin $K_2$'s job.)

In those who do supplement, bone scans often show improvements in bone density. But bone density is no guarantee of better bone health. Women who supplement still suffer a high rate of bone fractures because their bones, though mineralized, are brittle. Too often the problem of bone density is viewed through a microscope (one tiny part) instead of as a panorama (the wider view).

Magnesium is crucial. Far too many people are deficient in this mineral through a combination of inadequate intake, poor absorption, and depletion. To add to the problem, an overwhelming majority of older adults and people receiving chemotherapy are placed on proton pump inhibitors, such as omeprazole (Prilosec), which are known to deplete magnesium stores, contributing to osteoporosis. Unfortunately, the problem is compounded by a generally poor understanding in conventional medicine of how much magnesium we actually need. Part of this is due to the fact that most health care practitioners test blood levels instead of tissue levels. A more robust test assesses red blood cell magnesium.

The ratio of calcium to magnesium is also very important. For now, aim to make your ratio fall between a 2:1 and 1:1 ratio, using calculations from foods and any supplements you may be using. (Note that you can easily track your dietary and supplement intake of these and all other nutrients with Cronometer.)

One last note: Clinical studies have thoroughly documented the fact that people with insulin resistance (a characteristic of type 2 diabetes) have too much calcium and too little magnesium in their cells. Interestingly, this is also attributed to "normal" aging.

# Choosing Calcium and Magnesium Supplements

Here are some things to keep in mind when choosing calcium and magnesium supplements.

CALCIUM BASICS:

Calcium carbonate is the least expensive form but reduces stomach acid, which interferes with digestion. And impaired digestion can interfere with the availability and absorption of vitamin $B_{12}$. The calcium carbonate from supplements (but not from foods) may increase the risk of cardiovascular disease by contributing to calcium buildup in blood vessels, especially at amounts more than double the magnesium intake. It's added to many products, such as antacids, orange juice ("calcium-fortified"), and even almond milk (if calcium is listed in the ingredients).

Calcium citrate is a good choice. You can buy it as a pill, but these are difficult for some people to swallow and may contain a lot of fillers. I prefer to use calcium citrate powder, which gives me the option to titrate my intake based on how much calcium I'm consuming from food. Consider supplementing with 200 to 250 mg twice a day, recognizing that you're likely to get another 400 to 600 mg from foods.

MAGNESIUM BASICS:

While magnesium enhances calcium absorption, the two minerals compete for the same sites. If you take magnesium with your calcium, don't take more than 200 mg of calcium per dose.

Be careful with magnesium oxide. You may use it if you need a stool softener, but it's poorly absorbed as a nutritional supplement.

Magnesium citrate is well absorbed and may also work as a gentle stool softener. Go easy on the dosage until you have an idea of bowel tolerance.

Some chelated forms are less likely to have as pronounced gastrointestinal effects. Glycinate is an inexpensive option. Threonate is pricier but may be better for the brain; it may also more readily cross the mitochondrial membrane.

Magnesium chloride (Slow-Mag) is yet another option (and the personal choice of researchers Jeff Volek and Stephen Phinney).

A liquid magnesium chloride supplement, ReMag, has been developed by Dr. Carolyn Dean. It has an odd salty taste, but I like the fact that it's ionic and very bioavailable.

Some people supplement further with transdermal magnesium, either through use of a magnesium chloride oil or cream, or as a magnesium sulfate soak with Epsom salts.

Magnesium can lower your blood pressure. Discuss the risks and benefits with your health care team.

Also, if you have a history of renal disease, it is essential that you consult with your renal specialist before adding a magnesium supplement.

### HOW TO INCLUDE CALCIUM AND MAGNESIUM IN YOUR KETO PLAN:

Calcium and magnesium supplements can usually be taken together at mealtimes, although magnesium citrate (or Natural Vitality's Calm) is usually taken close to bedtime.

Divide the dose to ensure better absorption. Follow the general guideline of balancing total supplemental calcium to magnesium in a 2:1 or 1:1 ratio. (If the balance is off, too much calcium may remain in circulation.)

Magnesium has statin-like actions without the adverse side effects. It may lower your blood pressure, which is not a problem if your pressure is normal or high. If you have low blood pressure, however, consult with your medical team first.

Note that many drugs, including proton pump inhibitors and some anticancer drugs, can deplete magnesium. This requires an even higher amount of supplementation.

### Potassium

The RDA for potassium is quite high, but there are many scenarios in which supplementation is not advised. Talk to your doctor before adding a supplement. If you have a personal or family history of kidney stones, ask your doctor about a prescription for a citric acid or potassium citrate supplement such as Polycitra-K, which is sometimes prescribed prophylactically.

## No Iron or Copper

Most people, even those without cancer and especially those who are past mid-life, may benefit by reducing their iron intake. Iron overload is a cancer promoter and has other negative health impacts as well. In addition to looking at red blood cell counts and hematocrit, all preventive exams should include a ferritin test. (I'll go into more detail later.) The exception is premenopausal women or people with anemia. These individuals need to discuss the risks and benefits of iron supplementation with their team.

Copper-rich foods are plentiful in this diet, so adding a supplement may create an unhealthy zinc to copper ratio (another built-in calculation tracked by Cronometer). Also, copper has been implicated as a possible cancer promoter, though this is not yet well established.

### Trace Minerals: Zinc and Selenium

These other important minerals, needed only in small amounts, can be obtained through either diet or supplementation. However, they both have a sweet spot: Too little is associated with poor immune function, but too much may be problematic as well, especially with cancer. Check all supplement labels to be sure you're not overdosing with these two minerals. (If you eat two or three Brazil nuts each day, then you are getting enough selenium through your diet.)

### Manganese, Cobalt, Chromium, and Molybdenum

Another trace mineral, manganese is essential for many biochemical processes. It's also important to bone health. There are a number of factors that either increase or decrease absorption, but they are not specific to cancer and are beyond the scope of this book. Cobalt, chromium, and molybdenum round out the list of trace minerals. You may find these listed among the nutrients in your multivitamin/mineral supplement, but true deficiency is rare and ideal levels have not yet been identified.

## Other Nutritional Supplements

There are a large number of other supplements that are promoted for general health or as specific interventions for cancer. I certainly can't adequately address all the questions and issues about them here, but some supplements stand out as they appear to offer true benefits to most people. I touch on those here.

## Fish or Krill Oil

Consider taking 1,000 to 2,000 mg of *purified* or molecularly distilled fish oil, or krill oil, with EPA/DHA (e.g., Nordic Naturals Ultimate Omega). Note, though, the omega-3s from fish or krill may have an anticoagulant effect. Talk to your doctor first if you have low platelets or a bleeding disorder. Also, it's standard to discontinue use at least two weeks before a scheduled surgery. Note that krill oil is derived from crustaceans, so people who are allergic to that class of foods should use fish oil instead.

## Oxaloacetate

Oxaloacetate is a compound that is part of the essential first step in the Krebs cycle. It is also important to the gluconeogenic pathway. There is preclinical mouse model research suggesting that supplementation may be beneficial in brain cancer but no conclusions can be drawn from this. I mention it here because you may see it included in some experimental protocols.

## CoQ10

This is also known as ubiquinone, or its reduced form, ubiquinol. Although there is no established RDA for CoQ10, it is on my short list for a number of reasons, particularly for general mitochondrial health. CoQ10 is a cellular antioxidant, but its primary purpose is to accept and then pass electrons from one complex to another in the electron transport chain. Ubiquinol, the reduced (in this case, that

### A Caveat about Supplemental Antioxidants

Supplemental antioxidants, including CoQ10, can potentially work against prooxidant therapies, either conventional (chemotherapy and radiation) or alternative (hyperbaric oxygen, intravenous vitamin C). Definitely talk to your health care team before including even small amounts of any antioxidant supplements.

means "better") form of CoQ10, has already accepted its maximum number of electrons, so its only job now is to pass them down the chain. Supplementation here appears to be especially important for those who are taking cholesterol-lowering statin drugs, as these are known to also lower your levels of CoQ10.

## L-lysine

Consider adding L-lysine, one of the essential amino acids, as a supplement. Although it's found in foods, there are many potential benefits to supplementation:

- Unlike most other amino acids, L-lysine cannot be converted to glucose by the liver. It's strictly a ketogenic amino acid.
- Lysine combines with methionine (another amino acid) to make carnitine, a compound that transports fatty acids across the mito-chondrial membrane. Normally, you consume enough carnitine in a few servings per week of meat, but levels can be low in people on a ketogenic diet since more carnitine is used to maintain those higher levels of fatty acid oxidation.
- Supplementing lysine to improve carnitine status is an interesting, though untested, theory.
- Lysine has antiviral activity that targets some herpes viruses. Almost all adults have had exposure at some point in their lives to herpes viruses, and many people take supplemental L-lysine to suppress virus reactivation. Some cancers (such as brain tumors) have a herpes viral component. Will lysine prove helpful? (Note: There is zero research here.)
- Lysine can greatly reduce the occurrence and duration of mouth sores. That was originally found to be true with sores due to the herpes virus, but now research is showing a benefit for chemothera-py-related mouth sores as well.
- Animal proteins are naturally high in lysine, but nuts are high in argi-nine. This can disrupt the lysine to arginine ratio. You might want to maintain a good ratio by timing your lysine supplement to coincide with a higher intake of nuts (including nut butters or flours).

Consider 1.5 to 3 grams per day, in a divided dose. I believe that it's best to take it with food rather than on its own. Most people take it in tablet form, but I prefer the powder. I mix it into a few ounces of water, add some powdered calcium citrate (my calcium supplement), and top it off with a splash of cream.

It tastes just like milk! Another bonus to this blend is that lysine improves the absorption of calcium from the intestines.[2]

## Boosting Ketosis

Ketone supplements come in a variety of forms, both as foods and as synthesized salts and esters. They do have a place in a ketogenic diet, but the research is thin when it comes to cancer. Dr. Dominic D'Agostino's lab at the University of South Florida has published research that points to a survival benefit using a specific class of ketone supplements combined with a ketogenic diet in a mouse model of metastatic breast cancer.[3]

### Coconut Oil: The Most Affordable and Least Engineered

Coconut oil is touted as a "ketone supplement," but it's important to examine that claim carefully. Coconut oil is a complex blend of saturated fatty acids; over 50 percent of them can be formally classified as medium-chain triglycerides (MCTs) of varying lengths:

- 6-carbon caproic acid (no dietary value and only a tiny amount present in coconut oil)
- 8-carbon caprylic acid (most readily converted to ketones)
- 10-carbon capric acid (also ketogenic)
- 12-carbon lauric acid (Lauric acid is known to have antibacterial, antifungal, and antiviral properties, so I give it a plus in that department; however, it is not as ketogenic as caprylic and capric acids.)

The most ketogenic of these are the caprylic and capric acids (referred to simply as C8 and C10) but they make up a relatively small percentage (approximately 14 percent) of all the MCTs in coconut oil. Let's look at the properties that distinguish coconut oil from its more sophisticated cousins:

- It is inexpensive and readily available.
- It is mildly ketogenic.
- It is solid at room temperature.
- It can be used as either a cold oil or a cooking oil (medium heat).
- It is well tolerated by most people, even those with a compromised gastrointestinal tract.
- There are no contraindications for light to moderate use.

- Good-quality oil has a light and very pleasant aroma.
- It has antimicrobial properties, a definite bonus!

Look for "virgin" and "cold-pressed" on the label. Skip past any that indicate that they've been refined. If it smells like chemicals instead of coconuts, return it and try a different brand. Mix it into nut butters, add it to shakes, or stir a spoonful into your coffee or tea. You can make delicious curries with coconut oil as well.

## MCT Oil: Coconut Oil's Fractionated First Cousin

Caprylic and capric acid are separated from the other fatty acids in coconut oil (or in red palm oil), usually through a process known as fractionation. MCT oil is considered a supplement, not a cooking oil. You won't find it in supermarkets; instead, look for it in specialty stores or online. Make sure you read the label: You want 100 percent MCT, not a blend of MCT with flavorings or sweeteners. These isolated oils have been used for decades to boost ketones in an MCT version of the ketogenic diet developed to treat pediatric epilepsy. Pure caprylic acid, the most ketogenic MCT, is available now from several sources.

## Why Is MCT Oil So Ketogenic?

MCTs (specifically capric and caprylic acid) bypass the normal pathway for fat digestion. They don't require enzymes or bile. Instead, they diffuse through the membranes of the small intestine, collect in capillaries, and are sent to the liver via the hepatic portal vein. (Since MCTs don't require bile for digestion, they may make your stool lighter in color.) Once in the liver, MCTs are converted to ketones and returned to the bloodstream for distribution throughout the body, including the brain and central nervous system.

The liver has a limit as to how much it can handle at any given time and this amount varies widely between individuals. Some people experience bloating and diarrhea after ingesting even small amounts. That's why it's important to start with a low dosage, such as a teaspoon per meal. Take note of your tolerance, and if you can, gradually increase the amount over time. If you experience gastrointestinal issues, back off to the previous dosage and hold it there for a day or two before attempting to increase it again. Eating it at the same time as a fatty food, such as avocado or nuts, can improve tolerance for some people.

Limit your daily dosage to a maximum of three to four tablespoons a day. Unlike fat or carbs that can be stored in the body as energy, ketones are "use it or lose it": Those that are not used for energy are excreted in the urine or lost through sweat or respiration. If you are unintentionally losing weight, or losing weight too rapidly, then I recommend that you only count the first two tablespoons as part of your fat intake for the day.

Recently, the popularity of these oils in low-carb and ketogenic diets has exploded, due in large part to Dave Asprey's promotion of Bulletproof coffee. Now, many people start their day by adding MCT oil and some combination of ghee, unsalted butter, or coconut oil to their morning cup of coffee. You can make up your own variations using other hot beverages as well. You can also add MCT oil to broths or use it as one of the oils in salad dressings. (I usually advise against using MCT close to bedtime, as it may stimulate brain activity. Although this is a positive daytime side effect, it can interfere with your sleep.)

A powdered form of MCT is now available. (Quest Nutrition makes one that consists of MCT oil bonded to soluble corn fiber.) I see this powder listed among the ingredients in proprietary ketone supplements (more on those later). The advantage of this powder over straight MCT oil is that the fiber allows it to be absorbed at multiple points along the digestive tract, which enhances tolerability and sustains the ketogenic effect. I use this powdered MCT in keto muffins and in crackers. You can also add it to shakes.

One important caveat here: I suggest cutting back on consumption of MCT oil if your liver function is compromised or your liver enzymes (ALT, AST) are extremely high (indicating damage to the liver). While MCT does not cause liver damage, your liver must do the job of converting it to ketones. If your

## A Closer Look at MCT Oil

MCT oil has some unique properties that (if well tolerated) make it an important part of a ketogenic diet:

- It is a liquid at room temperature and remains liquid even when refrigerated.
- It is a saturated fat, which means it is fairly resistant to oxidation (though it should be kept away from light and heat).
- MCT oil has no taste or odor, so you can take it straight from a spoon.
- MCTs help ease constipation.
- MCTs raise HDL (good) cholesterol.

liver is damaged, that puts an extra load on all of its other tasks, including detoxification, gluconeogenesis, and glycogen storage, as well as converting triglycerides into free fatty acids. Give it a much-needed break!

## Exogenous Ketones

Coconut oil and MCTs may soon be overshadowed by the proprietary blends of ketone salts and esters that are entering the market, collectively referred to as "exogenous ketones" (i.e., ingested, not made by the body). To date, these newcomers are marketed primarily as weight-loss supplements or as sports drinks that can improve athletic performance. But importantly, the anecdotal evidence supporting the use of ketone esters in neurodegenerative disease is compelling, and at the time of this writing, they may be entering the commercial market as a sports drink that (of course) will also be available to people who choose to supplement with ketones for other reasons.

One of many questions I have is, "Will these supplements prove to be useful adjuncts to anticancer treatments in which therapeutic ketosis is the goal?" In time, I believe that this question will be answered, but for now, their benefit is mostly speculative. We know from reports and n-of-1 studies that the rise in ketones seen with these supplements is greater in those people who are already in nutritional ketosis (defined by Drs. Jeff Volek and Stephen Phinney as blood levels of βHB in the range of 0.5 to 5.0 mmol/L). In people already following ketogenic diets, the addition of exogenous ketones may boost levels into what is believed to be a therapeutic zone for cancer (blood glucose levels in a 1:1 to 2:1 ratio with blood levels of βHB—Dr. Thomas Seyfried's work).[4] Although this appears to be the case in the mouse model of cancer studied by Dr. Dominic D'Agostino's lab at the University of South Florida, a similar beneficial effect in humans is still only speculative.[3]

These supplements may provide a potential benefit for people with liver damage who want to boost ketone levels without involving the liver. Whereas MCT oil must be converted to ketones by the liver, salts are simply digested, and the ketones are delivered directly into the bloodstream. Talk to your doctor about this option before making the decision to supplement and take the time to carefully read the supplement label and full list of ingredients; you will want to choose a product (and dosage) that is a good match for your needs. Feel free to ask questions through the company websites. This is a more reliable approach than depending on hearsay posted on online forums. (Also please verify that the company you choose has purity and potency tested by a third party.)

Don't misunderstand what I am saying here: I don't believe for a single moment that ketone supplements on their own can provide all of the benefits of adopting a low-carb or ketogenic diet. Remember that cancer thrives on glucose, insulin, acidic microenvironments, inflammation, and the disruption of normal cell signaling. Although exogenous ketones will make an impact here, most of the factors contributing to disease will not change significantly unless you also change what you eat. My hope is that in time ketone supplements will play a role in liberalizing the diet, allowing for greater intake of vegetables and small portions of fruit. There certainly is the potential for a therapeutic effect (for example, if ketone supplements can reduce inflammation, improve the GKI, or temporarily boost ketones just prior to receiving a metabolic therapy, such as hyperbaric oxygen), but we need research—in humans—to test these possibilities.

## Potential Issues with Ketone Supplements

I've seen clear cases of overuse of these products. *More* is not necessarily *better*, especially if you take more than the recommended amount in combination with caloric restriction. This can severely limit your intake of nutrients from whole foods and backfire miserably, placing you at risk of developing a whole crop of new issues, including nutritional deficiencies. Additionally, several exogenous ketone supplements are marketed primarily to enhance athletic performance or facilitate weight loss. As such, they may include ingredients that are problematic in a cancer diet. Read the labels carefully!

The upside: For many people, βHB salts (βHB compounded with one or more of the minerals sodium, calcium, magnesium, or potassium) may not only boost ketosis but also help maintain electrolyte balance. Check the label to see how much of each kind of mineral is present. There are a couple of restrictions: Potassium salts can be problematic for people taking potassium-sparing drugs (such as lisinopril or losartan), since the combination may raise serum levels of potassium too high. (If in doubt, have your potassium levels checked and interpreted by your doctor). In fact, you should first check with your doctor if you are in active treatment or taking any prescription medications.

Another valid concern is whether overconsumption of these salts is capable of pushing ketone levels high enough to induce metabolic acidosis. After all, there's no easy way for an individual to determine what his or her ketone levels are beyond a certain point: If blood ketone levels surpass 8 mmol/L, the meter readout simply flashes "High." My colleagues versed in the science of exogenous ketones believe that it is indeed possible to reach acidotic levels with ingestion of ketone *esters*, but gastrointestinal intolerance of ketone *salts* is likely to limit intake of these (too much will cause diarrhea). Another biological safety net is that your body will excrete excess ketones in the urine, and this should help keep levels in check, especially if you stay well hydrated.

Finally, I have read a few heated exchanges about whether or not "racemic" ketone bodies in these new proprietary blends have a downside, at least in some scenarios. "Racemic" refers to both the form of βHB that our bodies synthesize (the D- form) along with its mirror image (the L- form), which is not metabolized in the mitochondria's ketogenic pathway. Instead, L-beta-hydroxybutyrate is oxidized as a fatty acid within the mitochondria. At present, home meters do not test for levels of L-beta-hydroxybutyrate, so if you are using racemic ketone supplements, your total ketone levels will actually be higher than what is shown on your meter. At what point might this pose a risk? Again, I would expect—but can't assume—that your body will excrete any excess ketones. I've listened to the debate on both sides of this issue, and I agree with Dr. Dominic D'Agostino's position that arguments against the use of racemic ketone supplements at present represent opinions, not research. Stay tuned!

## Prioritize Your Gut Health

We have evolved along with our gut microbiome, the collection of microorganisms that literally lead a life of their own, protecting their self-interests while serving ours as well. In fact, without a dense and healthy population of gut bacteria, our bodies are limited in their ability to kill pathogens that enter through the gastrointestinal tract, break down foods and fiber, and produce the vitamins, such as $B_{12}$ and $K_2$, that help maintain our body's functions and tissues. But only recently have we gained a deeper understanding of the complexities of this symbiotic relationship. Poor gut health is linked to more chronic diseases than I care to list, and there is an emerging body of evidence suggesting that a healthy microbiome is important to brain health as well. (For a deep dive here, read Dr. David Perlmutter's *Brain Maker*.)

If you have cancer, you can expect to experience a major disruption of your gut microbiome as a side effect of conventional treatments (chemotherapy, antibiotics, proton pump inhibitors, just to name a few). Your conventional oncology team can't offer you support—not because they don't want to, simply because they have no understanding of the problem or the solution. That means you'll need extra vigilance here. I include a few general suggestions below, but the best tip I can offer is to seek advice and support from a naturopathic integrative oncology specialist who can assess and address your unique situation.

## My N-of-1 Experience with Exogenous Ketones

I've tried many forms of exogenous ketones, including 1,3-butane-diol, βHB salts (both liquid and powdered), and an ester that may be coming to market if the developers can mass-produce it at a reasonable cost. The 1,3-butanediol, an alcohol, is harsh (and generally not available for purchase), but it does raise my ketones (by about 0.5 to 1 mmol/L at 40 minutes, depending on dosage). The liquid form of the salts was too caustic for my digestion, even if I diluted it with an acid, such as lemon. I've also tried powdered supplements from two of the leading suppliers (Kegenix and Pruvit). The ones I tried are a combination of βHB salts (sodium, calcium, magnesium, and potassium) together with MCT oil or MCT powder. These are very tolerable, and in the current formulation they provide not only βHB salts, but also ketogenic amino acids. They also raise my blood ketone levels by about 0.5 mmol/L even though I've chosen to limit my current use to one-quarter of a suggested serving at any given time.

I tested each of these exogenous ketone products prior to a hike, sticking to the same route and distance each time. They all seem to make a slight difference in my energy level and endurance, but I can't say for certain just how much of that can be attributed to the supplement as opposed to other variables, such as air temperature or the quality of my prior night's sleep.

I've also sampled a pre-market ketone ester. I did note a much more substantial bump in ketones (to over 4 mmol/L when taken at the full dosage), but not much change in overall energy. Interestingly, though, I did experience a very noticeable improvement in my vision; this was reported by a few others in my circle as well. (I have yet to

## Prebiotics and Probiotics

You might already understand the distinction between prebiotics and probiotics. If so, that's great. If not, here's a quick primer.

Prebiotics are fermentation by-products produced by allowing certain species of bacteria (usually lactobacilli) to "digest" the sugar in foods, such take a full dose of any of the other supplements, so I can't say if they would improve visual clarity as well.)

Moving beyond experimentation, I've found a few great applications that work for me personally:

- I'm a stress non-eater. When I'm under pressure, such as working on a presentation or under the gun to meet a deadline, I seldom take the time to eat a proper meal. In fact, I honestly can't eat. But I can drink a tasty beverage instead, so for me personally this is a great option.
- Exogenous ketones most definitely give me a brain boost, above and beyond what I already enjoy from staying in nutritional ketosis. Recently, I've begun timing my drink to fill in the brain energy gaps when I'm intent on my work.
- When I work out, I add one-quarter of a package of ketone salts to my water, along with 5 grams of BCAAs. I drink this *before* and *during* my strength training. (Yes, you *can* build muscle mass, even as an older adult!) Remember, this is my n-of-1. You may do better with more (or less).
- I now bring packets of these salts with me when I travel. It's so simple to add them to my water bottle, and they help provide the energy I need to slog through airports and deal with changes in routine forced on me by travel commitments and time zone changes.

It's clear that ketone supplements are here to stay. Over time, they will become more refined and perhaps more targeted to uses beyond fitness training and weight loss. I see this happening already in the athletic performance world where a ketone ester has been used by ultra-athletes, with promising results.[5] I hope to see similar funding for research specific to cancer.

as cabbage. In this process, the bacteria that live on the cabbage feed on the sugars found there. Then, when you eat unpasteurized fermented cabbage (sauerkraut and kimchi), you populate your gut with these friendly and beneficial bacteria, which help crowd out the less beneficial species that also live there. These "good" bacteria continue to thrive by fermenting the sugars in the soluble fiber found in your foods and supplements. The waste product of this fermentation includes short-chain fatty acids, such as butyrate, that nourish the colonocytes, the cells that line your colon. Healthy cells thrive on butyrate; cancer cells prefer glucose. Hmmm. . . . (If you need a refresher on fiber, refer back to chapter 12, "The Scoop on Fiber," page 213. If you want to dive deeper into the science regarding your body's microbiomes, read Ed Yong's *I Contain Multitudes*.)

In most circumstances, eating lacto-fermented foods, like sauerkraut and kimchi, is an excellent way to keep your gut's microbiome humming along, especially if you've experienced a major disruption. (Honestly, who among us has never taken antibiotics or suffered an intestinal flu?) Food allergies and sensitivities also have ramifications, and if you are currently receiving chemotherapy, that's a virtual guarantee that your intestinal lining is taking a huge hit. Sauerkraut may help restore the beneficial microorganisms. There are other health benefits of probiotics as well, along with some evidence of an anticancer effect. (Note: If you respond poorly to fermented foods, you may have FODMAP issues, histamine intolerance, or small intestinal bacterial overgrowth (SIBO). These issues need to be addressed by an experienced naturopath or integrative medicine doctor.)

Probiotics, traditionally taken in capsule form, provide your gut with basic lactobacilli and bifidobacteria species of beneficial bacteria. These support the growth of good bacteria while suppressing overgrowth of pathogenic bacteria, such as *Clostridium difficile*. There is also growing evidence that *Lactobacillus acidophilus* (the species found in most yogurt and in Floragen) nourishes healthy vaginal bacteria, which in turn keep vaginal pH in a better range. This can lower the risk for infections experienced by many postmenopausal women.

There is an ever-expanding number of probiotic options, offering a wide range of lactobacilli, bifidobacteria, streptococci, and saccharomyces species. My recommendation is to research which combination will best address your specific issues—such as histamine intolerance—and then acquire them from a reputable supplier. (Be aware that some cancer drug protocols weaken the immune system to the extent that a probiotic might not be advisable. Please check first with your oncology team.)

## Digestive Enzymes

Some people following a ketogenic diet benefit by using digestive enzymes. High-lipase options, such as Pure Encapsulations Pancreatic Enzymes, can certainly help with fat digestion. They also contain proteases, which aid in protein digestion. Non-GMO sunflower lecithin can also aid in fat digestion, plus there is the added benefit of the phospholipids, which appear to benefit brain health.

## Herbs and Botanicals

Botanicals have potent medicinal effects. In fact, several widely used chemo drugs are derived from botanicals. The vinca alkaloid drug vincristine, which disrupts cell cycles in cancer, is derived from a member of the periwinkle family. Another common chemotherapy drug, paclitaxel (Taxol), was refined from the bark of the Pacific yew tree. So when someone tells me that they want to use botanicals instead of drugs, I remind them that botanicals *are* drugs and as such they need to proceed as carefully as they would with any new medication. It's important to understand that just because a drug is closer to its "natural" form, it doesn't mean that it will work better or be less toxic. (And, of course, there's the issue of purity and potency in using natural versus FDA-approved drugs.)

In conventional medicine, you have access to health care practitioners and pharmacists who understand the biochemical pathways of prescribed medications. They also have data regarding various routes of introducing the drug (oral, extended release oral, injection, and IV). They can access information on common and rare side effects, half-life, common dosages, contraindications to its use, potential interactions with other drugs, and how the drug is cleared or detoxified by the liver.

This body of knowledge is not as well defined in the alternative world, and there are few professionals that you can rely on for this kind of information. I know many excellent integrative and naturopathic doctors who do possess the skill, but it is extremely challenging for a layperson to discern the difference between a practitioner who really has a grasp on this and one who may hold the same certifications but hasn't a clue or, worse yet, offers alternative protocols based solely on a profit motive. Buyer beware.

Lack of professional oversight is a huge problem when it comes to botanicals. This is true not only in cancer, but also with herbals used to treat other acute diseases. But keep in mind that even the best-qualified herbalists can't guarantee that your body will respond positively to a given substance any more than your conventional doctor can predict who will or won't respond to a given drug. Potential issues with botanicals to keep in mind are as follows:

- adverse side effects (including liver toxicity, lowered blood counts, and bruising—either from megadoses or from the synergistic effect of combining supplements that have an anticoagulant effect)

- exacerbation of autoimmune disorders
- cross-reactions tied to allergies or sensitivities, including environmental allergens
- contraindications that have yet to be identified
- drug–herb or herb–herb interactions
- questionable purity and potency (look for suppliers that offer third-party testing or genetically test their products)
- questionable or missing dosage recommendations
- contamination with heavy metals or other toxins
- antioxidants that negate the effects of prooxidant therapies

Resist the urge to pile on supplements just because you read a testimonial claiming that it cured someone's cancer, or a marketing piece claiming that it was used in a "clinical trial" (multiple interpretations of that). If you are reading research literature, make sure it's peer-reviewed and published in a reputable journal. It's becoming more common for charlatans to self-publish promotional materials and then claim they have "published research" to support the benefits of their product.

Now let me climb down from my soapbox and share a summary of just a few (of many) botanicals with good science behind them.

### Boswellia

Research shows that boswellia (frankincense) reduces vasogenic edema associated with radiation therapy for brain tumors.[6] It may also limit brain metastases in some cancers, such as breast cancer.[7] Choose your source carefully to ensure purity and potency.

### Melatonin

Melatonin is a pineal gland hormone that also acts as an aromatase inhibitor, similarly to some standard chemotherapy drugs used to treat certain types of breast and ovarian cancers.[8,9] It may also slow disease progression in other cancers as well.[10] Note that the *pharmacological* (drug) dose is much higher than the *physiological* (hormone replacement) dose (20 to 40 mg compared to 1 to 5 mg). Melatonin is contraindicated in people with lupus or other autoimmune disorders. Discuss the risks and benefits with your health care team.

### Turmeric/curcumin

Studies too numerous to cite here have proven time and again that turmeric and curcumin (a substance in turmeric) have anti-inflammatory and/or anticancer effects. Caution, though, as many formulations are not as pure or potent as advertised. Much of what is available, especially budget brands, is poorly absorbed. The brands Meriva and Theracurmin have both been used in research, so these may be your best options. If you prefer to derive your turmeric from foods (such as turmeric root or powder), add some pepper to increase bioavailability. Curry contains both turmeric and pepper.

## Cannabinoids

Although cannabinoids (CBD) from marijuana are not legal in many states, CBD from hemp is readily available. Both types are used to alleviate pain and ameliorate side effects of cancer and cancer treatment, including loss of appetite.[11] CBD might also improve seizure control in people with brain cancer. Some also appear to have a direct anticancer effect, at least in animal models. But at the time of this writing, only one trial in the United States (dexanabinol in patients with brain cancer) is looking at their effect in humans, and this trial is not yet recruiting participants.[12] Unfortunately, all marijuana extracts are Schedule I drugs in the United States, which has stalled research that could identify both the benefits and risks.

## Berberine

Berberine is well known for its potent glucose-lowering effects. It increases activity in the AMPK pathway, which in turn alters cellular signaling related to energy balance. One of the major actions of this enzyme is to suppress

## Do More Research

These are just a few of the public databases offering online information about a limited number of supplements.

- NIH Dietary Supplement Fact Sheets[13]
- Memorial Sloan Kettering Cancer Center[14]
- WebMD[15]

And, as I've mentioned before, I highly recommend Dr. Nasha Winters and Jess Higgins Kelley's book, *The Metabolic Approach to Cancer*. Some of these supplements are included in the discussion.

gluconeogenesis while increasing hepatic fatty acid oxidation and ketogenesis. It is also involved in mitochondrial biogenesis. But there are some notable side effects and contraindications to this botanical, so be sure to check the databases listed below. Also, ask your medical team for advice, especially regarding its potential to interact with other botanicals or medications.

## The Case against Antioxidant Supplements during Active Treatment

The use (or, should I say, overuse) of antioxidants is a controversial topic in oncology. Generally, I stay out of the fray, as this discussion does not relate directly to a ketogenic diet. That said, it is absolutely necessary that you understand the potential pitfalls with supplementation, as there is a veritable mountain of information on antioxidants, and at every turn an overwhelming set of diverse opinions, conflicting advice, and compelling testimonials. My intent here is to lightly touch on a very few but nonetheless significant points that I feel are especially important to people with cancer.

It's a fact that antioxidants help protect cells by scavenging and inactivating free radicals (unpaired electrons) while also facilitating needed repairs to damaged DNA. Certain radicals and certain vitamins (A, C, and E) are essential to this process, supported by a dizzying array of other vitamins, minerals, cofactors, and enzymes as well as other constituents either found in foods or synthesized within the body. This scavenging of free radicals is active in our bodies every second of our lives. Without it, we wouldn't survive.

Environmental factors, such as radon and cigarette smoke, can contribute to the production of excessive free radicals and resulting oxidative stress. Cellular metabolism also creates free radicals by mixing nutrients with oxygen carried by red blood cells. However, under normal conditions, this is quickly diffused by antioxidants made within the cell. Cellular protection and repair are part of any living organism's adaptation to the environment. So is apoptosis, the process by which a diseased cell identifies itself as damaged beyond repair and voluntarily triggers cell suicide.

Cells have multiple antioxidant pathways. Some protect the cytoplasm or nucleus, while others are specific to the mitochondria. Antioxidant therapy, properly applied, may help protect normal cells during conditions that are known to produce high levels of oxidative stress or when cells become less able to diffuse what was once considered normal—one of the declines in cellular activity commonly associated with aging. Given this knowledge, doesn't it seem logical to supplement with antioxidants? For example, we know that

CoQ10 acts as an antioxidant and, among other effects, may protect cardiac tissue from the oxidative stress associated with some chemotherapy drugs.

But here's the dilemma: Cancer is a "game changer." In other words, changes you make to your diet or environment that might have lowered your risk of developing cancer (i.e., prevention) may actually interfere with your response to treatment.

Please understand that I'm not singling out CoQ10! Instead, I'm shining a light on the conflicting messages you may hear regarding antioxidant *supplementation*. Note that I stress *supplementation*, as I want to be clear that I do believe that *foods* containing antioxidants and other cancer-fighting compounds definitely have a role to play in ketogenic metabolic therapy. An oncologist who states that "diet doesn't matter; eat what you want" should have no problem with your choice of foods, but across the hall may be a doctor in the same practice who is so concerned about the possible impact of antioxidants that you are instructed to refrain from eating a handful of blueberries or drinking a cup of green tea. So even when you seek medical advice, don't expect consensus between members of your team.

Frankly, you're between a rock and a hard place, and you have to choose what you believe to be the right path for you. If you commit to the standard protocols, understand that supplementing with antioxidants (particularly high-dose oral vitamin C, glutathione, vitamin E, selenium, and especially n-acetyl-cysteine) may jeopardize your chances for the best outcome that conventional medicine can offer. On the other hand, if you do nothing to protect yourself from the ravages of toxic therapies, you may find yourself cancer-free and thinking, "This isn't how I wanted to spend my golden years."

To add to the confusion, there is also some evidence that a supplement that might benefit one person may fuel another's cancer. For example, look at the increased risk of lung cancer in smokers who supplement with beta-carotene (the pre-vitamin found in deeply pigmented foods, such as carrots, beets, and spinach). What's happening there? Are these supplemental antioxidants actually rescuing as-yet undetected cancer cells, allowing them to slip past cell surveillance that would normally lead to apoptosis? Or is it possible that factors other than chemotherapy, such as certain prescription medications unrelated to smoking, are what contribute to the higher risk of cancer seen in the smokers? In any scenario, this reminds us that antioxidant supplements cannot be viewed as a "Do no harm" therapy. The following abstract from a group of USDA researchers summarizes the possible health consequences of supplemental antioxidants:

Antioxidant foods and ingredients are an important component of the food industry. In the past, antioxidants were used primarily

## The Acid/Alkaline Debate

I mentioned this debate briefly in chapter 6 ("Comparing Keto to Other 'Anticancer' Diets," page 81). Let's dive a little deeper here.

The acid/alkaline diet debate arises from misinterpretation and oversimplification of the science linking pH to cancer, which in turn has led many people to the erroneous conclusion that manipulating the alkalinity of their diet will prevent or reverse the disease. I wish it were that easy, but food and water alone can't accomplish this at the cellular level.

### MISCONCEPTION #1: CERTAIN FOODS, ESPECIALLY RED MEAT, MAKE THE BODY TOO ACIDIC.

Food can significantly alter urine pH, but this alone does not promote cancer.[16] In fact, urine pH has no impact on blood pH or on the acidity of the tumor microenvironment (a known cancer promoter). Acidic urine may increase the risk of kidney stones, but does not promote cancer.[17] Your blood and body pH are under tight internal controls that are not altered by diet. This is crucial given that the processes that support life can only occur within a narrow pH range. If you are still uncomfortable with the idea of acidic urine, you can opt for these keto-friendly foods that can make your urine slightly more alkaline:

> **Vegetables:** Asparagus, celery, chard, collard greens, cruciferous vegetables, cucumbers, eggplant, garlic, lettuce, mustard greens, onions, parsley, parsnips, peppers, pumpkin, sprouts, turnips
> **Fats:** Avocados, flaxseed oil, olives
> Lemon and vinegar, although acidic, produce alkaline ash.

### MISCONCEPTION #2: YOU NEED TO PURCHASE A TOP-OF-THE-LINE WATER ALKALIZER AND/OR IONIZER.

Good clean water free of viruses, bacteria, pharmaceuticals, heavy metals, and other contaminants is much more important than the alkalinity. You can accomplish this with a variety of inexpensive water filters. In fact, expensive alkalizers may do more harm than good by removing minerals from the water that your body uses to buffer acids.

The cancer and pH connection is not about water, but instead is tied to the acidification of the tumor microenvironment: that is, the acidity that tumors create in their immediate environment through an increase in fermentation of glucose. Lactic acid, the by-product of glucose fermentation, is pushed out of the cells. One of the potential benefits of a ketogenic metabolic therapy is that it disrupts this excessive fermentation. (Note that this elimination of lactic acid from cells is not the cause of lactic acidosis, a life-threatening medical condition.)

Actions that raise pH (alkalinize) the microenvironment may alter disease progression. Interestingly, there have been a few studies using a mouse model of metastatic breast cancer that showed reductions in the number and volume of metastases from something as simple as adding sodium bicarbonate (baking soda) to the diet.[18,19] However, more research is needed to confirm that this effect would be true in humans as well (and to arrive at the ideal dosage and timing).

My colleague William LaValley, MD, provided a compelling contribution to this debate that is so clear and well grounded that I've chosen to include it here verbatim (from an email exchange in April 2017):

A basic understanding of pH in the body is required to debunk the fuzzy-thinking assertions of this diet. The variability of pH within cells, within cellular organelles, within organs, within "compartments" in the body is widely flexible, dynamic, and in constant finely managed perturbations. The idea that a range of foods can induce overall alkalinity or acidity throughout the body—and can be identified by pH strip readings of urine and saliva is not rational. I think of a metaphor about weather that is just as irrational: like saying that measuring rain or wind speed at the shore of the Pacific Ocean in San Diego and the Atlantic Ocean in Boston can tell you about the weather in all the locations in between. pH is tightly regulated in each of the cellular compartments and in each organ. While dietary intake can change the pH in the stomach (temporarily), gastrointestinal tract (temporarily), and GU tract (temporarily) due to normal metabolic activity, the assertion that such a diet with a specific list of foods is an alkaline-producing anti-cancer diet is illogical and confuses causation and attribution of observable effects.

to control oxidation and retard spoilage, but today many are used because of putative health benefits. However, the traditional message that oxidative stress, which involves the production of reactive oxygen species (ROS), is the basis for chronic diseases and aging is being reexamined. Accumulating evidence suggests that ROS exert essential metabolic functions and that removal of too many ROS can upset cell signaling pathways and actually increase the risk of chronic disease. It is imperative that the food industry be aware of progress in this field to present the science relative to foods in a forthright and clear manner. This may mean reexamining the health implications of adding large amounts of antioxidants to foods.[20]

The bottom line: Although there is evidence that antioxidants may be problematic in cancer, there is no consensus on the science. Time and research may uncover some general truths but that will still leave plenty of gray area requiring individualization due to an overwhelming number of variables. If you decide to include antioxidant supplements, please work closely with the best integrative specialist you can find. Most likely, this will be an integrative or functional medicine doctor or a naturopathic doctor (ND) who specializes in integrative oncology.

# CHAPTER 15

# Other Health Challenges and Keto

I've learned a tremendous amount by listening to my clients' stories and observing the challenges they face. I've also learned a great deal by working through the process with health care practitioners who want to offer the ketogenic diet as an adjunct therapy for their patients. Thankfully, not everyone experiences unwanted side effects. But you may be among the many people who have layered on other health challenges over decades and need more tools to help you to integrate ketogenic metabolic therapy into your personalized treatment plan.

If you are already receiving conventional therapy, make your concerns known to your team even if you fear sounding "weak" or "whiny." Negative self-talk has no place here and will keep you from getting the support you need. But understand that many oncologists rely primarily on lab tests and scans for their assessment of how well you are responding clinically to therapy without acknowledging broader quality-of-life issues unless you bring them up. Remember that oncology nurses are an integral part of your team and are skilled at working through some of the more familiar health-related issues. They can also help you to identify issues that need to be addressed by your oncologist or another health care professional.

## Poor Appetite, Impaired Digestion, and Malabsorption

Whether I'm speaking to health care practitioners or new clients, I always stress the need to be proactive with workarounds to address the gastrointestinal side effects of the standard-of-care cancer treatments. Some of these are quite easy to implement, such as staying well hydrated and keeping electrolytes in balance with salted bone broth; but others are far more complex and require a team approach. Unfortunately, when it comes to dietary advice, your conventional team is most likely to offer you a conventional solution: Avoid fatty foods in favor of consuming easily digestible carbohydrates in the form of sugars and starches. In fact, many chemotherapy infusion centers stock their refrigerators with Ensure and Boost. Obviously, this runs counter to a ketogenic plan!

I wish I could offer you a one-size-fits-all solution to these issues, but that is simply not possible. Instead, let me stress how important it is to have a general practitioner, internist, or integrative oncology specialist who can problem-solve your particular set of challenges with you. This may be as simple as a change in medication type or dosage used to treat a chronic disease, such as diabetes or high blood pressure. They may also suggest alternative therapies, such as acupuncture, to help alleviate symptoms.

## Constipation

Constipation merits its own discussion here as it is a common problem even in those who are cancer-free and following conventional diets. Tune in to any national news program, and you are bound to see at least one advertisement for a prescription or over-the-counter treatment for constipation. According to the Mayo Clinic's website (www.MayoClinic.org),[1] risk factors include:

- age (Constipation is more common in older adults.)
- gender (Women experience more constipation than men.)
- dehydration
- inadequate fiber intake
- lack of physical activity
- certain medications, including sedatives, narcotics, or medications to lower blood pressure

Constipation can become more of an issue when you are receiving chemotherapy. Both the chemotherapy drugs themselves and the medications used to treat side effects often contribute to the problem. For example, anti-nausea medications, though very effective in controlling nausea and vomiting, often list constipation as one of the most common side effects. Without a doubt, though, the most intractable constipation is associated with opioid use. Pain medications, such as hydrocodone and morphine, slow gastrointestinal motility and interfere with peristalsis. Resulting constipation is a medical problem that often requires stool softening and peristalsis-inducing treatments. Note that it is potentially dangerous to add fiber or other bulking agents to your diet to counter opiate-induced constipation, as this can lead to bowel obstruction from fecal impaction. Remember those commercials I mentioned? One now directs the viewer to "ask your doctor" about a new prescription drug for opiate-induced constipation (of course this has its own set of side effects).

Medications aside, you are likely to notice a change in bowel habits once you begin a ketogenic diet, notably that you may no longer experience daily regularity. This is not true constipation unless you are straining to pass hard, dry stool, and regularity may return once you are up and running with your new plan. For now, your goal is to keep your stool "comfortably soft" so you are not straining. Ways to address the problem include:

- Drink plenty of water and other no-carb fluids! Add a cup or two of salted broth.
- Choose keto-friendly foods that have a laxative effect, such as avocados, aloe vera juice, and MCT oil.
- Lightly wilt spinach or sauté greens over medium heat using olive or avocado oil (or an animal fat such as bacon grease). This can have a laxative effect.
- Add fiber-rich foods.
- Improve your gut's microbiome by using pre- and probiotics. (If you are in active treatment or know that you are immune-compromised, you need to consult with your health care team prior to adding these.)
- Switch from calcium carbonate to calcium citrate. Read product ingredient lists carefully for the type of calcium they contain; as an example, most boxed almond milk contains up to a third of the RDA for calcium, but it's in the form of supplemental calcium carbonate.
- Consider using milk of magnesia, magnesium oxide, magnesium citrate, or a proprietary magnesium blend. Adjust the dosage to achieve a comfortably soft stool without diarrhea. (If you have pre-existing renal disease, don't take magnesium without talking to your doctor first.)
- Drink a cup of senna tea. (This is not advised for women who are pregnant or lactating or for those with certain bowel diseases, electrolyte imbalances, or heart disease; be sure to check with your medical team first.)
- If possible, get regular exercise, such as walking, that gently works your abdominal muscles.
- Change the way you use your toilet so that you are squatting rather than sitting. This can be as simple as keeping a footstool near the toilet.[2] Squatting is our evolutionary default for elimination; if you

need convincing, talk to anyone who's spent time in the backcoun-
try—or just watch the way that dogs relieve themselves!

- For the more adventurous, you can also self-apply perineal acupres-
sure to improve rectal tone and bowel function. It's important here
to receive instruction on proper technique.[3]

Notice that I didn't include enemas on this list. If you resort to enemas to
relieve constipation, do so only when necessary and under the most sterile
conditions possible. There is significant evidence that enemas can rupture
the colon wall and/or introduce unwanted pathogens into your body.[4] Frequent use of enemas may also reduce colonies of beneficial bacteria and
deplete electrolytes. Regarding the belief that a coffee enema will flush toxins by stimulating dilation of the bile duct, I have yet to see any convincing
evidence of this.

## Issues with Liver Function

Your liver is the primary site of ketone production, which makes it a key player
in a ketogenic metabolic therapy. Your liver is also responsible for a dizzying
array of other functions, such as maintaining glucose homeostasis and recycling metabolic waste (i.e., glycerol and lactate). It detoxifies oral medications,
including botanicals, as they take a "first pass" through this organ. Unfortunately, all these activities also mean that the liver is vulnerable to many kinds
of insults, including:

- primary liver cancers
- cancers that have metastasized to the liver
- toxicity from chemo drugs and medications used to treat side effects
  of these drugs
- toxicity from medications such as statins or acetaminophen overdose
- too much of the wrong kind of vitamin A
- megadoses of some botanicals or combinations of botanicals
- viral hepatitis and other diseases (both viral and autoimmune) that
  cause liver inflammation
- hemochromatosis (a genetic disease that causes an overload of iron
  in the blood)
- pancreatitis
- alcohol (primarily as cirrhosis and fatty liver disease)
- fructose (by contributing to non-alcoholic fatty liver disease)

When I'm assessing whether or not someone is a good candidate for the ketogenic diet, I always look for a major red flag: elevated liver enzymes. These appear on a blood test as alanine transaminase (ALT), aspartate transaminase (AST), and alkaline phosphatase (alk phos). A slight elevation above the normal range is common and not usually a concern, but it does mean that you need to keep a close eye on any changes in these values over time. This is easily accomplished since most oncology protocols call for the routine evaluation of liver enzymes.

Other tests are also used to assess liver function, including the level of serum albumin. Albumin is a protein produced in the liver that the body requires to help transport drugs, vitamins, hormones, and other substances throughout the body. Low albumin levels are common in cancer due in part to the fact that so many substances compete with one another for transport. Low albumin may also be an indication of poor nutritional status, including cancer cachexia. This is yet another reason to have medical oversight, even if your team is not supportive of your diet or other choices in treatment. (You can learn more about your blood test results from https://LabTestsOnline.org.[5])

Be advised that your nutritionist is *not* the person who should determine whether your lab test results mean that you shouldn't move forward with the diet. Although I ask about "red flags," this is only so that I can redirect people back to their medical teams if I run across any of the issues I've described. Unfortunately, too few health care practitioners understand the ketogenic diet, so asking them for advice about its effect on your liver may not be very helpful to you unless they express concerns about liver failure. That puts the decision back in your lap. If you want to move forward with the diet at that point, please work with an integrative oncologist, especially if you plan to add herbals and

## The Ketogenic Diet Does Not Cause Liver Damage

While this statement is true, you may not be able to reach therapeutic ketosis if you already have liver damage. Ketone supplements may prove beneficial here. MCT oil, however, is not a good choice as it needs to be converted to ketones in the liver. While some of the newer ketone products, such as ketone salts and esters, do not need any action by the liver, remember that's no guarantee that they are safe for you to use under all conditions.

botanicals that have potential adverse effects on your liver. And don't count on "liver flushes," including coffee enemas, to help restore your liver to health. You're better off simply drinking your coffee!

## Pancreatic Structure and Function

There is a common but misplaced belief that individuals with pancreatic cancer are not good candidates for a ketogenic diet. This belief stems from the fact that pancreatic cancer, along with colon cancer, can quickly progress to cancer cachexia *Please note: If you are already experiencing refractory (late-stage) cachexia, you cannot begin the diet without intense medical management from a keto-savvy team.* Unfortunately, I have few resources (other than ketone supplements) to offer at this time, but research is ongoing, so check my website for updates as more information becomes available.

### Cleve's Pancreatic Cancer Success Story

My first client with pancreatic cancer was one of my beloved cousins. Cleve had been aware of symptoms for months, but initially didn't take any action to identify what was causing them. By the time he received a diagnosis, the cancer had metastasized and was inoperable. He was told that he had only six to nine months to live if he opted for treatment with chemotherapy (which he did). But he also asked me for help because he'd seen for himself what the ketogenic diet had done for my son, Raffi. Honestly, what did Cleve have to lose? His appetite was good and his other health issues were minor, even though he was 78 years old at the time. In the past he'd followed the Atkins diet for weight loss and was hopeful that a simple change in diet might allow him to retain a decent quality of life. He opted for Modified Atkins.

Cleve did amazingly well while combining his Modified Atkins plan with gemcitabine (Gemzar), a standard chemotherapy for pancreatic cancer. His oncologist, though not an outright supporter of the diet, didn't object to it, except to warn Cleve not to lose weight. (Cancer cachexia is one of the most intractable and deadly issues in pancreatic cancer.) So instead of swigging down Ensure or Boost, my cousin chose creamed soups and other high-fat foods lovingly prepared by his family.

However, it can be a much brighter picture if the diet is started early on, preferably at diagnosis or well before the onset of symptoms, such as loss of appetite. Even with this dire disease, ketogenic metabolic therapy has the potential to improve quality of life, and perhaps the potential to extend survival as well.

Pancreatitis can also complicate or even preclude adoption of a ketogenic diet. This disease has many possible causes:

- pancreatic or bile duct cancer
- gallstones, or complications stemming from gallbladder disease
- lifestyle factors, such as alcoholism or smoking cigarettes
- prior personal or family history
- drugs used to treat diabetes
- abdominal surgery or injury
- high triglyceride levels

Cleve lived an extraordinary 19 months past his diagnosis, *far* beyond the original predictions of his team and, I suspect, far beyond his own expectations as well. For most of that time he was able to live his life, spending quality time with family and friends. He even kept up with golfing, his favorite pastime. His death was ultimately caused by complications from a single dose of a new chemotherapy drug.

Unfortunately, many people diagnosed with pancreatic cancer never consider a change in diet until they've been dismissed to palliative care. By this time they are very compromised by their disease and its treatment, which often includes surgery to remove the duodenum, the site of fat digestion, along with part of the pancreas. Once chemotherapy fails, cancer quickly hijacks the functions of the liver as well as the pancreas. Opiate medications used to control pain contribute to anorexia, nausea, vomiting, and constipation.

The cachexia cascade begins at this point; most people are able to eat only a fraction of what they need to stay alive, while the cancer continues to thrive. For most people in this situation, a high-fat diet would not be tolerable at this stage. That said, perhaps there is benefit from supplementation with exogenous ketones. Only time and research will determine if that is indeed true.

## Q: How Do You Decide If You're Still a Candidate for the Diet?

**A:** Simple. You thoroughly discuss all of these issues with your team. Some risks can be reduced—for example, you can talk to your doctor about changing the medication that you use to treat your diabetes. (Remember, too, that adopting a ketogenic diet is very likely to improve your blood glucose control.) Sadly, there is little you can do to change the picture if you have a pancreatic disease related to conditions such as cystic fibrosis or hyperparathyroidism.

- infections
- other health conditions, such as cystic fibrosis or hyperparathyroidism
- certain medications, including those commonly prescribed for people with cancer (antibiotics, blood pressure medications, diuretics, corticosteroids, valproic acid, and antidepressants)[6]

## Hyponatremia and the Syndrome of Inappropriate Antidiuretic Hormone (SIADH)

Low sodium is a common problem in people with cancer due to the loss of electrolytes through vomiting or diarrhea. However, cancer brings with it a higher risk of chronically impaired sodium levels, or SIADH, an acronym for the endocrine disorder syndrome of inappropriate antidiuretic hormone, which causes a drop in serum sodium levels.[7] This syndrome can't be reversed with sodium supplementation, although it's still important to be sure you're taking in adequate amounts. Also, SIADH has a different origin than that of the decrease in sodium levels that may occur in the first few weeks or months of the diet. If you do notice a dip in sodium in your lab results, please be sure to discuss with your medical team.

## Diarrhea

Diarrhea is another common side effect of several chemotherapies and other anticancer drugs. Since dehydration and a loss of electrolytes are common consequences of diarrhea, it's important to take steps to remedy this. Talk to your team. If diarrhea is caused by an autoimmune bowel disease, you will need to coordinate the efforts of your oncology team with those of the practitioners who are involved in helping you manage your disease.

Sometimes diarrhea is caused by taking too much of certain magnesium supplements. I'm sure you're familiar with the stool-loosening effects of milk of magnesia, but did you know that magnesium oxide and even magnesium citrate can have a similar laxative effect? If you are using one of these forms as your magnesium supplement, then I suggest you switch to another type, such as magnesium glycinate, that does not draw water into the colon. (Another bonus: The magnesium in magnesium glycinate is much more bioavailable than that in magnesium oxide.)

## Challenges Introduced by Other Chronic Diseases

Many of the people I work with are dealing with multiple health issues in addition to cancer—as if that wasn't enough. There is a constellation of issues, some of which require only awareness and monitoring but others that can complicate adherence to the diet or even bring it to a screeching halt.

### Gallbladder Issues

Your gallbladder is a storage compartment for bile produced by the liver. During digestion the gallbladder is stimulated to release a portion of the bile by a hormone secreted by special cells in the duodenum. In the most common type of gallstone, the bile becomes supersaturated with cholesterol, forming a solid, crystalline mass that blocks the bile duct, the opening in the gallbladder. This obstruction can cause excruciating pain and lead to necrosis of the gallbladder. This blockage can also cause pancreatic enzymes, which travel down the bile duct, to back up into the pancreas, resulting in pancreatitis. The prevalence of gallstones in the United States is approximately 10 to 15 percent of adults, and surgical removal of the gallbladder (cholecystectomy) is a common procedure.[8] The myth surrounding gallstones would lead you to believe that fatty foods are at fault but the evidence doesn't support this. In fact, your risk of gallstones is greater if you are obese, experience rapid weight loss (which I discourage), or consume a diet high in calories and refined carbohydrates.[9] Is it any wonder that rates of this disease have climbed so high?

If you have suffered attacks or have had your gallbladder removed, the conventional nutritional advice is to eat a low-fat diet. And you might believe that the cholesterol in your diet had something to do with the cholesterol that caused the development of your stones. But in truth there is no connection between dietary intake of cholesterol and the formation of gallstones. Many people who could benefit from adopting a ketogenic diet do not believe it's an option for them, but this is simply not true. Instead, the appropriateness of a ketogenic diet should be determined on a case-by-case basis, mostly dependent on what symptoms you are currently experiencing. If you do decide to adopt the plan, I would advise against fasting and discourage rapid weight loss, given that both of these situations can precipitate gallstones.

## Obesity Medicine Surgical Procedures

Both gastric bypass surgery and gastric banding (placement of a lap band) require you to follow lifetime dietary restrictions along with intensive nutritional supplementation. In a new, less invasive procedure for weight loss, a balloon is placed into the stomach and then filled with saline. This process may present less of an issue in adopting the diet. Still, if you have undergone any procedure that alters the amount of food that you can consume at one time, check with your obesity medicine specialist before making the decision to adopt a ketogenic diet. (Dr. Eric Westman, director of the Duke Lifestyle Medicine Clinic, is an obesity medicine medical doctor and a strong advocate of very-low-carbohydrate ketogenic diets. He is also a trusted resource for those who have undergone surgical procedures. I have included his contact information in the resources section.)

## Renal Disease

This covers a broad spectrum of diseases, some of which require tight medical management and others that can be monitored through simple blood or urine tests. Talk to your team! Impress upon them that your ketogenic diet is not a high-protein diet. In fact, you can reassure them by stating that the recommended protein intake is in the neighborhood of 0.8 grams per kilogram of ideal body weight. If you have renal disease, it is essential that you review the details of this diet (along with any supplements you plan to use) with your renal specialist.

Do you have a personal or family history of kidney stones? The ketogenic diet can lower urine pH, which can raise your risk of developing a stone. There is some debate about whether or not the oxalates in foods, such as spinach, kale, and almonds, can raise your risk as well. Stay hydrated! Alkalinizing your urine may also lower your risk for stones. You can test your urine pH with specially developed test strips or paper before you start the diet and then monitor it regularly moving forward. You can also talk to your doctor about adding a buffer, such as a prescription supplement (Polycitra-K) or an over-the-counter product. (Remember that potassium supplements are contraindicated if you are taking potassium-sparing drugs. Sometimes doctors will overlook this, even if you give them a list of the supplements you are taking.) If you have a personal history of stones, you'll also want to be sure that your blood levels of vitamin D stay in a range that supports overall health while not being so high as to create other issues. (Ask your doctor for details.)

## Gout

Gout is a complication that arises from high blood levels of uric acid and the subsequent formation of uric acid crystals. These crystals characteristically accumulate in joints, causing the pain and inflammation associated with gout. In the first few weeks of a ketogenic diet, uric acid competes with ketones

### A Potential Therapeutic Effect of βHB in Gout

Dr. Vishwa Dixit and his colleagues (Dr. Dominic D'Agostino among them) have conducted fascinating mouse model research that they describe in a letter to *Nature Medicine*. In their work with mice, they were able to suppress a major inflammatory pathway (NLRP3) associated with many chronic illnesses and forms of cancer.[10] Dr. Dixit and colleagues also researched the effect of infusing βHB to relieve gout flares induced in rats.[11] Dixit's team introduced uric acid crystals into rats, and, as expected, these crystals activated an inflammatory response known as crystal-induced peritonitis. (They used this technique because rats do not develop gout.) The rats were then infused with the ketone bodies βHB and acetoacetate. βHB (but not acetoacetate) attenuated the inflammation. The important takeaway: βHB, a substance that the body makes in those who follow a ketogenic diet, resulted in a desirable anti-inflammatory systemic effect, at least in this animal model. This is wonderful news when you think that the current standard of care in gout is reliant on drugs to resolve symptoms—and these drugs all have many adverse and even life-threatening side effects.

for excretion in the urine, so it is common for blood levels of uric acid to rise, approaching the high end of normal. If you don't have a history of gout and you are not symptomatic, then you may not need to treat the increased level. (Of course, ask your doctor for advice here, as each person and situation are unique.) Levels usually drop back to your baseline once you become keto-adapted. If you have a history of gout, it may ease your concerns here if you limit your intake of purines, especially in the early weeks of the diet. There are also a few foods, including coffee and cherries, that can lower uric acid levels. Vitamin C may have this effect as well.

## Diabetes

Since diabetes is a disease characterized by high blood glucose levels, it makes sense that reducing the dietary intake of carbohydrate will provide benefit. Yet as of this writing, the American Diabetes Association continues to recommend that people with diabetes consume at least 130 grams of carbohydrates per day! This guideline is based solely on the faulty assumption that the brain's energy requirements must be met in the form of glucose. But now you know that up to 70 percent of the brain's energy needs can be met by ketones. If you have diabetes or prediabetes, the good news here is that your symptoms are likely to improve once you initiate a well-formulated ketogenic diet that lowers glucose levels. In fact, the authors of a paper entitled "Dietary Carbohydrate Restriction as the First Approach in Diabetes Management: Critical Review and Evidence Base," published in 2015 in the journal *Nutrition*, state that the evidence is "sufficiently compelling that we feel that the burden of proof rests with those who are opposed."[12]

More good news: Recent research has shown that in a mouse model of diabetes (both type 1 and type 2), the ketogenic diet has the potential to reverse diabetic nephropathy, a dire complication in diabetes that can lead to renal failure.[13] But there's a caveat here: You must work with your doctor before you make any dietary change, *especially* if you are taking prescription drugs to manage the disease. (Spoiler alert: There are a few diabetes drugs that are definitely not compatible with any low-carbohydrate plan, so you will need to switch medications a few weeks before you start.)

Even if you are a good candidate, you still need to educate yourself about all the nuances of implementing this diet for diabetes. One issue is a condition known as "hypoglycemic unawareness"; if you suffer from episodes of this, then you'll be happy to hear that the ketogenic diet may offer protection here. Ellen Davis and Dr. Keith Runyan, a physician who enjoys an excellent quality of life despite living with type 1 diabetes, have coauthored two books on the subject: *The Ketogenic Diet for Type 1 Diabetes* and *Conquer Type 2 Diabetes with a Ketogenic Diet*. Let me again stress that you need to involve your endocrinologist in your diet decisions, as all of the medications you currently take are likely to need adjustment as you adapt to the diet, and this requires medical oversight.

## Polycystic Ovary Syndrome (PCOS)

Some obesity medicine doctors are now using ketogenic diets to treat PCOS, an endocrine system disorder characterized by the overproduction of androgens (male hormones), resulting in an imbalance in sex hormones. PCOS is associated with insulin resistance, type 2 diabetes, obesity, and infertility. In a study conducted at a clinic in North Carolina, five women with PCOS completed 24 weeks on a low-carbohydrate ketogenic diet. All saw significant improvements in the levels of their sex hormones, and two of the women—both with a history of infertility—became pregnant during the study.[14] What a delightful side effect of this diet therapy!

## Elevated Triglycerides

First let's define the problem: Elevated triglycerides are one of several markers that are associated with poor outcomes in diabetes and heart disease. Generally speaking, a rise in triglycerides is unexpected in those following a ketogenic diet. In fact, carbohydrate restriction is associated with improvements in many of the markers of metabolic health, including lower levels of triglycerides and higher levels of protective HDL cholesterol.[15] Despite this generally favorable picture, you may experience a slight rise in triglyceride levels. This is often temporary and may be linked to the rapid weight loss that can occur with a calorie-restricted ketogenic diet. No worries there. Understand that when I say "high triglycerides," I'm talking about levels that are two to three times greater than the high end of normal. If triglycerides rise that dramatically, I look for non-diet causes. Did you neglect to fast for the test?

If these possibilities seem unlikely, then I look at another possible cause: carnitine deficiency. This is discussed shortly as it is usually accompanied by symptoms such as fatigue and muscle weakness. If none of this helps you to troubleshoot persistently high triglyceride levels, even with the help of your medical team, then perhaps you need to reassess whether or not the diet is a suitable option for you.

## Persistent Fatigue or Muscle Weakness

As noted in the prior section, high triglycerides may be a symptom of low carnitine, but persistent fatigue and weakness can also signal carnitine deficiency. Carnitine is a chemical compound found primarily in meat. As discussed previously, carnitine's primary role is to shuttle long-chain fatty acids across the mitochondrial membranes into the matrix, where they can be utilized for energy. It makes sense that more carnitine is needed to support the increase in fatty acid oxidation associated with ketogenic diets: In most people, the extra need can usually be met by consuming a few meals a week that include red meat. Carnitine is also synthesized in the body through reactions involving the amino acids L-lysine and L-methionine. However, if you are taking valproic acid as an antiseizure medication, it's important to know that this drug interferes with the biosynthesis of carnitine.[16]

If you have chosen not to eat red meat or you are experiencing fatigue, ask your team to order a carnitine panel (total, free, and acyl only). Even if levels of free carnitine are low, I am reluctant to recommend the customary high-dose supplementation here (1 to 2 grams a day); the jury is still out on whether this may provoke disease progression in people with certain cancers. The best advice I can offer at this time is to weigh the potential risks versus the benefits of supplementation and, if supplementing, to choose the lowest dose that will move your free carnitine levels back into the normal range. (Use prescription Carnitor or over-the-counter L-carnitine fumarate.) After a few months, retest. (My nutrition colleagues who specialize in use of the diet for epilepsy in children are more likely to be tracking carnitine levels and have shared that total carnitine, or the esterified ratio might be slightly elevated but of no concern.)

Persistent fatigue can also be due to insufficient production of ketones. Test your blood levels of ketones consistently over a period of several days to ensure that you are not slipping in and out of ketosis. If ketone levels are low despite strict adherence to your plan, you might want to consider supplemental (exogenous) ketones. If these improve your energy level or lift your brain fog, then you may want to take them regularly, but any formal recommendation here is beyond the scope of this book.

Persistent fatigue may also be due to underlying metabolic problems. Many naturopathic and functional medicine doctors evaluate mitochondrial health and function through assessment of organic acids excreted in urine. Ideally, this test is performed both prior to starting the diet and again as a follow-up after several months.

## Hashimoto's Thyroiditis

A disproportionately large number of people who contact me for help with the diet list low thyroid activity as one of their ongoing health issues. In most cases, they're referring to the fallout from a condition called Hashimoto's thyroiditis, an autoimmune disease that wreaks havoc with thyroid function. Most people derive some benefit from oral hormone replacement of thyroid hormone, but this cannot replicate the temporal pattern of the spurts of the hormone that are secreted from a normally functioning thyroid gland. Drugs used to treat this disease (and other thyroid disorders as well) may disrupt glucose homeostasis. This may be why some people with Hashimoto's thyroiditis don't feel well when they fast. Diet modifications, such as easing into ketosis with a higher intake of carbs (20 to 25 grams) and smaller, more frequent meals, may be a more balanced approach for people with this disorder.

## Crohn's Disease and Ulcerative Colitis

Diseases that involve bowel inflammation compromise nutrition and often limit intake of some keto-friendly foods. People with these diseases may also have difficulty consuming the amount of fat needed to maintain a ketogenic diet. Furthermore, medications taken to reduce bowel inflammation and other symptoms may not be compatible with the diet. If your disease is under control, consider sticking to the dietary pattern that works best for you while very gradually testing the effect of increasing the amount of fats and oils per meal (or between meals). Ask your gastroenterologist to recommend the type and amount of fiber (if any) to add to your diet.

## Autoimmune Disorders

If you have an autoimmune disorder in addition to cancer, I highly recommend that you read Dr. Terry Wahls's book *The Wahls Protocol*. Dr. Wahls has a personal history of multiple sclerosis and developed her comprehensive and multi-layered plan as an integrative treatment. Her most rigorous diet plan, Wahls Paleo Plus, is a ketogenic diet with an emphasis on maximal intake of cruciferous vegetables, while eliminating vegetables from the nightshade family (including tomatoes and eggplants). When I work with someone with an autoimmune disorder, I suggest that they take a few weeks to ease into their keto plan, keeping their carb intake at around 20 to 25 grams of net carbs per day.

## Issues That Can Impact Food Choices

As you can imagine, there are numerous other health issues that either arise from or affect your food choices. Some of these may be struggles you have had to deal with over the course of your life, and others may have popped up as a side effect of cancer. Either way, it's important to consider these issues in your journey toward optimal health. The list below is not complete, but it touches on a few of the more common challenges I see with my clients.

### Food Allergies

Some allergens, such as peanuts, are known for provoking full-blown ana-phylactic reactions. Other food allergies are more subtle and may include an increase in asthma symptoms unrelated to your usual triggers. The ketogenic diet eliminates many of the more common food allergens (such as wheat, corn, and soy), but emphasizes intake of others (such as eggs, fish, and tree nuts). Overall, though, the diet reduces systemic inflammation, which typically leads to an improvement in most symptoms related to food allergies. If you suspect a food allergy, it's best to visit with an allergy specialist before beginning the diet. Also, be aware of the cross-reactivity of latex and avocado: That is, if you have an allergy to latex, you are more likely to react to avocado as well![17] The protein that you react to in latex is very similar to a protein in avocado—bananas and kiwi, too, but the latter are not usually consumed as part of a ketogenic diet. This is not likely to be much of an issue if you have a simple dermatitis reaction to latex, but it's certainly worth keeping in mind, especially if you experience any airway symptoms with latex exposure. Ask your doctor to help you identify other possible cross-reactions between environmental and food allergens. This is especially important if you are considering botanical supplements, including herbal teas.

### Food Intolerances and Sensitivities

Food intolerances and sensitivities are commonly seen in most people with chronic illnesses and cancer, and they can worsen during cancer treatments that affect the gastrointestinal tract. If you are in active treatment, you may not have many options to improve your gut health. For example, many people develop temporary lactose intolerance as a side effect of certain chemother-apies. FODMAP issues are also very common. (FODMAP is an acronym for a group of carbohydrates that are often poorly absorbed from the small intestine and instead are fermented, causing gastrointestinal distress.) These intolerances may improve once you are past active treatment, so you may want to experiment with reintroducing foods later that you don't tolerate well now. Sensitivities due to poor gut health or a disrupted gut microbiome may also improve on their own, but it is likely that you will need individualized support here. Naturopathic oncologists and functional medicine doctors can be an enormous help!

## Histamine Intolerance

Histamine issues run along a continuum from intermittent episodes triggered by food containing high levels of histamine to living with the threat of full-blown mast cell degranulation and anaphylactic shock due to an allergic reaction. Symptoms include headaches, postnasal drip, asthma, hives, gastrointestinal distress, and more. As it relates to diet, you may have a low threshold for histamine-containing foods due to insufficient production of the enzyme needed to break it down, or you may be choosing foods that increase the histamine load in the gut. A viral illness or a disruption in your gut microbiome may also trigger episodes, making you temporarily less tolerant of certain foods. How food is handled, prepared, and stored ultimately affects gut histamine levels as well. Get to know the symptoms so you don't mistakenly write them off as due to some other cause, and take action to reduce your histamine load. Buy frozen fish and cook it before it's fully thawed, and avoid foods with a high histamine content, such as sardines and ground meat. (Even avocado may not be tolerated if you have histamine intolerance.) There are also steps you can take during your allergy season to reduce your total body histamine load.

If you suspect you have histamine issues, I highly recommend that you work with a specialist to learn how best to control your particular set of symptoms and triggers. (Don't expect much help for gut issues from conventional allergists. They are not usually trained in this.) My friend and colleague Dr. Georgia Ede, a psychiatrist, has an excellent post about histamine intolerance on her website (www.DiagnosisDiet.com).

## Antinutrients

*Antinutrients* are compounds found in plant foods that can interfere with the absorption of nutrients. Most antinutrients are part of the plant's defense against pests and certain diseases, and, for the most part, we have evolved alongside these compounds. Ironically, your body's reaction (called a "hormetic response") may actually contribute to your overall health at the cellular level. But in many people, these compounds, especially in excess amounts, can cause some problems. Many plants high in antinutrients, such as grains and legumes, are not part of the keto plan, but others, such as those from the nightshade family (tomatoes, eggplants), may be included in small amounts. Antinutrients are also found in keto-friendly foods that we generally view as healthy, such as nuts and seeds. Even flavonoids can act as antinutrients.

## Oxalates

Many keto-friendly foods—including avocados, spinach, raspberries, and almonds—are high in oxalate, also known as oxalic acid. Normally our bodies excrete oxalic acid in stool and urine, but at high levels—whether from ingested foods or from endogenous production (yes, our bodies do make it)—it can also bind to minerals and precipitate a type of kidney stone. If you have a personal or family history of oxalate kidney stones, please discuss this with your renal specialist, as your urine oxalate levels can be monitored. Check the resources section for a link to my current favorite list of high oxalate foods. My general recommendation for those without oxalate issues is to limit nuts on this list to two to four servings per day and high-oxalate veggies on the list to two or three servings per day.

## Phytic acid

Phytic acid is a natural compound found primarily in nuts and seeds. It stores phosphorus for use by the sprouted seed. However, it can bind to important minerals such as zinc, iron, and calcium in your digestive tract and interfere with their absorption. This can create some nutritional deficiencies in certain people who are highly reliant on foods that contain a lot of phytic acid. Fortunately, phytic acid does not interfere with the minerals found in animal proteins, so it is not a major concern for people following a ketogenic diet that includes meat, poultry, or fish. If you have concerns and want to lower the phytic acid content of your foods, you can soak, ferment, or sprout many raw nuts and seeds.

## Glucosinolates

Glucosinolates interfere with the uptake of iodine from the diet. These are present in large numbers in the very same cruciferous vegetables that are generally viewed as essential in an anticancer diet. Yes, they can alter thyroid function, and yes, poor thyroid function is common in people with cancer, but this concern is definitely overstated in the press and on blogs. Also, steaming cruciferous vegetables, even lightly, reduces the level of some of these compounds. (Consider replacing some of that raw kale with steamed broccoli.)

## Blender Ketogenic Diets

I've worked with a number of people who use feeding tubes, either for themselves or with a child. Yes, there are keto formulas—developed mostly for children on the diet for epilepsy or for individuals with inborn errors of metabolism who require a special diet—but these are costly and most of them contain inferior oils and synthetic vitamins. There is an alternative: a blender keto diet. Beth Zupec-Kania, consultant nutritionist to The Charlie Foundation for Ketogenic Therapies, has written a short guide to the safe and proper preparation of keto meals using wholesome foods and a blender. This is ideal for those who need a soft or liquid diet, or who receive their nutrition via a feeding tube. Her guide, *Blender Keto*, is filled with recipes and tips for meal preparation. (It may be purchased through The Charlie Foundation's website.) Blender meals are a wonderful idea if you are recovering from surgery or radiation that has affected your ability to chew or swallow.

# CHAPTER 16

# Evaluate Your "Response to Treatment"

In the conventional oncology world, you will become familiar with the term "response to treatment" that describes how your cancer has changed since you initiated therapy. Your team will use objective criteria, such as CT scans and evaluation of blood markers, and then assess their findings using standardized terminology:

**"Complete response"** or **"no evidence of disease"** (but let me remind you that this is not the same as "cure").

**"Partial response"** reflects a positive change from baseline (such as a reduction in tumor size or a decrease in the level of blood markers of disease).

**"Failure to respond"** requires no explanation.

Since response to treatment varies greatly between individuals, even among those with very similar cancers, there is no way that your team can objectively evaluate the actual benefit of a ketogenic diet or other adjunct therapies. Of course you'll be thrilled to hear that you've had "an amazing response to treatment," but don't expect your doctor to attribute any part of that response to your change in diet. It may not sound fair that your team excludes any possible role that diet or other therapies might have had on the course of your disease, but until we have some objective measures (which, given research constraints, will be slow to happen), we must accept the fact that any benefit derived from ketogenic metabolic therapy will be viewed by conventional oncology as purely speculative—at best. But don't let that discourage you or in any way detract from your accomplishment. The science is there, but practice lags behind. This has always been true; just look how long it took for the fact that the earth was round to catch on!

Fortunately, there is movement forward here, and there is a mounting body of preclinical evidence—many very compelling case reports along with animal model research. And it's heartening to see how many doctors are now occasionally telling their patients, "Whatever it is you're doing, keep it up." These are small steps, but at least they are moving in the right direction.

## Assess Your Response to Foods

In the first few days or weeks of a ketogenic diet, your blood glucose and ketone numbers are likely to bounce around quite a bit as your body adapts to the metabolic shift. During this time, you may see glucose levels ranging from a low of 50 mg/dL to a high of 90 mg/dL. As you move beyond the transition period, you will begin to spot daily trends. If you are young and metabolically flexible (meaning free of metabolic challenges such as insulin resistance), expect to see low and steady glucose levels (approximately 55 mg/dL to 75 mg/dL), with ketones consistently in the mid-range of nutritional ketosis.

But if you're past mid-life, you are not likely to see the same numbers as a younger person, even if you are eating identical meals. This may not be evident from reading the research, but think about this for a moment. Are you aware of any ketogenic diet study conducted on an aged animal model? Of course not! All of the research is conducted on young, healthy animals that are free of insulin resistance and systemic inflammation.

Keep in mind that any blood glucose measurement taken shortly after a meal will be higher than the measurement taken before the meal, but these higher levels are not considered a spike unless glucose has increased more than about 20 mg/dL. And never underestimate the impact of stressors that are associated with your disease: Anxiety, poor sleep, depression, financial pressures, and disruptions in routine, to name just a few, all have an impact on blood glucose control. Be realistic in your expectations. Look for positive trends over time and resist the urge to hold yourself to measurements you read about in the research. In addition to those I've just noted, there are a few other common situations affecting glucose and ketone numbers, including:

- steroid hormones prescribed to lower inflammation associated with side effects of treatment or to reduce inflammation associated with edema in brain cancer
- "fight or flight" reactions to circumstances (or even thoughts) that keep your sympathetic nervous system on high alert
- shifts in the hormones associated with menstrual cycles

- functional issues with your gastrointestinal tract, treatment side effects, or a compromised liver or renal function that interferes with diet compliance and/or acts independently to keep glucose high
- metabolic issues caused by a large tumor load or compromised liver or kidney function
- effects of surgery, radiation, or chemotherapy (These are "injuries," and your body responds by raising glucose.)
- vigorous or strenuous exercise that causes swings in blood glucose or ketones (in contrast to gentle or moderate exercise that can lower blood glucose)

What's important to remember is that your body is a dynamic system, constantly responding to both internal and external signals. Stressors are an inevitable part of this system, and you have considerable control here.

In chapter 11 ("Track Your Blood Glucose and Ketones," page 189), I suggest a blood glucose and ketone testing schedule for your first few weeks on the diet along with a recommendation to keep careful records. But testing doesn't stop there. Recordkeeping helps compliance by keeping you accountable. It also provides you with great feedback that you can use to fine-tune your plan.

Unfortunately, home blood meters are only accurate to within 20 percent of what your actual blood glucose might be at any given point in time. So what does this mean to you personally? Say you test a drop of blood and your meter reads 75 mg/dL. Just out of curiosity, you immediately retest using a different drop of blood from that same finger. Your second reading could fall anywhere between 60 and 90 mg/dL and still be considered within acceptable tolerances! Thankfully, most meters are not quite that erratic, although it is common to get an unusual reading now and then. There are many reasons why that can happen, but rather than guessing and stressing, just thoroughly wash and dry your hands and retest.

Also understand another limitation of home blood glucose meters: The strips contain a reagent that reacts with the glucose in your capillary blood. You may want to compare this reading to the result of a test done in the lab, which assesses the amount of glucose in venous blood (drawn from a vein). If you're curious about the difference in readings, take your meter to the clinic and compare a finger prick reading on your meter with your lab draw. The point in doing this is to look for consistency in the variation, not accuracy; so you'll want to repeat this on several occasions before drawing any conclusions about the accuracy of your meter. If the difference is significant, contact the manufacturer of your meter. It may offer to replace your device or send you some control fluid that you can use to see if your meter falls within the manufacturer's tolerance.

## Are You Practicing Daily Intermittent Fasting?

If not, now is the time to integrate this into your plan. Narrow your eating window to around 8 to 10 hours by delaying your first meal of the day and steering clear of food for at least 3 hours before bedtime. Now, check to see what is happening in the time between when you first awaken and take your fasting blood glucose (FBG) and when you are ready to eat your first meal. Take a few readings within this time span. If you are on the right track, you'll see a drop from your fasting levels.

For example, if your FBG is in the low to mid-80s, your immediate pre-meal number might be in the low 70s. That's the pattern I see in myself. I attribute the higher FBG to the dawn effect (as a reminder, this refers to the rise in pre-dawn cortisol and reflects a natural and normal circadian rhythm; your body makes cortisol to prepare you for awakening, and this in turn stimulates gluconeogenesis). That's the reason why your FBG is likely to be higher than other readings during the day (provided that you are not comparing FBG to post-meal glucose levels).

So why does the medical community, and now even the keto community, make such a big deal about FBG? Simple: It's an easy way for health care practitioners to monitor overall blood glucose control over time, as it is typically the only measurement of the day that doesn't reflect a variable, such as food intake or physical activity.

You can use FBG to assess your daily intermittent fasting plan. If your pre-meal number is higher than your FBG, this might be an indication that your fast is too long, and your stress hormones are kicking in to increase glucose production in the liver. If you notice this pattern, you may need to reduce the amount of time before your first meal. (In other words, you may need a wider eating window.) But don't depend on a single day's results. Track the values over several days; then, if you continue to see this pattern, widen your window by an hour or two and repeat the testing.

During the first few weeks, you were consistently testing your fasting blood glucose. Continue with that. By now you should have an understanding of your trends. Also continue bedtime testing. Typically both these numbers will be lower than they were when you first started, but you can expect your fasting blood glucose to rise slightly over time. This is not a sign that you've lost control. Instead, it appears to be more of an artifact associated with lower fasting insulin levels.

Once you are keto-adapted, kick up your testing a notch. Pick one meal on a day when you plan to be at home and are able to test often. This should also be a time that you are not planning to exercise, as this will cloud your results. Record what you eat, preferably by entering the details into Cronometer. Add notes, such as the exact time of your meal, how many hours it has been since your prior meal, and how you are feeling (mood, energy, stress level). Other testing tips are as follows:

☐ Test your blood glucose and ketones right before your midday meal.
☐ Test your blood glucose at 30 minutes, one hour, and two hours after the meal.
  • How much of a rise did you see at 30 minutes? Was it small (15 to 20 mg/dL) or large?
  • What do you see at one hour? Did it rise even further? If so, how does this number compare to your pre-meal number? (FYI: Post-meal blood glucose usually peaks within 1 hour.)
  • What do you see at two hours? Is the number still higher than pre-meal, or has it dropped back down? (If it is still more than 10 mg/dL higher than your pre-meal number, then test again at 3 hours.)
☐ Test blood ketone levels as well at two hours.
  • How does this level compare to your pre-meal level?
☐ Calculate your glucose ketone index using Dr. Seyfried's formula described later in this chapter ("Monitoring Your Glucose Ketone Level [GKI]," page 306).

Repeat these same steps on another day, choosing a different meal, such as dinner. Compare your results.

## Test Your Response to Snacks and Beverages

On occasion, test your response to snacks and beverages. Allow at least three hours between your last meal and the food or beverage that you want to test. Take a pre-snack blood glucose measurement, then test again 45 minutes afterward. If the rise is minimal, you're done with testing that food or beverage. If you see a spike, tweak the snack or beverage to make it more keto-friendly (add fat? cut portion size?) and test it on another day. For example, you can take a teaspoon or two of MCT or coconut oil along with the food to see if that improves your numbers.

People usually assume that they have to give up coffee on a ketogenic diet. If you feel strongly about this, please complete your caffeine withdrawal before you start the diet, as you are likely to experience symptoms, such as migraines or low morning energy. If you want to continue with a caffeine drink, such as coffee or tea, test your response: Take a pre-drink measurement, then test again at 30 minutes and one hour after. If you don't see a spike, leave the drink in your plan.

Personally, I love my morning cup of coffee! I've tested its effects on several occasions. Fortunately for me, coffee with cream doesn't spike my glucose. I also tested my tame version of Bulletproof, which is simply adding some coconut oil and MCT powder. That combo actually lowers my blood glucose! For the sake of science and in the spirit of an n-of-1 trial, I also tested coffee with cream and a teaspoon of sugar. At 30 minutes, my blood glucose had shot up over 30 points! Granted, that seemed extreme to me, but I was never willing to retest, since sugar has no place in my life—or in your keto plan.

Fasting blood glucose and post-meal measurements provide only a piece of the puzzle. There are many reasons aside from foods for spikes in your blood glucose. Is it exercise? Illness? Injury? Stress? Remember that glucose spikes provoke insulin spikes as well. If that wasn't damaging enough, insulin also suppresses ketogenesis. Your goal in lowering carb intake and moderating protein is to keep glucose and insulin levels low and steady, allowing gluconeogenesis to replace insulin and glucagon control in maintaining glucose homeostasis, but be aware of the role stress hormones can play as well.

## Can You Liberalize Your Plan?

Your keto plan can—and should—evolve over time. Your decision to reassess your plan will rest on key issues, such as your overall health and nutrition status as well as changes in your treatment protocols. Your glucose and ketone responses to foods are also likely to change, pointing to opportunities to assess and possibly liberalize your plan, especially if you are resolving some long-standing metabolic issues, such as inflammation or insulin resistance.

Let a few months pass to allow yourself to become fully keto-adapted, then test your body's response to some slight changes. For example, you might want to double up on fibrous vegetables at one of your meals, or add a few tablespoons of a low-glycemic favorite like hummus with added olive oil. If you've been longing for berries or fruit, this might be a good time to introduce them (or to increase portion size slightly), always with some fat, as in berries and cream. Test the change using the protocol at the beginning of this section, and let your test results guide you. Remember, though, that there is no room in your plan—now or ever—for sugar or refined carbohydrates. In my opinion, these poor-quality foods increase activity in all the wrong pathways and introduce temptations that may cause you to abandon your goals. In essence, they have great potential to "feed" your cancer or other chronic disease without providing any nutritional benefit to your healthy cells. Why play with fire?

## Your Response to Exercise

How your body responds to exercise is even more individualized than how it responds to food. Some of that depends on how much of a stressor exercise is for you. Does it stimulate your stress hormones or leave you breathless, sweaty, or exhausted for hours afterward? If so, back off for now and wait at least until you're keto-adapted. Chances are excellent that your exercise tolerance will be better than it was prior to adopting the diet, especially with activity that doesn't require anaerobic bursts of activity. A potentially damaging downside to vigorous exercise before you are keto-adapted is that, in the absence of dietary carbohydrates, your body will break down more muscle tissue so it can divert those amino acids to the liver for gluconeogenesis. You want to avoid that scenario. Also, the more metabolic waste you create, the more need there will be to recycle lactate into glucose in the liver.

## Your Response to Stressors

As you know, your emotional state can ramp up production of stress hormones, leading to increased blood glucose levels. Chronically high levels of these hormones create other health problems as well. Illness, fever, nausea, and vomiting are a fact of life with many cancers and cancer treatments. Poor sleep patterns take a toll. Physical injuries (including surgery and radiation) also add to your burden. It's critical that you understand and address your personal stressors, or your dietary changes may not be enough to keep your glucose level low and steady. You may say, "Of course I'm stressed; who wouldn't be?" and you'd be absolutely correct! It's true that you can't change many of your stressors, but you *can* develop more awareness of their impact and learn to change the way you respond to these signals.

To increase your awareness of the impact of stress, test your blood glucose several hours after a meal when you've spent that time reading or socializing with friends. Compare that with your glucose measurement taken shortly after an argument with your partner or child (or other stressful event, such as

## How Does Exercise Affect Your Glucose and Ketone Levels?

Regular exercise is without a doubt a healthy habit, and gentle to moderate-intensity exercise can lower stress and improve your mood and appetite. But you also need weight training or resistance training to help you retain (or even gain) muscle mass. (Loss of muscle mass associated with "normal" aging has a devastating impact on quality of life.) However, high-intensity exercise, especially when you're in a compromised state, can have negative impacts, so save that for when you are keto-adapted.

For those of you interested in exercise physiology, you may already know that your body will run efficiently on fat until you surpass 70 percent of your maximal oxygen uptake (VO2 max). Beyond that, your body will need to access your stored liver glycogen; and at that point even ketone supplementation may not supplant glucose as a fuel. (Fuel is a separate issue from the potential beneficial effects that ketones, whether endogenous or exogenous, have on cellular signaling and inflammation.) While running on glucose from glycogen, additional energy needs will be met by a hormone-mediated stress response that supplies metabolic substrates that can be utilized for energy even in the absence of oxygen (anaerobically). This perfectly normal response to intense bouts of activity can prolong the period of time needed to become keto-adapted.

I've worked with several top athletes with cancer who refused to cut back on their pre-diet routines despite this obvious downside. It took extra guidance in optimizing food choices to move beyond the fatigue and the less-than-ideal glucose and ketone levels that they experienced during adaptation, but ultimately, even they made the switch and were soon hitting their stride again. How rewarding for them (and affirming for me as a nutritional consultant) to see first-hand that the advantages of running on fat as fuel weren't just hype—but instead, for these individuals, reflected personal experience grounded in science.

To get a taste for recent research in this field, read the 2016 article entitled "Metabolic Characteristics of Keto-Adapted Ultra-Endurance Runners," published in the journal *Metabolism*.[1] In their work, Jeff

Volek and colleagues observed that a group of keto-adapted athletes who consumed a low-carbohydrate diet (roughly 10 percent of calories from carbohydrates) oxidized 2.3 times the amount of fat compared to a group that consumed a traditional high-carbohydrate diet (roughly 60 percent of calories from carbs). This stands as a clear example in the scientific literature of some of the amazing metabolic adaptations that occur in response to low-carbohydrate intake in elite athletes.

To better understand what type and duration of exercise are ideal for your own glucose and ketone management, test your blood glucose level just before you begin your activity, then again immediately afterward. Most likely, gentle activity will bring down your glucose level while high-intensity exercise will drive it up sharply. If that occurs, you may opt to spend an extra 30 minutes engaged in a gentle activity to help lower blood glucose (by directing it to working muscle), then test again. If your glucose levels do not return to pre-activity levels in that time, then your diet routine may not yet be adapted to your current level of exercise intensity. Give yourself a few more weeks to adapt to the diet, then test again. If you are interested in working toward more strenuous bouts of exercise, you can periodize (divide up) your workout routine to progressively increase the frequency, duration, and intensity of your activity. This should allow your body to adapt to elevated activity levels without triggering a stress response that hinders your keto-adaptation.

Once you are keto-adapted, you can also test your blood ketone levels before and after exercise, although even in seasoned athletes, these numbers tend to be highly variable from day to day, and I am reluctant to speculate on what factors might affect your results. Also, understand that even though muscles thrive on fatty acids and ketones under most conditions, your body may have difficulty keeping up with your needs during more intense or prolonged activity. If

a problem at work). Be aware of what time spent on the computer does to you as well and how that may vary depending on what you're doing. For example, if you're updating pictures on Facebook or watching a video of bear cubs paddling around a pool (Google it), your levels are bound to be lower than if you're researching your disease. And did you know that a single night of bad sleep can induce insulin resistance or lower immunity?[2,3] It can also cause brain you notice that you drop out of ketosis with exercise, consider ketone supplementation 45 minutes to an hour prior to heavier workouts, then test your levels to see how this affects your post-workout glucose and ketones. Of course, subjectively assessing your energy levels is a huge part of optimizing a personal plan!

You may also want to consider supplementing with branched-chain amino acids to stimulate protein synthesis in muscle. For now, consider limiting your workout supplementation to 5 to 7 grams of these amino acids mixed in water that you drink prior to and during your workout. However, understand that research specific to such supplementation in people with cancer is scarce, and it is non-existent in people with cancer who follow ketogenic diets! The best advice I can offer is to keep up with new developments by periodically searching the web for news from Dominic D'Agostino and Jeff Volek.

Outside the world of elite athletes, most of us mere mortals should at the very least engage in some form of gentle exercise, such as walking, slow lap swimming, or gentle cycling, all of which provide tremendous benefit in directing blood glucose to working muscle while preserving muscle mass. Gentle exercise can also relieve stress and improve mood, and there is strong evidence that physical activity improves quality of life and overall survival in many cancers, including those of the breast and colon. Bonus: You can get your nature fix at the same time if you choose to engage in these activities in natural surroundings. And as I noted at the beginning of this discussion, resistance training, weight training, and high-intensity workouts should all be folded into your health improvement plan.

*Many thanks to Andrew Koutnik, cancer researcher, and Dominic D'Agostino, PhD, for their review and edit of this important information.*

fog and problems with concentration, which often means that your tasks take longer and are more challenging to complete.

Illness and injury are also potent stressors, yet so often people fail to truly recognize these as the cause of a rise in glucose. Reminding them is one of my many roles as coach. In fact, when a client tells me that their blood glucose is running a bit higher than normal, I ask a lot of questions: How do you feel?

## Pre-MRI Syndrome (or, as Some Would Call It, PMS)

When I was smack in the middle of our journey with Raffi, I would notice that my anxiety level would skyrocket the week before Raffi was scheduled for an MRI. This was no surprise given the number of times that we'd been blindsided by bad news. (Early on, we learned that it was best to schedule Raffi's scan first thing in the morning, then follow up with an appointment with his oncologist in the afternoon. By then, he always had the preliminary report in hand.) I quickly learned that I wasn't alone. One forum I belonged to (almost entirely mothers of children with brain tumors) even had a name for it: pre-MRI syndrome (PMS). More recently, I've seen the term "scanxiety" circulating.

We all experience some anxiety, but each of us expresses it in different ways. Some direct it outward, growing angry or impatient with loved ones. Others get lost in negative thoughts. One mom in my group reported a near-accident on the highway due to her preoccupation with a scheduled scan. There are many different ways to cope with this added stress. Now I would use breath practice to calm my mind, but my go-to at the time was to attack the clutter around me. I had no control over the results of the upcoming scan, but I could definitely micromanage a small part of my surroundings. Mind you, I'm not a neat person, so it's almost comical to think back to my attack on that hallway closet overstuffed with coats and boots or the pile of toiletries that suddenly demanded my attention—but only for that week. So when I get a text or email out of the blue from someone stressing over a non-issue such as a single high blood glucose reading, I might ask, "When are you scheduled for your next MRI?" Then we can discuss the real issue at hand.

Scanxiety is heightened post-imaging if you are kept waiting for unacceptably long periods of time, often a week or more, before you receive your results. I understand that the reading of your scan shouldn't be hasty or rushed, but often the only obstacle between you and your results is a busy office that will respond to a gentle reminder that you are anxiously awaiting news.

Are you nauseous or running a fever? How did you sleep? What woke you up during the night? Are you in pain? These are all stressors of one kind or another.

Another situation that may go unrecognized is the lingering impact of conventional therapies. Even at its best, your body is going to react to surgery with inflammation, and—you guessed it—a rise in blood glucose. When you are treated with chemotherapy and radiation, the intended outcome is mass destruction of cancer cells, and there is *always* collateral damage to normal tissue as well. Of course this is going to cause inflammation! Your body reacts to this by creating its own steroid hormones, and on top of this you may be given steroid drugs as well to quench the flames. Be kind to yourself. Understand that even if your diet is perfect, your numbers may still be higher than you want them to be. Imagine what your numbers might look like if you weren't following a ketogenic diet!

Awareness of your stressors, both mental and physical, along with an understanding of how they affect your glucose levels, is an important first step. In chapter 17 I'll offer some tips to reduce stress that I've picked up during my own continuing journey.

## What Laboratory Tests to Order, and Why

Most lab tests obtained by oncology teams are used to monitor your disease and any potential side effects of your treatment. As one oncologist bluntly stated, "We don't run tests because we're curious." Far from it. Even if your team is more curious than most, they are still not very likely to order a test that you might feel is important but is not part of the protocol for your disease. If they do agree to order it for you, your insurance company may still refuse to pick up the tab.

Baseline testing is used to determine your health status before beginning any cancer therapy, and these tests are repeated as you progress through treatment. Always ask for a paper copy of the results, unless you are absolutely certain that you can access and print the complete report through your online health portal. Organize these paper copies in a binder. You should also become familiar with what these tests are tracking and why. Look for explanations on the web at https://LabTestsOnline.org.

HERE'S A LIST OF RECOMMENDED TESTS,
FOLLOWED BY MORE DETAIL, INCLUDING WHY EACH IS IMPORTANT:

- complete blood count
- comprehensive metabolic panel
- cancer biomarkers
- thyroid panel
- vitamin D
- magnesium
- HbA1c
- fasting insulin
- carnitine panel
- lipid panel
- hsCRP
- homocysteine

## Glucose Levels and Physical Injury

I saw the perfect example of the consequences of a physical injury in an incident involving Raffi. Normally, his glucose levels stayed in a very tight range (upper 60s to low 70s). So when he got smacked in the head with a soccer ball, I decided to test the "injury" theory. I tested his blood glucose within the hour. It was over 100 mg/dL. When I retested a few hours later, it was still in the 80s.

Understand that recent injury or surgery, especially in a contained space such as the skull, is going to cause swelling and, with it, a rise in glucose. Too many people experiencing this issue wrongly attribute that rise to some failure in their diet.

## Complete Blood Count and Comprehensive Metabolic Panel

A complete blood count (CBC) and comprehensive metabolic panel (CMP) are tests that are part of standard preventive health screenings and are also universally monitored in people with cancer. The CMP may also be called "blood chemistries." Different hospitals may use different names. These tests are used to detect any underlying issues, such as anemia or liver inflammation. Moving forward, these tests provide feedback on how your body is handling the treatment. Keep in mind that you may see lower sodium, higher uric acid, and possibly even lower $CO_2$ shortly after you start the diet, but these are usually still within the range of normal. Discuss these findings with your medical team, and make them aware that levels may represent the norms for people who follow a ketogenic diet. If you fail to do this, you may find yourself taking new medications that you may not need. If your team is curious, suggest that they read Volek and Phinney's Art and Science of Low Carbohydrate Living.

## Cancer Biomarkers

These tests are specific to the various types of cancer. For example, certain proteins have been found to correlate with a change in status (typically an increase or decrease in tumor burden). One of these proteins, CA-125 (CA stands for cancer antigen), is used as a marker of ovarian cancer; another, CA 19-9, tracks progression in pancreatic cancer. Elevated levels of lactate, indicating tissue damage or cancer progression, can be assessed by looking at levels of the enzyme lactate dehydrogenase (abbreviated LDH or LD).

## Thyroid Screening

If your team has reason to suspect that thyroid function may be compromised as a result of treatment, they will order a thyroid screening prior to starting. This should include a full thyroid panel (including reverse T3, triiodothyronine), not solely thyroid-stimulating hormone (TSH). On follow-up testing, there may be some changes in your numbers that lead your team to believe that there's been a change in thyroid function, but in most cases, these numbers return to baseline on their own within a few months. Also, it can be extremely challenging to separate out symptoms related to thyroid function from those that occur as side effects of conventional treatment. (Note that nivolumab [Opdivo], a newer anticancer drug, is one of the drugs known to affect thyroid function.)

## Vitamin D (as 25-Hydroxyvitamin D)

Maintaining sufficient stores of the active form of vitamin D is crucial to maintaining health. Most likely, your team will approve this test, since it's become increasingly clear that low vitamin D status is linked to a higher risk of many diseases, including some cancers. Stay on top of the reported results, though; your doctor may tell you that your levels are "normal" if they are at or above 30 ng/mL, whereas it is now believed that optimal levels are more likely to be in the range of 50 to 70 ng/mL.

## Magnesium

Levels of this mineral should also be tested. More than likely, you have no issues obtaining the standard serum test, but this value does not give you information about your more important tissue levels. That said, if your serum levels are in the low end of the range and/or you are taking any of the medications that are known to deplete magnesium (such as omeprazole, a proton pump inhibitor), then you can assume that your tissue levels are also low and you need to supplement. Settle for that or step it up a notch and ask for an RBC magnesium test. This may be a "send out" lab (not evaluated on-site at the hospital), and its cost may not be covered. (In my opinion, unless your doctor has specific restrictions regarding magnesium, supplement this important mineral.)

## HbA1c (Glycosylated Hemoglobin)

This test offers a panoramic view of how well blood glucose has been controlled over time (spanning several months). It's a standard test for people with diabetes and can be easily obtained if you have prediabetes. However, it is now so inexpensive that you should ask for it even if it's not covered by insurance. Keep in mind that there are a number of conditions that may interfere with the accuracy of this measurement. These include (but are not limited to) recent surgery, high red blood cell turnover, anemia, ethnic variation in red blood cell size, and a recent history of vitamin C infusions.

## Fasting Insulin

This value provides valuable information on your degree of insulin resistance. In my opinion, as well as the opinion of many of my colleagues, only the very low end of the normal range is optimal. Given that levels bumping up against the high end of this range are still considered normal, you can begin to understand why diseases of insulin resistance are not diagnosed until there is obvious disease progression. Fasting insulin should be retested a few months after implementing your ketogenic diet. If the level is still at the higher end of the range, then you need to troubleshoot this with an obesity medicine doctor or other health care professional who understands the underlying causes of persistent high fasting insulin levels.

## Carnitine

Carnitine is a substance that transports fatty acids across mitochondrial membranes. Ask your team to order a carnitine panel (total, free, and acyl only). Your baseline will likely be normal; the value in testing is to be able to compare the baseline to a retest six months later if you are experiencing symptoms of carnitine deficiency, such as fatigue, or a rise in triglyceride levels. (Refer back to chapter 15, "Persistent Fatigue or Muscle Weakness," page 282.)

## Lipid Panel

Often referred to simply as a "cholesterol" test, this is another lab that is routinely included in preventive health screening. The panel typically includes an evaluation of total cholesterol, triglycerides, LDL, and HDL levels. Most likely, you already have fairly recent results that you can use as a baseline. Most people with high triglycerides (one of the markers of prediabetes and diabetes) who start a ketogenic diet notice a favorable drop in these levels. However, you may also notice a rise in LDL, and most conventional care doctors view this as undesirable. But before you grow concerned that a ketogenic diet is pushing your cholesterol in the wrong direction, I urge you to seek out a more advanced lipid test, which (at a minimum) should include an LDL particle count and density (referred to as Pattern A or Pattern B). A high particle count is one indication that your cholesterol is oxidized, which puts you at a higher risk for heart disease. A calorie-restricted ketogenic diet usually results in lowering of LDL particle counts, while a ketogenic diet without calorie restriction may result in a temporary rise. Any ketogenic diet should also lower the density of LDL particles; that is, you should see more of the healthy "Pattern A" (large, light, fluffy) than the disease-promoting "Pattern B" (small, dense, atherogenic). Although these advanced lipid panels are now widely available, not every doctor sees the value in the details, so you may need to pay for it out of pocket. With any lipid testing, ask for the following two tests to be drawn at the same time, as these may be better indicators of cardiovascular risk than LDL:

**High-sensitivity C-reactive protein (hsCRP)** is a good general marker of inflammation. While this test is used mostly to assess heart disease risk, other inflammatory conditions and diseases (such as rheumatoid arthritis) can cause hsCRP to be elevated. The ketogenic diet reduces systemic inflammation, so you should see a downward trend here. Note that chemotherapy and radiation induce inflammation, so you are likely to see an elevated hsCRP until you fully recover from your therapies. Conventional oncologists do not routinely monitor hsCRP, so work closely with your integrative clinician if your hsCRP level remains stubbornly high.

**Homocysteine** is an amino acid with a bad reputation. High levels are associated with arterial plaque formation and an increased risk of Alzheimer's disease. In fact, people at risk for Alzheimer's (and that includes most of us) are often advised to take action that will bring homocysteine levels down into the low end of the normal range. High homocysteine can also be a sign of poor methylation, suggesting the need for supplemental vitamin $B_{12}$ and folate. That said, people with cancer need to approach this problem cautiously as hypermethylation, especially during active treatment, might not be wise. Seek out an integrative doctor for advice. (My friend and colleague Dr. Kara Fitzgerald has a special interest in methylation issues and has coauthored an eBook about this that she offers on her website, www.DrKaraFitzgerald.com.)

## Be Careful with the
## Oral Glucose Tolerance Test (OGTT)

The oral glucose tolerance test is *not* part of standard labs for cancer. In fact, it's a highly specialized test used primarily to detect gestational diabetes, but it can also be used to check for diabetes or prediabetes. What's important to be aware of is that this test can be dangerous if you are following a low-carb or ketogenic diet, as carbohydrate restriction typically results in a generally benign condition referred to as physiological insulin resistance. This is very different from the insulin resistance associated with type 2 diabetes and appears to be a metabolic adaptation that keeps glucose in circulation as backup for the needs of the central nervous system.

If your doctor does order this test, she or he needs to be informed of your diet regimen and should advise you to eat at least 150 grams of carbohydrates per day for three days prior to the test. If your doctor suggests this test, please ask why it needs to be performed and be sure all parties understand what needs to be done to keep you safe.

This list of recommended labs is far from complete. Instead, it is what you can expect to be offered from conventional medicine. If you want to dive deeper, find a responsible and ethical integrative or naturopathic doctor who will order additional testing. At a minimum, they may suggest (urine) organic acids, fatty acid profiles, ferritin, and nutrients (including selenium, vitamin B$_{12}$, and folate). They may also suggest blood tests to check levels of circulating tumor cells (CTC). Before you end up paying thousands of dollars out of pocket for testing, ask questions and decide for yourself if the results will provide you with information that you can use to guide decisions. (The same is true for infusion therapies, which can also run up a big tab. You want to target your cancer and improve your health without mortgaging your home.)

## What Imaging Studies Tell You

I'm often asked if a particular cancer will respond to a ketogenic diet. Of course I can't answer this question, but I do look at how individuals with cancer are routinely scanned, either to detect cancer or to monitor disease status. Clearly some cancers are extremely glucose-avid; that is, the tumor cells take up glucose at a much higher rate than surrounding normal tissue. This can be evaluated using a non-metabolizable glucose analog, a modified form of glucose that cannot be utilized for energy. Other imaging scans use tracers or contrast that is injected or infused to allow the radiologist to identify changes in metabolic activity. Check with your team if you have questions about imaging. Typical scans include:

**FDG-PET (fluorodeoxyglucose positron emission tomography):** This uses a radioactive glucose analog as a tracer to identify sites of elevated metabolic activity. This material is readily taken up by glucose-avid tumor tissue, as well as sites in the body that are expected to be more metabolically active. (Only a minuscule amount of glucose is used, so you are not feeding your cancer.)

**MRI (magnetic resonance imaging):** This technique uses a contrast material, or dye, that is most often injected into the bloodstream and concentrates in regions with higher metabolic activity. Brain tumors are commonly followed with MRIs rather than FDG-PET because even healthy brain tissue takes up glucose at a high rate. MRI spectroscopy is a more sophisticated scan but rarely offered.

**CT (computerized tomography):** This imaging method combines x-rays and injected contrast material to identify tumors or other abnormalities, mostly within body cavities. Because of the radiation involved, some people opt to have this test done less frequently than is generally recommended by most standard of care protocols. Limiting these scans has both benefits and risks, so please be sure to discuss your concerns with your team before deciding to agree to or to reject the suggested schedule.

Some new tests, such as one that detects metabolic activity associated with glutamine, are in development.

## Once Again, I Encourage Self-Advocacy

Always ask for a copy of your scans on a compact disk (CD) on the day of your study. It is much easier to have the imaging department make you a copy right then than it is to track it down later from the hospital's medical records department. Also always ask for a copy of the scan report when you meet with your oncologist after the test. It may be only a preliminary report at that point, so ask them to email you the final report when it's ready. If your provider uses an online health portal, sign up for access and make sure your report is loaded in a timely fashion. (You may need to follow up on your request.) Look for key words in the report, those dog whistles that radiologists use to communicate information to your team. A couple of examples:

**"not conclusive"** (This may leave it open to interpretation. If you are treated at a small local center, I urge you to send it out for a second opinion at a center that reviews hundreds of similar tests per year.)

**"possible artifact of surgery or radiation"** (Calling it an "artifact" is akin to hedging the bet—in other words, the radiologist isn't stating with certainty that it's an artifact in case it turns out to be something more serious.)

When recent scans are compared to older ones, you may begin to see more definitive statements, such as **"stable from the prior study"** or **"no interval change."**

Also note the name of the radiologist interpreting your scan. Over time you may notice certain patterns, such as Radiologist A always includes specifics, such as precise measurements, while Radiologist B notes only interval changes. There is no one right way to interpret scans, but these variations in interpretations make it more challenging for you to understand these reports. Again, I suggest a second opinion; no harm in having a second set of eyes looking these over.

Finally, always look for errors in the report. Sometimes these are inconsequential and nothing to worry about. But if you see something major, as we did on two occasions, ask to have the error corrected and make sure that the revised copy is the one that is included in your medical records.

## Monitoring Your Glucose Ketone Index (GKI)

Dr. Thomas Seyfried and colleagues have developed a tool for assessing the potential therapeutic efficacy of the ketogenic diet, called the glucose ketone index (GKI).[4] What he's noted from his research—which appears to be true anecdotally as well—is that people with cancer derive the most benefit from the diet when their GKI falls somewhere between 0.7 and 2.0 (0.7 to 1.0 may be more therapeutic for those with brain cancer).

Follow these steps to calculate your GKI. You'll need to test blood ketone levels using your Precision Xtra monitor. (You cannot use urine strips or breath analyzers for this calculation.) Glucose levels must be tested at the same time as ketones. In the United States, the unit of measurement for glucose is expressed as milligrams per deciliter (mg/dL), and the unit for ketones is millimoles per liter (mmol/L). This means you'll first need to convert mg/dL into mmol/L, accomplished by dividing the glucose measurement by the numeral 18. You then divide that result by the ketone measurement to arrive at your GKI.

## Raffi's Scan and X-Ray Errors

The detailed text of one of Raffi's scan reports stated incorrectly that there was "interval increase" in the size of his tumor, yet in the summary it was correctly stated as "no interval increase." Raffi's oncologist wasn't concerned about the discrepancy, but I asked for a correction anyway since I never wanted to have to explain the contradiction to a third party. (Mom's word doesn't mean much compared to what's documented in these reports.)

On another occasion, Raffi had a wrist x-ray to check his bone age because his tumor type and location was known to affect endocrine function. X-rays of both hands and wrists were taken since Raffi had what was diagnosed at the time as Poland's syndrome: his right hand was much smaller and the bones were less developed than those in his left hand. Astonishingly the radiologist reading the x-rays missed this, and in his report noted that there were no abnormalities. I was blown away! There is no way that anyone could arrive at that conclusion if they were actually comparing the images. We asked for a second opinion because what we were really interested in was bone age, and we couldn't trust the radiologist's conclusion on that front either given the outrageous error he made in the comparison.

EXAMPLE #1: GLUCOSE 72 MG/DL; KETONES 4.0 MMOL/L

First convert mg/dL into mmol/L:

72 mg/dL ÷ 18 = 4 mmol/L

Now divide glucose units by ketone units:

4 mmol/L glucose ÷ 4 mmol/L ketones = GKI of 1.0

EXAMPLE #2: GLUCOSE 83 MG/DL; KETONES 2.7 MMOL/L

First convert mg/dL into mmol/L:

83 mg/dL ÷ 18 = 4.6 mmol/L

Now divide glucose units by ketone units:

4.6 mmol/L glucose ÷ 2.7 mmol/L ketones = GKI of 1.7

At its core, ketogenic metabolic therapy aims to lower blood glucose and insulin and raise ketones. Since glucose and ketones exist in an inverse relationship to one another, once you have made the shift to ketosis a rise in ketones further reduces your need for glucose, which in turn affects how much new glucose is made by the liver. The opposite is true as well: If you take additional actions (either physiological or pharmacological) to lower your glucose levels, ketones will rise in order to meet more of your body's energy needs.

This book is designed to guide you in the proper implementation of a ketogenic diet as a targeted nutritional strategy to reach and maintain ketosis. However, there are some non-dietary tweaks that can influence your glucose and ketone levels and improve your GKI. Mind you, this is no guarantee that your new and improved GKI will be more therapeutic, but I want to share what I know, and you can take it from there. (This is *not* medical advice!) Here's my short list:

Metformin, a drug commonly prescribed to treat type 2 diabetes, can lower blood glucose, which will result in an improvement of your GKI. There is a great deal of research that shows a strong link between the use of metformin in people with diabetes and a reduced risk of cancer. As is often stated, however, correlation is not the same as causation, and it is not yet clear if adding metformin to your protocol may translate to better outcomes in cancer. Any potential benefit may also be limited to certain types of cancer. An analysis of data from the Women's Health Initiative concluded that, compared with users of other diabetes drugs, post-menopausal long-term users of metformin were at a lower risk of developing invasive cancers and dying from their disease.[5] These women were following standard diets and were obviously insulin resistant (as evidenced by the fact that they had diabetes), so the effect could be due primarily to metformin's role in increasing insulin sensitivity. Thankfully, there is more research currently going on. Dr. Dominic D'Agostino at the University of South Florida has posted some information on metformin and cancer on his blog: http://ketonutrition.blogspot.com.

You can also search www.PubMed.gov for the latest research. Understand that metformin must be prescribed and monitored by a medical professional, usually your general practitioner, not your oncology team. (Recall that metformin interferes with the absorption of vitamin $B_{12}$, so you may want to monitor your blood levels or consider a supplement!)

Berberine is one of many botanicals that can lower glucose. Berberine excels at this, but there are others that may also be good adjuncts to your diet. Do your homework, though, as several botanicals can interfere with the metabolism of certain drugs. Ask your pharmacist to review your medications.

Ketone supplementation can raise blood levels of βHB, which will also improve the GKI. In some people, ketone supplements also lower blood glucose levels (since ketones are glucose- and protein-sparing). To date, there is minimal research here, though there is an intriguing study using a mouse model that showed a profound benefit when a ketone supplement was given to mice fed a ketogenic chow versus mice fed a ketogenic diet alone.[6]

Fasting can improve your GKI as well. I prefer daily intermittent fasting (that 8- to 10-hour eating window. It is less stressful on your body than prolonged fasts.

Not everyone will find it possible to keep their GKI below 2.0. Illness, injury, even age, all play a role. This does not automatically mean that the diet has no effect, especially if you are using it as an adjunct to other treatments. Troubleshoot your numbers as best you can, but don't allow GKI to become an additional stressor!

# CHAPTER 17

# Your Anticancer Life

Coping with your disease often involves making profound changes that impact your quality of life. Treatment side effects may leave you too fatigued to maintain your normal routine, or you may need to change your work hours to accommodate your treatment schedule. Loss of income and/or cancer treatment costs may deplete your savings. You may even need to put a temporary hold on pleasurable activities, such as walks in nature or bike rides with your children. Unfortunately, these unwelcome modifications are often a necessary part of the new norm: your cancer lifestyle. But there's a flip side: Your diagnosis can be a catalyst for positive lifestyle changes. Balance your new norm by developing your own unique anticancer lifestyle.

Anticancer doesn't just happen. You need to take an active role in initiating these changes. Here are just a few of your many opportunities:

- Act to improve your physical and social environment.
- Get moving with gentle physical activity.
- Strive to get enough of the right kind of sleep.
- Spend time outside, preferably in natural surroundings.
- Begin (or upgrade) a restorative mind/body practice.
- Identify and reduce toxins in your environment.
- Develop strategies to deal with day-to-day challenges.
- Anticipate and address upcoming challenges.
- Look for support from family, friends, community, and mentors.
- Keep momentum rolling by building on each success.
- Monitor your progress: Record, assess, correct, recommit.

There is no single best anticancer lifestyle. The changes you make need to fit your values, personality, and unique set of circumstances. You are more likely to succeed if you approach this with intention, commitment, and a readiness to change. And remember to go easy on yourself. Change doesn't happen overnight.

# Reduce Stress!

How you handle stress can make or break your anticancer lifestyle, so cultivate a heightened awareness of your personal stressors. "Living every day" is not just a platitude: It became a way of life almost from the day of our son's diagnosis. Stress has an enormous impact on the immune system and overall resilience. It also has a direct impact on blood glucose levels. Now let's look at some practical ways to reduce stress in your life. Start with the low-hanging fruit.

## Scale Back on Multitasking and Overscheduling

Do you ever feel that you're not doing enough? Chances are good that you're already doing too much! In addition to meeting the demands of the people in your life, you may also be placing unrealistic expectations on yourself. Face this issue head on. It's not too late to change old habits, especially given your new motivation! Take it from me: It feels so good to slow down, focus on your breath, and make some decisions about what you can let go. Since I'm a prime offender here, let me share what has worked best for me: I ask myself, "If I knew this was my last day on earth, what would I be doing right now?" You can bet it wouldn't involve multitasking, making lists, or striving to meet the expectations of others.

## Turn Down the Volume on Negative World News

Uncertainty is a way of life, and naturally we expect the media to report on issues that keep us informed and involved. But in recent years, the dosage of negative news has skyrocketed—in part because it is no longer delivered only in the morning paper or during a half-hour segment in the evening news. It's everywhere and constant, and it has become much more polarizing over time. Look for ways to limit your exposure, both online and from television. And don't fall into the trap of responding to every political posting from Facebook friends or relatives; in most cases, you are just throwing fuel on the fire without engaging in productive debate. (Consider getting your news from PBS or the BBC; they present a more global view with less hype and none of those annoying pharmaceutical ads.)

## Recognize Negativity

We all have negative thoughts and emotions. Acknowledge them as they pop into your consciousness and then move past them so that they don't end up hijacking your day. This is the main lesson I've learned from mindfulness practice. If you already have a practice—such as meditation, yoga, or tai chi—nurture it and take note of how much it gives back to you! And remember that you don't need to dedicate hours you may not have. I have a core group of simple yoga poses (asanas) that take only minutes to move through but are incredibly restorative.

Yoga and other mind/body practices, such as tai chi and qigong, not only subjectively improve vitality and well-being, but also have been shown to lower markers of inflammation.[1] Even the conventional medical community is waking up to this. Create balance between restorative and energizing practices. You need both! Start with breath practice. There are countless variations: Some calm the autonomic nervous system, some are restorative, and some are invigorating; but they can only help if you actually practice on a regular basis. So next time you're in a line that's not moving, quiet your mind and breathe (here, choose a method to calm your nervous system). It sure beats fidgeting or getting angry. I've included a few of my favorites in the resources section.

Other mind/body practices can open you up to a deeper appreciation of your own existence, such as practicing gratitude, reflection, visualization, relaxation, and yoga nidra. Get a massage or receive a Reiki treatment, or work with a Feldenkrais or Hanna Somatics movement practitioner. Others find it helpful to pray or ask for spiritual guidance. Do whatever resonates with you.

For me, personally, practicing gratitude was my lifesaver. I learned this from my son, and share it whenever and with whomever I can. Watching him draw closer to his essence, still expressing his gratitude for a beautiful day or a roof over his head even as his life was slipping away, made it impossible for me to hold on to my selfish "why him, why me?" thinking. This was just one of Raffi's many gifts to me, and one that will remain with me as long as my feet touch this earth.

## Set Limits on Screen Time

I'm sure you are already well aware of at least some of the health benefits of cutting back on your screen time (this includes your smartphone, laptop, tablet, TV, and/or video games). If you haven't made a change here, now is the time to set some limits. Start by cutting back on TV, especially violent programs that serve no useful purpose in your life. From there, consider a screen-free hour or two prior to bedtime. It may help your resolve if you set a curfew. Screen-free evenings have many benefits: Your mind settles into a nighttime rhythm, you let go of an activity that overstimulates, and you reduce the amount of blue light that you are exposed to in the evening. (Blue light from the sun is normal and natural, in contrast to the blue light emitted from devices and LED bulbs, which is known to disrupt the circadian rhythm and may even accelerate vision damage.)

## Spend Time in Nature

I can't imagine a life in which I couldn't spend time in nature! Being close to the natural world is what motivated me to move from the busy East Coast to a remote mountain valley. Even if a move isn't an option for you, or you enjoy your present surroundings, I urge you to get outdoors whenever you can—even if you're simply sitting on a bench. If you are physically able, enjoy some restorative activities, such as gentle walks or bike rides with family or friends. Time spent outdoors can help to relieve tension, elevate mood, improve blood flow and digestion, and promote better sleep. Remember: We evolved as part of the natural world, a truth that is only too easy to forget when we spend most of our time cloistered in our comfortable homes.

There are plenty of other activities to help you enjoy life and reduce your stress:

- Spend time socializing; we're hard-wired to connect!
- Listen to music, sing, or play an instrument.
- Watch a comedy or read a lighthearted book.
- Laugh. A lot.
- Express your creative side through painting, pottery, crafts, and textile arts (among others).
- Volunteer!
- Travel for pleasure.
- Write, or keep a journal.
- Enjoy a spa day!
- Acknowledge a special person in your life who is a source of strength and support, then call or send the individual a text expressing your appreciation.

Never refuse an offer of help! Even if you can't think of anything at the moment, you can circle back to this when the need arises. Keep a list of names and numbers. Family or friends can run errands or preview resources for you online (this will cut down on your own screen time). Some families ask adult children to help with food shopping and meal planning. And if you're struggling to get up to speed with Cronometer, a teenager or young adult can help you with your profile settings.

## A Note to Caregivers about Stress

Stress reduction applies to caregivers as well. When you take care of yourself, you are better able to care for your loved one. As you are aware, I've walked in your shoes and know how important—and challenging—this is. It's tempting to think that you don't have time, and the truth is, some days don't allow for a shower or proper meal, let alone a night out with friends. Even so, keep looking for ways to carve out time for yourself. You need to recharge your batteries! You may not have an hour for a nap or a walk, but there is always time to follow your breath for 20 or 30 cycles. If you have a whole 10 minutes to spare, watch the video on yogic breathing listed in the resources section. After all, you have to breathe; you might as well make the most of it! Encourage your loved ones to join you in this. Each situation is unique. (Raffi loved breath work: a special connection to Mom, especially since it was followed by some cuddling and heart-to-heart talks.)

Check out a few online support groups. Look for those that are a good fit with your own needs as a caregiver. They can be cancer-specific, such as Facebook groups or forums at www.Inspire.com, or more general, such as those you can find through such organizations as AARP. You can also seek out local support groups in the newspaper or on hospital message boards. Meeting face-to-face with others in situations similar to yours can help you feel connected and reduce the isolation that so often accompanies caregiving. If you're not finding what you need, ask your medical team for help: Most hospitals and clinics employ a social worker who can connect you with resources.

## Get Good Sleep

Good sleep is critical to health and well-being, yet so few people, especially those who are older or in active treatment, get enough restorative sleep. Even one night of poor sleep can have a negative effect, and no one operates at their best when sleep-deprived. There is already so much written about this that I don't feel the need to reinvent the wheel here; it's easy to find information online about how to optimize your sleep by improving what's known as "sleep hygiene." I've already covered a few of the many tips you'll find, such as reducing screen time, avoiding blue light in the evenings, and limiting your exposure to negative news reports. What you do during the day counts as well. Get out for a stroll, work out at the gym, practice yoga, or meditate. The more active you can be, the better. Other suggestions include darkening your room and avoiding alcohol close to bedtime. An Epsom salts bath in the early evening can also be incredibly relaxing.

If you do need (or choose) to spend time online in the evenings, you can download an app, such as Iris or f.lux, install Twilight on your Android devices, and use Night Shift with iOS—these all help to control the amount of blue light emitted by your screen. And consider switching to a print book if you currently read a Kindle at bedtime. For those who have more of a challenge with staying asleep, use your breath practice to replace those thoughts that spin through your mind like caged mice on an exercise wheel! Biohackers may want to purchase an Oura ring. (This is not an endorsement. In fact, I've never tried one. But friends who have used this sleep and activity–tracking ring appreciate the feedback it gives them about the length and quality of their sleep.)

## The Benefits of Moderate Exercise

Despite the many physical and emotional benefits of regular exercise, you may not feel like you can begin or maintain a regular routine. However, once you are keto-adapted, you may find that you feel better and have more energy than expected. The metabolic changes that accompany the shift to ketosis can improve your well-being even as you move through treatment. This improved quality of life is one of the surprising and very desirable side effects of anticancer ketogenic metabolic therapy.

Make some type of movement or exercise a priority even if you have a heavy schedule of treatments and other appointments. Almost everyone can find a few minutes scattered here and there. Here are some tips on being ready to move:

- Keep your walking shoes and water bottle near the front door.
- Bookmark your favorite yoga video, or leave a DVD near your TV.
- Store your yoga or exercise mat and light weights in an easy-to-access space.

You may need to start by simply visualizing what you want to do. Is it a walk in the woods? Smell the leaves and feel the earth beneath your feet. Is it yoga practice? Run through the Sun Salutation in your mind.

Now, kick it up a notch. Maybe all you can manage right now is a five-minute walk. But that's a great start! Keep it light. The goal is to move, not to exercise to the point of exhaustion. In fact, if your routine leaves you feeling worse rather than better, it's time to ease up on your expectations. Do you have an exercise buddy? It's a great way to combine socializing with physical activity and may even strengthen your commitment!

# How Long Should You Remain on the Ketogenic Diet?

You may be wondering, "How long do I have to stay on this diet?" I'm asked this question frequently. My answer? The ketogenic plan is much more than just a diet, so try to change the way you view it. There are so many potential health benefits to the changes you've made, not only in sidestepping diseases, but also in improving the way you approach aging. Of course you are welcome to look at liberalizing your diet plan over time (as I have done), using a glucose meter to test your body's response to specific foods or meals. Remember that the first weeks are the most challenging, and research tells us that it typically takes us several months to develop new habits. Relief from symptoms or an amazing scan will strengthen your motivation and resolve, which will undoubtedly help to shift your attitudes toward food. I would urge you to stay on "The Diet" until you are keto-adapted. After that, commit to a ketogenic plan that serves you for a lifetime.

## Fully Commit to at Least 12 Weeks before Changing It Up

Twelve weeks is about how long it takes for the vast majority of people to see results. Once you're keto-adapted, you may decide to play with the plan to see if minor variations affect your glucose and ketone numbers to any significant degree. At this point, you most likely have learned how to dine out, and know how to sidestep the common food traps (including hidden sugars in sauces and too large a portion of protein) that may have kicked you out of ketosis in the past.

Now is also the time to look through those low-carb recipes you passed on during the first few months. If you have the book *The Ketogenic Kitchen*, check out Domini Kemp's contributions—she emphasizes quality ingredients, then uses a variety of spices and seasonings to add interest to the meals. The nutrition information included with each meal will help you to customize the recipe to meet the macro targets you've set for yourself.

Adopting a new way of thinking about food as nutrients rather than food as comfort allows you the freedom to grow and change, making better choices and more informed decisions as you continue on your journey. I am not suggesting that you allow non-keto foods to sneak back into your diet or to take extended keto holidays. In fact, you should periodically test to be sure that your ketone levels are staying above the threshold for nutritional ketosis (0.5 mmol/L), indicating that you are consistently using fat and ketones as your major source of cellular energy.

## My Experience with Keto as a Long-Term Lifestyle

My son, Raffi, followed the ketogenic diet for almost three years. We adopted the strict model used for kids on the diet for epilepsy and micromanaged every bite he consumed, carefully dividing his recommended protein/carbs/fats into three equal meals and a couple of snacks. We acted as diet police. We sent food with him wherever he went. It was rough at the start, but it certainly got easier over time.

As we passed the two-year mark, we realized that we could lighten up on some aspects of it. We relied less on blood testing and more on urine sticks. We learned to "go with the flow" (Raffi's words). Out of MCT? Use more coconut oil. Fish smells bad? Toss it out and pull some shrimp from the freezer. Got one more errand to run? Fill in with an extra snack that we brought with us.

Another lesson we learned: Raffi's ketogenic lifestyle improved our lives as well as his. We were no longer tethered to a hospital or expecting miracles from clinical trials. Raffi's anticancer diet became a family lifestyle. We lived our lives as fully as we could, and I will always be grateful for the extra time granted to us by this diet.

My husband and I both still follow a ketogenic pattern. Not because we have to, but because we are so aware now of what it means to eat well that we simply can't imagine going back to our old ways. It doesn't feel limiting, and neither of us is tempted to indulge in pizzas or fast-food burgers. Now, we view food-industry marketing in the same negative light that we view the direct marketing of pharmaceuticals. So do we believe that sugary cereals are a "good source" of fiber or vitamin D? Of course not! Instead we choose to get our nutrients from whole foods. In fact, for us one of the best parts of traveling is returning home so we can go back to eating fresh, high-quality foods.

I urge that you remain true to these basics:

- Consume no grains, sugars, or refined carbohydrates.
- Eat only small amounts of berries and certain low-glycemic fruits.
- Keep protein portions low but adequate to meet your needs.
- Limit dairy proteins to condiment-sized portions.
- Always include lots of healthy fats and oils!

## Navigating Sick Days

Glucose and ketone levels fluctuate as a result of illness or injury. This is a given, and it's important that you fully comprehend this. Thankfully, uncomplicated illnesses rarely require medical intervention, but if you are in doubt, please err on the side of caution and seek medical care.

**Nausea and vomiting** are common in people receiving conventional cancer care. Talk to your team about ways to address these side effects proactively. Also, review the research on short-term fasting in chapter 7 ("Short-Term Fasting as an Adjunct to Chemotherapy," page 102). If you do choose to eat on chemotherapy days, you may feel more comfortable if you reduce fat, increase protein, and divide meals into smaller portions.

**Diarrhea and/or constipation** can be a complication of certain cancers (e.g., colon cancer, pancreatic cancer, and lymphoma). Some cancer treatments, such as chemotherapy and radiation, may also initiate or exacerbate these issues. Talk to your team about how to address this problem.

**Flu viruses** may cause vomiting and diarrhea, which can quickly lead to dehydration and the loss of electrolytes. Keep well hydrated! Sucking on ice chips can help. Salted broth is an excellent option if it is well tolerated.

### A Great Homemade Electrolyte Drink

Beth Zupec-Kania, consultant nutritionist to The Charlie Foundation for Ketogenic Therapies, has suggested this home remedy for electrolyte replacement.[2]

½ teaspoon Morton Lite salt
½ teaspoon baking soda
4 cups water

Dissolve salt and baking soda in water. Drink 1 cup every two hours. Test blood glucose frequently. If it drops below 55 mg/dL, sip 1 to 2 tablespoons of apple juice. When you are able to eat again, start with small meals of bland foods. Add small amounts of mayonnaise, butter, or coconut oil. Good food choices include avocado, soups, or keto shakes (almond or coconut milk, cream, vanilla, stevia).

You can also use sugar-free sports drinks (such as Propel Workout Water), but most of these drinks have colorings and artificial sweeteners. Pick the purest ones you can find and keep a few bottles on hand.

## Emergency Care

It is far better to have your personal medical information with you at all times and never use it than to find yourself at the emergency room, struggling to access your records. If your treatment team offers you access to a patient portal, sign up and make sure that your medical records are uploaded in a timely and complete fashion. Also be sure that you can access the portal from your smartphone, so that your records are never more than a click away. If you keep paper copies or compact disks, store them in a clear plastic ziplock bag that you can keep on your person or in your car. Also keep a summary with you at all times that includes:

- details of your ketogenic diet plan
- normal-for-you blood glucose and ketone measurements
- normal-for-you sodium levels (especially if levels are on the low end)
- your health care team's contact information, including names, phone, fax, and email

If you are the parent of a child on the diet, ask your child's health care practitioner to print and sign several copies of your child's summary on office letterhead.

Communication between hospitals can be cumbersome at best, so carry a copy of your latest scan on a disk, and make sure to keep a list of your current medications and supplements, noting daily dosages.

### If You Need to Go to a Hospital or Clinic

Share the information above regarding normal-for-you glucose and ketones with your hospital treatment team. Although what is considered normal is highly variable, you risk being treated for hypoglycemia if your glucose levels dip below the norms, even if you don't have symptoms. You or your advocate will need to stress how important it is for you to receive saline-only intravenous fluids whenever possible. Ask the nurse to place a reminder on your chart.

Of course you know that most hospital meals are a train wreck! If you can't find a workaround, err on the side of eating more protein (or drinking a protein shake) rather than giving in to rolls, desserts, sugary yogurts, or ice cream. If hospital policy allows, ask friends or family to bring you fresh salads, steamed veggies, avocados, and broth. You can usually get a few pats of butter, but it's best to bring your own high-quality olive oil, coconut oil, and mayo.

If you are placed on steroid medications, remind your doctor or nurse that you would like the lowest effective dose for the shortest period of time. If you are given opioid pain medications, expect to become constipated and ask if you can begin taking stool softeners, such as milk of magnesia. (You can go back to using your preferred methods once you get back home.)

## Vacations

I hope you have the luxury of squeezing in a vacation despite your cancer treatment, especially if you are tolerating your protocol well and feel like this would be a treat, not a burden. Mini-vacations may be easier. Take advantage of a scheduled treatment break to enjoy a special time with family or friends. Anticipate challenges and think about how you'll address them, such as learning what keto-friendly foods are available at your destination. You should already know your options if you are in familiar territory, but if travels take you to places with different foods, customs, and languages, you will need to do some homework! Will you be staying in hotels or in a vacation rental? Hotels mean that you'll be dining out more often. Rentals give you the option to bring your favorite keto recipes, go shopping, and prepare your own meals.

If you make a conscious decision to suspend the plan while you're away, don't let this become a feeding frenzy. A few slices of apple with cheese is a much better decision than mindlessly chowing down on a bag of potato chips on your way to the beach. Grain-based desserts combine two evils: flour and sugar. And most snacks can trip you up as well. While you're away, you may decide to indulge in more protein (to make up for the inevitable shortage in fats) or even to allow for a limited amount of starchy vegetables or fruits. Find fats where you can, though: Butter, heavy cream, and cream cheese can be found just about anywhere in the world.

Whether you're planning a two-hour or a two-week trip, never venture far from home without several ziplock bags filled with your favorite snacks. For longer trips, pack a cooler with keto meals stored in small plastic containers. Don't forget the fats!

## Long-Term Rewards

It's too early to know for certain what the long-term rewards will be for those who opt to follow a ketogenic diet for cancer. In fact, it would be challenging indeed to attempt to separate out the effects of the diet from the impact of other lifestyle improvements. Still, it's worth zeroing in on many of the benefits that we already see and a few that we expect to learn more about in the near future. These include:

- weight loss (if this is a goal)
- improved blood pressure
- improved metabolic health
- improved insulin sensitivity
- lower levels of inflammation
- more consistent energy and better endurance
- less reliance on scheduled meal times
- improved mitochondrial health
- a sharper mind
- an amazing quality of life
- the potential for a longer lifespan
- the knowledge needed to make better food choices
- all the other benefits that come with understanding the role that nutrition plays in health and disease

I've been following a low-carb ketogenic plan for several years now and am solidly keto-adapted. It is no longer a diet; it's a way of life for me, and a satisfying one at that! Over time I've conducted more than a few experiments with foods and find that my body responds best when I add some fruits or berries at my first meal, include beet or carrot or peppers at lunch, and keep my dinner protein light. I vary my diet seasonally: I prefer slow-cooked meats with rutabagas in the winter and spicier salads in the summer. I add butter, coconut oil, and olive oil wherever I can and try to include some ginger and turmeric every day, whether in the meal itself, as an infused vinegar, or in a hot drink. I track glucose only occasionally, more out of curiosity than for any other reason. Occasional testing also provides me with indirect feedback on my insulin sufficiency and sensitivity. (Insulin is important not only for glucose control, but also for its role in cellular signaling, so I want it to stay within the normal range.) If you are not content with your present plan, or feel that it is no longer serving you well, you certainly have options. This comes with a warning, though, for those with brain cancer. Here, adherence to a rigorous ketogenic diet may be the only nutritional strategy that helps you manage your disease. That means tight limits on carb intake as well as low overall protein intake coupled with only enough fat to maintain your weight on the lean side. This approach is likely to be the only way to keep glucose low and steady while also maintaining ketones in the zone assumed to be therapeutic (using the GKI as a measure). On the other hand, if you are following a ketogenic diet for an early-stage and less aggressive cancer, such as some types of breast cancer, then a more liberal low-carb plan adopted alongside other lifestyle improvements may be all you need moving forward. May I stress, though, that there is nothing to be gained and too much to lose by letting sugar and starches sneak back into your life.

When all is said and done, the ketogenic diet is simply a different mix of familiar foods, and ultimately you are the one who gets to decide what you eat. Where that takes you is an unknown. We are on a journey of discovery, and like the early explorers, we will uncover new worlds as we keep putting one foot in front of the other.

# Raffi's Gift of Life

In the summer of 2011 Raffi was in very rough shape, despite no observable changes on his MRI. He'd been in a downward spiral for 10 months when we finally decided to have a feeding tube placed. Because of his deteriorating neurological status, eating and drinking had become too much of a chore, and we were hoping that his condition would improve if he received sufficient food and water. The tube did improve his nutrient intake, but this didn't help to reverse his decline. His doctor suggested home hospice. We were reluctant to get hospice involved; it felt too much like we were abandoning hope for our son. Nevertheless, we agreed to talk to the hospice team. They laid out their case, and we signed on.

Part of what hospice workers do is to prepare the family for each step of the dying process. The workers who came to us were compassionate but frank in their assessment. The countdown began. Three weeks. Two weeks. I panicked when they predicted that we had less than a week left with our precious son.

Throughout this time we continued to make trips to Raffi's favorite hot spring, holding him in our arms as he floated on his back. By this point he was noncommunicative, so it was impossible to know what he was thinking, but the look on his face was so peaceful that I was sure he was experiencing some level of bliss. But on the long drive home, he would slump in his seat, unable to hold himself up.

After one such visit, I laid him down on the couch in our living room. Suddenly, he struggled to sit up, something he hadn't done in at least a month. Clear as a bell, he said, "I have the feeling that someone is looking for me." I was stunned. This was more than he'd been able to say in several months. But that moment of clarity was over in a flash and down he went again.

The following week we made what I thought might be our final trip to the hot spring. When we returned, I put him in his bed and lay down next to him. He dozed for a few minutes, then suddenly opened his eyes and asked, "So what are we doing for the rest of the day?" I was thrilled to once again hear his beautiful voice and admit to being amused by his straightforward question. I gambled on, asking, "If you could do *anything* you want, what would it be?" I was afraid I wouldn't be able to meet some lofty expectation, but his request was simple. "Go to Kmart and buy a toy." I called my husband into the room. Neither of us could believe Raffi's clarity and determination. On the short ride to Kmart, he struggled to sit upright. Once we were in the store, he walked, with support, to his favorite aisle, the one with the remote-controlled cars. Within an hour, we were back home with his sporty new car, exhausted but exhilarated. We were also saddened to think of how quickly the time had passed, as we fully expected this to be Raffi's final rally.

But it soon became clear that this wasn't just a rally. Raffi grew stronger and chattier with each passing day, regaining his strength and wonderful sense of humor. The next time we went to the hot spring, he walked up the steps on his own and paddled around the pool. Within a few weeks, he was back to riding his trike to the farmer's market. It was so much fun to watch the shocked faces and warm welcome he received from our tight-knit community. The doctor who had admitted him to hospice was among the folks at the market, and it was especially rewarding to see the puzzled look on *his* face. I just smiled and shrugged my shoulders.

We hung in with hospice for several more weeks. Finally, they agreed with us that Raffi needed restorative therapies, which were not part of the hospice package. Raffi was officially dismissed—"kicked out" as we liked to call it! That was the beginning of a *full year* of extra time with our son before he started his final decline. Time to cuddle and talk. Time to ride bikes and swim at the pool. Time to camp and chill out in Mexico. Time to comfort one another with the certainty that our hearts were bound together—"with a big bow"—in this life and beyond. Raffi never tired of hearing that, and I never tired of letting him know how much he meant to me.

To this day we can only speculate on what took him down and what brought him back to us. But that final magical year with Raffi was the most special of times, an amazing gift, and I'm so grateful for every moment of it.

## Support the Research

In talking about our own personal journey, I used to say, "If we knew then what we know now. . . ." In the years since then, my thinking has evolved, and now I know that the game changer lies not in what we know today but in what we will know *10 years from now*. Progress in our understanding of whom this therapy may benefit is dependent on research, however, and research requires funding. Unfortunately, the current paradigm is profit-driven, and the pharmaceutical companies that support cancer research understandably have no interest in funding studies of an anticancer diet. Equally unfortunate, most funds raised by individuals driven by a personal passion also end up in corporate hands. But there are other options that can make a real difference, so if you feel as strongly as I do about supporting the research, you'll look into these two opportunities.

## The Foundation for Metabolic Cancer Therapies

If you are familiar with science writer Travis Christofferson's work (*Tripping over the Truth*), you've already been introduced to the foundation he created to fund metabolic research: Single Cause, Single Cure. Under its new name, the foundation continues to be the best conduit for supporting the important work conducted by some amazing and passionate researchers, including those at Dr. Thomas Seyfried's lab at Boston College. Dr. Seyfried's team has made huge strides toward developing new combination therapies that converge to exploit cancer's many vulnerabilities. You can donate here: http://www .foundationformetaboliccancertherapies.com/donate.

## University of South Florida

Dr. Dominic D'Agostino's lab at the University of South Florida (USF) also draws the best and the brightest to the study of ketogenic metabolic therapies. I am grateful for the core group of researchers there who have helped me every step of the way by sharing information and taking time from their own work to review parts of this manuscript. USF hosts the Annual Conference on Nutritional Ketosis and Metabolic Therapeutics, a Who's Who of the movers and shakers in the world of keto therapeutics. Keep an eye on the Conference website: http:// metabolictherapeuticsconference.com. You can donate to USF's research by following the links to the USF Foundation found at www.ketonutrition.org.

# APPENDIX A

# Troubleshooting

Troubleshooting is a huge part of what I do in my work with clients. As you might expect, answers to questions about the ketogenic diet, especially as it is used in cancer, are hard to come by and often highly individual. What I offer here is an overview of questions I'm asked most often.

*Are you feeling flu-like symptoms similar to those you may have experienced in the first few days?*

First and foremost, ensure that you're getting enough sodium. As your insulin levels drop, the kidneys excrete more sodium. If sodium levels become too low, you will begin to lose potassium as well. (Magnesium is also lost in the urine.) Replenish your electrolytes by drinking homemade broth with added Himalayan or sea salt, or by using Morton Lite (a combination of potassium chloride and sodium chloride) to salt your foods, at least in the short term. (However, a potassium-containing salt may not be appropriate for you if you take a potassium-sparing drug such as lisinopril.) Also keep in mind that Morton Lite contains iodine, so alternate it with non-iodized salts. Certainly, my suggestion here should not override your doctor's advice to limit your intake of either potassium or sodium.

*Are you hungry between meals?*

If you're still experiencing hunger, increase the frequency of ketone testing for a few days. Do you find times when you are dropping out of ketosis? If so, review your carb intake and look for hidden carbs in supplements and beverages.

*Do you still crave certain foods?*

If you find you crave a specific food, work to identify what it is you miss most about it. If it's a treat, can you find a keto-friendly substitute, such as a fat bomb or a keto sorbet? If you're craving a salty or crunchy food, will a handful of fried pork rinds do the trick? (Careful here, as these are relatively high in protein.) If you're craving protein, what satisfies you most? If it's cheese, it may be that the opiate sensors in your brain are still fired up, and casein is your fix. Cravings for protein may also indicate a genuine need, so heed this and double-check your macro calculations and food records to be sure you're meeting your target. Raise the amount slightly for a few days and see if the cravings stop. It also happens that some people have a more pronounced insulin response from certain animal proteins, especially dairy and eggs, and the down stream effect of that could be what's triggering your craving.

*Are you losing weight too quickly?*

This may seem like an odd question for people who view ketogenic diets as weight-loss plans. But for those with cancer, weight loss can be a problem if it is too rapid or unsustainable. If you are losing more than two pounds a week, or you are already at or below your ideal weight, it's time to put the brakes on weight loss. Exclude the MCT oil from your tally of total fat grams/calories for the day. Instead, consider it a bonus.

Another way to slow weight loss (or encourage weight gain) is to add a small serving (50 to 60 grams) of a food with a low GI as part of a meal; that is, one with a GI of less than 50—even better, less than 40. Legumes and select fruits are options. You can easily find GI information online, but don't get too caught up in the numbers. Instead, assess your response by testing your blood glucose just before the meal and again 45 minutes afterward. Expect to see a rise in glucose of about 25 to 30 mg/dL—this is higher than the usual recommendation but the purpose here is to stimulate insulin—briefly—to preserve your fat stores. If your glucose rises by more than 25 to 30 mg/dL, then reduce the portion slightly and test again on another day. Start by altering just one meal per day, so that you can determine the lowest level that keeps your weight where you want it while still maintaining ketosis.

A third method is to add a ketone supplement, such as one of the βHB salts available as powders. Use just one-quarter to one-half a packet once or twice per day; it is not likely to have an appetite-suppressing effect at this low intake. This is strictly a bonus: In other words, you can note it in your food diary, but don't count it toward your total macros for the day.

*Are you seeing spikes in glucose (a rise of more than 20 mg/dL)*
*with a meal or snack?*

Check the ingredients of any packaged foods or low-carb snack bars you're eating. (Hopefully, you're not relying very heavily on these!) Identify which ingredients might be causing the spikes. Look for sneaky sugars or problematic fibers, such as fructooligosaccharides (officially, oligosaccharides are indigestible sugars, but they can raise blood glucose in some individuals). Also, be wary of foods labeled "sugar-free" and marketed to people with diabetes, as these may not be keto-friendly.

### Are you taking steroid medications (e.g., prednisone, dexamethasone, or cortisone)?

Prednisone and dexamethasone are both commonly prescribed before and after treatment with chemotherapy to control inflammation, and cortisone can be prescribed as a replacement hormone if you are not producing normal levels of cortisol. All steroids cause glucose levels to rise, but they may be a necessary part of your protocol. Do not take yourself off of these drugs on your own—the results can be dire! Instead, ask your doctor for a weaning schedule.

### Are you dropping out of ketosis?

If you aren't already using it, try tracking with Cronometer for a few days. I think you'll find that it is a huge help in identifying foods that may contain hidden carbs. (It can also help you to keep to your protein target; too much protein is actually a bigger problem than you may think.) Remember, too, that you need to divide your macros fairly evenly over the day and not overeat protein, especially at dinner.

## Sometimes the Reason Is Right under Your Nose

I can recall a time that I dropped out of ketosis and wasn't sure why. I thought back through the previous day's meals, and there didn't seem to be anything out of the ordinary. Then I went to the refrigerator to get a bowl of broth with meat and rutabagas that my husband had made and noticed that the cooled liquid was more gelatinous than usual. When I mentioned this to him, he explained that he was experimenting with adding collagen to improve the consistency of the broth. Mystery solved! The amino acids in collagen are very glucogenic. Now I knew to limit the amount of broth I consumed. Within a few hours, I was back in nutritional ketosis.

*Are there hidden carbs in any of your medicines, supplements, or hygiene products?*

Look for sugars, starches, and sugar alcohols (aside from erythritol) in the ingredients list on food and supplement labels. You can also go to The Charlie Foundation website (www.CharlieFoundation.org) and download its list of low-carb and carb-free supplements and personal hygiene products (https://www.charliefoundation.org/resources-tools/resources-2/low-carb).

*Are you experiencing nausea? Vomiting? Constipation?*

All of these symptoms can trigger the release of hormones that stimulate glucose production, so they should be addressed! If your symptoms are treatment-related or due to your cancer, ask your doctor or oncology nurse for suggestions. (Be careful with natural remedies while in treatment. For example, ginger, while seemingly benign, has anticoagulant effects and may also interact with certain drugs.) If your symptoms are due to an illness, ride it out and know that your glucose will improve when you're feeling better. If your nausea appears to be diet-related, cut your intake of fats and oils down to a level at which you are comfortable, then gradually increase the amounts while maintaining your awareness of which fats you can tolerate and which create too much of a feeling of fullness. You can also opt to add a high-lipase pancreatic enzyme, such as Pure Encapsulations, that will aid in digesting fat. Other strategies include spreading your fat intake out over several small meals and/or snacks and widening your eating window to a place that allows you to comfortably take in the amount of fat that you need.

*Is your glucose still high?*

Is your glucose level still high (> 90 mg/dL), despite tight adherence to the diet? If so, work through these questions: **Is it just your fasting blood glucose that is high?** Recall that this can simply be due to the dawn effect, the normal circadian action that cortisol has on gluconeogenesis. High fasting glucose can also be due to too much protein at the evening meal, particularly if that meal (or other food) is eaten within a few hours of bedtime. Another possibility, but one that is poorly understood, may rest with what is now referred to as *physiological insulin resistance*. Put simply, a lower fasting insulin (a good thing) may result in less glucose uptake, resulting in a higher fasting number. Typically, high fasting numbers drop within a few hours of waking, even faster if you engage in some gentle movement that directs glucose to the liver. **Are you receiving chemotherapy or radiation, or recovering from surgery (all of which are "injuries")?** If so, understand that your body's response here is the same as for other illnesses or injuries. Expect your numbers to be higher than if you were not facing these additional challenges. Your efforts are not futile! Instead, realize that your glucose would be even higher on a standard diet.

**Do you have extensive metastatic disease?** A large tumor load anywhere in your body can create inflammation and produce metabolic waste that is converted back to glucose in the liver. Also, extensive liver metastases may interfere with your ability to make ketones. Ask your oncology team if they believe that your disease may be contributing to higher glucose levels. There is nothing to be done about this, unfortunately, but at least you will understand the cause.

**Are you insulin resistant?** If you have a long history of excess weight or other risk factors for metabolic disease, you may be insulin resistant. If so, your circulating levels of glucose and insulin might both remain higher than ideal because your cells are less sensitive to the insulin you secrete. The presence of insulin also suppresses ketone production, creating a vicious cycle. You need more time to adapt to the diet. Another option is to talk to your primary care doctor about adding metformin, a prescription medication that helps to lower blood glucose levels and restore insulin sensitivity in people with diabetes (or prediabetes). Although metformin is not a cancer drug, your doctor may already be aware of the lower cancer rates in people who have been prescribed this drug for diabetes. If you do take it, your doctor should monitor your HDL cholesterol and vitamin $B_{12}$ levels.

**Are you waiting too long between meals or taking in too few calories?** In some people, waiting too long between meals can signal the liver to fill in the energy gap by making glucose. Also, rapid weight loss (greater than 5 to 7 pounds in the first two weeks) can be a red flag that calorie intake is too low and, again, that can be a stressor that stimulates gluconeogenesis. Rework your calculations. You may need to relax the amount of caloric restriction.

**How well are you coping with stress?** Remember that stress stimulates the internal production of steroid hormones, which then stimulate your liver to make glucose. If your stress level appears to rise in the week before follow-up scans, acknowledge your apprehension, then plan some pleasant activities or create productive distractions.

### Are you bored or dissatisfied with your choices?

Change it up! If you're bored with bacon and eggs, you don't have to stick to traditional breakfast foods; any keto meal can take its place. If you need more variety, dive into your keto cookbooks for some new ideas. Also, there is an ever-expanding number of websites that offer a variety of keto-friendly recipes. I've included several recommendations in the resources section.

# APPENDIX B

# Recipes

## Pete's Sesame Cheese Crackers

YIELD: 48 CRACKERS

My husband is a very talented cook. For him, it's a bit of this and a pinch of that so when he comes up with a clear winner, I follow him around the kitchen, clipboard in hand, weighing every ingredient and making notes on his preparation technique. That's how we came up with the recipe for these delicious crackers!

I encourage you to adapt this recipe to include your favorite herbs and seasonings. You can adjust the amount of protein powder as well. The small amount used here adds "umami" (savory taste). It also acts as a binder, keeping the crackers from crumbling. (I usually eat these with butter, cheese, or cream cheese.)

NUTRITION INFORMATION.
SERVING SIZE: 1 CRACKER (APPROX. 14 G)

| | | |
|---|---|---|
| Fat | 5.3 g | (82%) |
| Protein | 1.8 g | (12%) |
| Net Carbs | 0.85 g | (6%) |
| Fiber | 1.0 g | |
| Calories | 57 | |

INGREDIENTS

80 g ground flaxseed
80 g sesame seeds
40 g coconut flour
42 g MCT powder (I use Quest brand)
28 g protein powder
   (calculated using Sunwarrior but
   other brands are options)

8 g garlic (granulated)
8 g onion (granulated)
8 g salt
80 g cheddar cheese, grated
110 g sour cream
120 g melted butter
   (salted or unsalted)

PREPARATION

Preheat oven to 250°F (275°F for convection oven). In a medium-size mixing bowl, blend together the dry ingredients and cheese. Spoon into the food processor, add sour cream, and pulse until blended. Add melted butter and pulse until stiff. (You may need to knock it down from the sides a few times.) Remove dough from processor and divide into 3 equal parts. Form each into a log (approx. 2.5" × 4.5"). To get 16 slices from each log, cut each log in half widthwise, then cut each of those in half widthwise, repeating until you have made 16 round slices from each log. Press slices onto a silicone baking mat or cookie sheet lined with parchment paper. Bake on one side for 30 minutes, then turn them over and bake for another 30 minutes. Cool crackers on rack.

## Keto Muffins (Lemon Poppy Seed)

YIELD: 9 MUFFINS

We've been enjoying what are known as "mug muffins" since we discovered them in 2008. Since that time, there's been an explosion of variations, and now if you search online for "keto mug muffins," you'll find hundreds of low-carb and keto recipes. Unless you can trust the source, always verify any nutrition data you find online by entering it into your own preferred database, either using an app or going directly to the USDA Food Composition Database (see resources section).

We've had a lot of fun coming up with new ideas for these keto muffins. We've experimented with many variations on this basic theme: for example, pumpkin nut, blueberry, cranberry-apple, zucchini, and carrot cake. We've even made a chocolate sour cream version and several dairy-free variations as well. Each version requires some tweaking to accommodate for our choice of spice or extract, or to adjust for the moisture content or sweetness of the fruit or vegetable we use. I'll lay out the basic recipe for a lemon poppy seed muffin, and you can take it from there.

We use baking *soda* instead of baking *powder*: The baking soda reacts with the acidic ingredients (e.g., sour cream, lemon juice, or vinegar in mayo) causing the batter to rise.

Note: The recipe yield is 9 muffins. We use a 12-muffin silicone mold that we cut down in order to fit it into our microwave. (Yes, we microwave these but you can bake them in an oven—with some tweaking to adjust for moisture.)

## NUTRITION INFORMATION.
### SERVING SIZE: 1 MUFFIN (APPROX. 32 G)

| | | |
|---|---|---|
| Fat | 9.8 g | (83%) |
| Protein | 3.2 g | (12%) |
| Net Carbs | 1.4 g* | (5%) |
| Fiber | 1.2 g | |
| Calories | 106 | |

* This includes the carb content of the stevia/erythritol blend (although it does not raise glucose levels)

## INGREDIENTS

32 g almond flour

30 g ground flaxseed

18 g MCT powder (I use Quest brand)

18 g Pyure Organic stevia/erythritol blend (adjust to taste)

10 g poppy seeds

1.4 g baking soda (rounded ¼ tsp)

2 large eggs

40 g mayonnaise (no soybean oil; read the ingredient list carefully)

20 g sour cream (for dairy-free version, substitute more mayo for sour cream)

5 g vanilla extract (you can use other extracts as well, such as lemon or orange oil)

15 g lemon juice

3–4 drops stevia (of course this is optional)

## PREPARATION

Mix dry ingredients in a medium-size mixing bowl. In another medium-size mixing bowl, whisk together the wet ingredients until smooth. Fold the blended dry ingredients into the wet ingredients. Optional: Add 30–40 g of fruit, berries, cooked pumpkin, or shredded zucchini or carrot. (Just be sure to include these extras in your food diary, along with any nuts, spices, or extracts that you use.)

Spoon batter into the silicone muffin mold. Microwave on "high" for approximately 2 minutes 45 seconds. Muffins should be sticky but not wet. Pop them out onto a cooling rack.

These muffins travel well, and I take them everywhere so I will have a filling keto food with me even if I'm stranded in a food desert. They will also keep well in the refrigerator for a few days.

Feel free to experiment, making sure to take notes on the weight of each ingredient. When you have a winner, enter it as a custom recipe in Cronometer (or other tracking tool).

# Miriam's Homemade Chocolate

YIELD: 3 SERVINGS

Why buy expensive chocolate bars with mystery ingredients? Instead, you can make your own in just minutes! I use a microwave, but you can also use a double boiler on the stove.

NUTRITION INFORMATION.

SERVING SIZE: APPROX. 28 G

| | | |
|---|---|---|
| Fat | 11 g | (87%) |
| Protein | 1.6 g | (6%) |
| Net Carbs | 2.1 g* | (7%) |
| Fiber | 1.6 g | |
| Calories | 113 | |

\* This includes the carb content of the stevia/erythritol blend (although it does not raise glucose levels)

INGREDIENTS

28 g of unsweetened baking chocolate (should contain only chocolate)

45 g (3 tbsp) heavy whipping cream

12 g (1 rounded tbsp) Pyure Organic stevia/erythritol blend

5 g (1 tsp) vanilla

Chop (or shave) chocolate into small pieces and set aside. Combine whipping cream, stevia/erythritol blend, and vanilla in a small microwavable mixing bowl. Microwave on "high" for a total of 1½ minutes. Watch it closely. The mixture will start to boil at 30 seconds and will continue to boil rapidly for close to a full minute. (Remove the bowl from the microwave as soon as the boiling slows down and the mixture starts to settle. This may take more or less than 1½ minutes depending on your microwave.) Be careful! Both the bowl and the mixture will be very hot. Let cool for a few minutes, then stir in chocolate pieces until melted.*

Customize it to suit your taste. For example, I like mine with a pinch of chili powder. You can also add cacao nibs, citrus zest, orange oil, salt, and caramel extract. . . . You get the picture, right?

Drop or spoon the mixture onto a silicone sheet or parchment paper. (Waxed paper works, too.) Spread it out to your desired thickness. I like it thinner than supermarket bars; it's easier to break into smaller pieces and not as hard on my teeth. Cool and store in the refrigerator.

\* Candy thermometers don't work well here, so you may need a few tries to find the Goldilocks zone for when to add the chocolate. If the chocolate doesn't melt completely, the mixture cooled for too long before you added the chocolate; if the end product is grainy or oily, the mixture was still too hot.

# Resources

## Ketogenic Metabolic Therapies

*Cancer as a Metabolic Disease: On the Origin, Management, and Prevention of Cancer* by Thomas N. Seyfried, PhD (Wiley, 2012)

Dr. Seyfried is a lead researcher at Boston College. Here, he presents a solid case for the science behind his theory that cancer is primarily a mitochondrial metabolic disease. He also introduces the concept of metabolic therapy; the use of the ketogenic diet alongside FDA-approved drugs, and other therapies that target energy metabolism in cancer.

*Fat for Fuel: A Revolutionary Diet to Combat Cancer, Boost Brain Power, and Increase Your Energy* by Joseph Mercola, DO (Hay House, 2017)

Dr. Mercola enthusiastically presents his structured plan for optimizing mitochondrial health. His metabolic management therapy nutrition plan features a whole-foods ketogenic diet that stresses the importance of choosing the highest-quality food sources.

*Fight Cancer with a Ketogenic Diet: Using a Low-Carb, Fat-Burning Diet as Metabolic Therapy* by Ellen Davis, MS (Gutsy Badger Publishing, 2017)

In *Fight Cancer,* Ellen Davis addresses every major question and concern for those who may be initially overwhelmed by what they may have read about the diet online. Using clear language, she offers the reader a simple and practical guide to initiating and monitoring a ketogenic diet for cancer. The format of the print version of this book (large print and easy to navigate) makes it an ideal resource for older adults.

*Ketogenic Diet and Metabolic Therapeutics* edited by Susan A. Masino, PhD (Oxford University Press, 2017)

Lead researchers and clinicians in metabolic therapeutics join together to present this scholarly collection highlighting the established and emerging applications of the ketogenic diet and other metabolic modalities.

*The Ketogenic and Modified Atkins Diets: Treatments for Epilepsy and Other Disorders* by Eric H. Kossoff, MD, et al. 6th ed. (Demos Health, 2016)

With this 6th edition, the pediatric epilepsy team at Johns Hopkins updates the science and application of ketogenic diet therapy for epilepsy and other neurological disorders. Fortunately, this practical and vetted information is applicable to the use of the diet for cancer as well. This is a valuable resource and a "must-have" manual for all parents with children on ketogenic diets.

*The Metabolic Approach to Cancer: Integrating Deep Nutrition, the Ketogenic Diet, and Nontoxic Bio-Individualized Therapies* by Nasha Winters, ND, LAc, FABNO, and Jess Higgins Kelley, MNT (Chelsea Green Publishing, 2017)

The authors expose the inadequacies inherent in the entrenched model of conventional cancer care. Looking beyond the manifestations of a body out of balance, they open the reader's eyes to the underlying metabolic changes that contribute to the development and progression of cancer. Also included here is a set of tools—including nutrition, lifestyle, and metabolic therapies—that offers an opportunity to bring body and mind back into balance.

*Tripping over the Truth: How the Metabolic Theory of Cancer Is Overturning One of Medicine's Most Entrenched Paradigms* by Travis Christofferson, MS (Chelsea Green Publishing, 2017)

Travis's book features background stories on the major players in the development of the metabolic theory of cancer. Entertaining, readable, and very informative! Watch his interview with Dr. Joseph Mercola to learn more about Travis, his book, and the Foundation for Metabolic Cancer Therapies, formerly known as Single Cause, Single Cure.

## Ketogenic Diet Classics

*The Art and Science of Low Carbohydrate Performance* and *The Art and Science of Low Carbohydrate Living* by Jeff S. Volek, PhD, RD, and Stephen D. Phinney, MD, PhD (Beyond Obesity, 2012)

No discussion of cancer here, but both of these books are excellent introductions to the science and practice of low-carb diets. *Performance* is a great manual for athletes who want to know the "why" and not just the "how" of low-carb performance. *Living* presents the science and clinical applications for health care professionals and science-savvy laypeople.

*Keto Clarity: Your Definitive Guide to the Benefits of a Low-Carb, High-Fat Diet* by Jimmy Moore with Eric C. Westman, MD (Victory Belt Publishing, 2014)

Jimmy Moore brings together keto experts to emphasize the many benefits of ketogenic living. This book is a great primer for those new to the keto world who want their many questions answered in a straightforward fashion, free of hype.

*The New Atkins for a New You* by Eric C. Westman, MD, Stephen D. Phinney, MD, and Jeff S. Volek, PhD (Fireside, 2010)

The Atkins diet has always offered a simple, do-it-yourself program for weight loss, but these same guidelines apply to other uses of the diet as well. *The New Atkins* offers online support with meal plans and recipes, including some vegetarian and vegan options. Phase I (Induction) is low carb (20 net grams). (Once the basics are mastered, it will be easier to advance to a keto-for-cancer plan by lowering protein, adding fat, and monitoring blood glucose and ketone levels.)

*The Wahls Protocol: How I Beat Progressive MS Using Paleo Principles and Functional Medicine* by Terry Wahls, MD (Penguin, 2014)

Although this book is not about cancer, it is a valuable resource for those who are coping with autoimmune disease and now have a new diagnosis of cancer. Dr. Wahls draws on her own personal experience to offer a stepped approach that covers both diet and lifestyle. Her Paleo Plus plan is actually a modified ketogenic pattern with an emphasis on cruciferous and highly pigmented vegetables.

## Keto Cookbooks and Recipes

*200 Low-Carb High-Fat Recipes* by Dana Carpender (Fair Winds Press, 2015)

In stark contrast to Emmerich's books, there are no illustrations here. Instead, you'll find no-nonsense, easy-to-prepare, field-tested recipes that are a snap to adapt to a keto-for-cancer plan. Although there are a few recipes that yield two servings, most yield four to six servings, which is a great option for those who want to limit actual cooking time to just a few days per week and store leftovers in the fridge. Carpender also offers tips on food prep and a backstory for each recipe.

*Blender Keto: A Guide to Making Blended Formula for Ketogenic Therapy* by Beth Zupec-Kania, RDN, CD (The Charlie Foundation for Ketogenic Therapies, 2016)

This pamphlet is a labor of love and a much-needed resource for those who must consume liquid or soft diets part or all of the time—or who receive their nutrition solely through specialized feeding tubes. These recipes are based on whole, fresh foods. Available only through The Charlie Foundation website.

*The Ketogenic Kitchen* by Domini Kemp and Patricia Daly (Chelsea Green Publishing, 2016)

This is my number one recommendation for those who want meal plans and recipes served up with great meal prep tips and other valuable keto-for-cancer information. Both authors are cancer survivors, and their book is divided into two distinct approaches: Patricia Daly's is ketogenic and Domini Kemp's is low carb. Daly offers meal plans that serve as a starting point for those who thrive on structure and are willing to use a scale to weigh foods (highly recommended). Some adjustments need to be made for those who wish to make single servings or who are not interested in including organ meats (which are more commonly consumed in Europe). Kemp's section reflects a more moderate view of a sustainable low-carb lifestyle— perhaps something to think of as a lifetime plan.

*The Modified Keto Cookbook* by Dawn Marie Martenz with Beth Zupec-Kania, RDN, CD (Demos Health, 2016)

Dawn Martenz is mom to a keto kid and Beth Zupec-Kania is the consultant nutritionist for The Charlie Foundation. This is their second collaboration, this time designed for those who desire a more liberal keto diet plan. The recipes included here are ideal for those who are easing into (as opposed to jumping into) a keto diet plan. All recipes include gram weights as well as standard kitchen measures, which also helps with a gradual transition. The major difference in presentation is that servings include information on diet ratios, not macros.

*Quick and Easy Ketogenic Cooking* by Maria Emmerich (Victory Belt Publishing, 2016) and *The Ketogenic Cookbook* by Jimmy Moore and Maria Emmerich (Victory Belt Publishing, 2015)

Both of these books are oriented toward healing the body through adherence to Paleo principles (though many recipes do include dairy). They are best suited for people who are comfortable with whole-food cooking and enjoy the process of meal preparation. The lavish illustrations are inspiring, and both books include charts and other aids. Choose the print versions.

*Sweet and Savory Fat Bombs: 100 Delicious Treats for Fat Fasts, Ketogenic, Paleo, and Low-Carb Diets* by Martina Slajerova (Quarto Publishing Group USA, 2016)

Fat bombs are a great way to incorporate more fat into the diet. Martina Slajerova's website, www.KetoDietApp.com, features "60 Amazing Fat Bombs," but you may prefer to purchase this compilation as a handy reference for your keto bookshelf.

Favorite Sources of Online Keto Recipes (most other "low-carb" recipes are too high in protein and/or carbs):

- https://www.charliefoundation.org/resources-tools/resources-2/find-recipes (all keto approved)
- www.KetoDietApp.com (source of "60 Amazing Fat Bombs")
- https://PatriciaDaly.com/recipes (recipes and meal plans from Patricia Daly)
- https://fiercefoodsacademy.wordpress.com (MaxLove Project)
- www.ruled.me (carbs are low, but protein may be too high)
- www.Ketogenic-Diet-Resource.com (low-carb recipes; may need to be tweaked for keto)
- Search online for several variations of the "Keto Mug Muffin." (Note: Not all are keto, and nutrition information may be incorrect. Double-check them!)

### Calling All Chefs

The keto world needs cookbooks that cater to dairy-free diet plans. Individual recipes can be found online, but it would be great to have a whole collection compiled into an easy reference book. The same holds true for egg-free. (Most egg substitutes contain starch.)

## Other Books of Interest to the Keto Community

*The Alzheimer's Antidote: Using a Low-Carb, High-Fat Diet to Fight Alzheimer's Disease, Memory Loss, and Cognitive Decline* by Amy Berger, MS, CNS (Chelsea Green Publishing, 2017)

*The Big Fat Surprise: Why Butter, Meat, and Cheese Belong in a Healthy Diet* by Nina Teicholz (Simon & Schuster, 2014)

*Brain Maker: The Power of Gut Microbes to Heal and Protect Your Brain—for Life* by David Perlmutter, MD, with Kristin Loberg (Little, Brown and Company, 2015)

*The Case Against Sugar* by Gary Taubes (Alfred A. Knopf, 2016)

*The Complete Guide to Fasting* by Jason Fung, MD, and Jimmy Moore (Victory Belt Publishing, 2016)

*Conquer Type 2 Diabetes with a Ketogenic Diet* and *The Ketogenic Diet for Type 1 Diabetes* by Ellen Davis, MS, and Keith Runyan, MD (Gutsy Badger Publishing, 2017. eBook online at www.ketogenic-diet-resource.com)

*Good Calories, Bad Calories: Challenging the Conventional Wisdom on Diet, Weight Control, and Disease* by Gary Taubes (Alfred A. Knopf, 2007)

*The Grain Brain Whole Life Plan: Boost Brain Performance, Lose Weight, and Achieve Optimal Health* by David Perlmutter, MD, with Kristin Loberg (Little, Brown and Company, 2016)

*I Contain Multitudes: The Microbes within Us and a Grander View of Life* by Ed Yong (Vintage, 2017)

*Misguided Medicine* by Colin Champ, MD (2nd ed, CDR Health and Nutrition LLC, 2016)

*Nourishing Fats: Why We Need Animal Fats for Health and Happiness* by Sally Fallon Morell
(Hachette Book Group, 2017)
*Power, Sex, and Suicide: Mitochondria and the Meaning of Life* by Nick Lane, PhD (Oxford
University Press, 2005)
*Radical Remission: Surviving Cancer against All Odds* by Kelly Turner, PhD (HarperOne, 2015)
*Surviving Terminal Cancer* by Ben Williams (Fairview Press, 2002)

## Integrative Oncology Practitioners

At the time of this writing, there are precious few practitioners that I know of who can provide
guidance for the clinical application of ketogenic metabolic therapy. Consider this list just the
beginning of what I expect to become a consumer-driven need for this specialty. Several national
organizations with an interest in medical nutrition therapy now include members who support
the integration of ketogenic metabolic therapies into cancer care protocols. These include:

- American Board of Naturopathic Oncology
- American College of Nutrition
- American Nutrition Association (keto certification course in development)
- Institute for Functional Medicine
- Oncology Association of Naturopathic Physicians
- Personalized Lifestyle Medicine Institute
- Society for Integrative Oncology

Check my website for updates (www.DietaryTherapies.com)

### J. William LaValley, MD (www.LaValleyMDProtocols.com)

Dr. Will LaValley has been treating patients in Austin, TX, and Nova Scotia, Canada, since
1988. Currently, Dr. LaValley serves as a professional consultant to physicians. His area of
advanced interest and expertise is in developing and communicating detailed evidence-based
and molecularly targeted treatment plans for cancer patients and their physicians to consider
as part of integrative care. His personalized protocols include scientifically evidence-based
recommendations for natural supplements and repurposed (off-label) pharmaceuticals as
adjuncts to—not in place of—conventional chemotherapy and radiation therapy. He is a
member of numerous medical associations, including the American Medical Association, the
Canadian Medical Association, and the Society for Integrative Oncology. More information is
available at https://www.Linkedin.com/in/LaValleyMDProtocols.

### Kara Fitzgerald, ND, IFMCP (www.DrKaraFitzgerald.com)

Dr. Fitzgerald is a skilled integrative and functional medicine doctor with a practice in Sandy
Hook, CT. She completed post-doctoral training in nutritional biochemistry and laboratory
science at Metametrix (now Genova) and has authored and edited numerous papers and
publications. She and nutritionist Romilly Hodges, MS, CNS, are experienced in the use of
the ketogenic diet for cancer and other metabolic diseases, and regularly educate other practitioners in the applications of the ketogenic diet. They follow Dr. Thomas Seyfried's work and
are quick to revise protocols based on the latest research. Dr. Fitzgerald and Ms. Hodges have
coauthored *Methylation Diet and Lifestyle*, available on the clinic's website.

Optimal Terrain Consulting (www.OptimalTerrainConsulting.com)

Find support for the ketogenic diet as an adjunct to other nutritional and oncological proto-cols. Optimal Terrain Consulting was founded by Nasha Winters, ND, LAc, FABNO, coauthor of the book *The Metabolic Approach to Cancer* (Chelsea Green Publishing, 2017).

Raymond Chang, MD (www.meridianmedical.org)

Dr. Chang is a physician-researcher, trained in both contemporary Western and traditional Eastern medicine. He supports the use of conventional therapies integrated with alternative modalities, including the ketogenic diet as part of a "cocktail" anticancer therapy for brain cancer. He also partners with Dr. Thomas Nesselhut's clinic in Duderstadt, Germany.

## Keto-for-Cancer Nutrition Specialists

**The Astro Brain Tumor Fund** (www.astrofund.org.uk/news.php) supports ketogenic diet and other adjunct therapies for the treatment of gliomas (a type of brain cancer) in the United Kingdom. Contact it for more information.

**Beth Winter**, a keto dietitian and long-term melanoma survivor, is also working with cancer clients. Contact her at beth.winter@comcast.net.

**The Charlie Foundation** (www.CharlieFoundation.org) has a group of dietitians and nutritionists with extensive experience in implementing ketogenic diet therapy, including the use of the diet for cancer. Learn more at www.KetogenicSpecialists.com. You'll find bios and links to their websites. At the time of this writing, six of these keto specialists are working with private clients (listed in alphabetical order by first name):

> Beth Zupec-Kania, RDN (specialist in enteral nutrition)
> Candy Richardson, RD, LDN, CNSC (clinical oncology experience—solid tumors)
> Denise Potter, RDN, CSP, CDE
> Jenny Kramer, MS, RDN
> Mary Beth Joy, MS, RDN, CSP, LD
> Sarah Jadin, MS, RDN, CSP, CNSC (includes vegetarian and vegan plans)

**Miriam Kalamian, EdM, MS, CNS** (www.DietaryTherapies.com), yes, that's me! I am a nutrition educator, consultant, and speaker, as well as the author of this book. I am avail-able to help people who have adopted a ketogenic diet for cancer connect with emerging ketogenic metabolic therapies. I am also a resource for health care professionals who want to learn how to implement a well-formulated ketogenic diet for their patients or clients.

Please understand that I am not endorsing any particular person. I'm simply sharing what I know at this time and will keep an updated list on my website.

## Ketogenic Diet Clinics (Not Specific to Cancer)

**HEAL Clinics** (https://HealClinics.com). Established for the treatment of diabetes and medical weight loss by Eric C. Westman, MD, an obesity medicine specialist and director of the Duke Lifestyle Medicine Clinic. There may be some flexibility here in accepting patients with dysregulated metabolism who are also cancer survivors.

**Virta** (www.VirtaHealth.com). A new start-up whose founders include Jeff Volek, PhD, RD, and Stephen Phinney, MD, PhD. Although the goal of this company is to reverse diabetes, its medical model is an inspiration to those with an interest in ketogenic metabolic therapy for cancer. I hope to see a similar start-up in the cancer world soon!

## Podcasts and Videos

**Dr. Colin Champ** is a radiation oncologist who supports ketogenic and calorie-restricted diets as adjuncts to conventional care. His IHMC video includes discussion of metabolic pathways in cancer that are targeted by diet: https://www.youtube.com /watch?v=ot96y5-D_K0.

**Dr. Dominic D'Agostino** was interviewed about his cancer research by Tim Ferriss (www.fourhourworkweek.com) in August 2015. (Here's the link: tim.blog/2015/11 /03/dominic-dagostino.) Settle in and listen to all three hours of this podcast! Ferriss has interviewed Dr. D'Agostino on two other occasions; you may want to listen to these thought-provoking interviews as well, even though they are not specific to cancer. You can easily find many more podcasts and videos of Dr. D'Agostino's interviews and presentations.

**Dr. Eugene J. Fine** is an internist and nuclear medicine physician with a keen interest in ketogenic diet therapy. He has published the results of a compelling pilot trial using a ketogenic diet in advanced cancers. The report included information on each patient's ketone levels as well as documentation of the metabolic response of the tumor to treatment as evidenced by a PET scan. View his video from the Ancestral Health Society meeting in 2012 where he discusses specifics of his human study: https://www.youtube .com/watch?v=04A5U6IlHqk.

**The Florida Institute for Human and Machine Cognition (IHMC)** offers an evening lecture series, videotapes of which it posts online. To see what's coming up in the near future, visit its website at https://www.ihmc.us/life/evening_lectures.

**Dr. Jeff Volek** is another leader in the community of low-carb researchers (though not focused on cancer). You'll find countless videos of his presentations online. For those of you who want to learn more about keto-adaptation, start with this YouTube intro: https://www.youtube.com/watch?v=GC1vMBRFiwE.

**Dr. Joseph Mercola** has a strong interest in ketogenic diets for mitochondrial health as reflected in his recent book *Fat for Fuel*. He has interviewed a number of leaders in the keto world as well as researchers and clinicians at the leading edge of ketogenic metabolic therapeutics. Visit www.Mercola.com for archived interviews.

**Dr. Thomas Seyfried** is a frequent presenter at scientific conferences and has been interviewed extensively about his research. Keep up with what's new by a simple online search of his name. For those of you new to keto, you may want to start by watching his short presentation at the Ancestral Health Society's 2012 symposium (available on YouTube at https://www.youtube.com/watch?v=sBjnWfT8HbQ).

**The University of South Florida** has hosted two well-received conferences on nutritional ketosis and metabolic therapeutics. Fortunately for the keto world, all presentations are videotaped and posted. Explore the archives at www.MetabolicTherapeuticsConference .com and, if you can, plan to attend the next annual conference.

## Websites and Blogs

**Allison Gannet's** brain cancer story: https://www.youtube.com/watch?v=x91vpkXCmH8.

**Alix Hayden**, a brain tumor survivor, has a lively Facebook page (https://www.facebook.com/alix.hayden).

**Andrew Scarborough** has a compelling personal story at mybraincancerstory.blogspot.com.

**The Charlie Foundation** (www.CharlieFoundation.org) is a nonprofit organization that I've referenced multiple times. It was originally focused on the use of the ketogenic diet for pediatric epilepsy, but has since expanded to include emerging applications of the diet as well. It's an amazing resource for general keto information, recipes, and food-prep videos. Matthew's Friends (www.MatthewsFriends.org), its British counterpart, is also a great resource.

**Dr. Dominic D'Agostino** has his own website (www.KetoNutrition.org) and blog (Keto Nutrition.blogspot.com).

**Dr. Georgia Ede** is a psychiatrist at Smith College in Northampton, MA. Her website, www.DiagnosisDiet.com, is a wonderful place to learn more about her passion and find information on the relationship between nutrition and mental health.

**Jimmy Moore** (www.LivinLaVidaLowCarb.com) has been a cornerstone of the low-carb and keto world since 2006. His list of guests reads like a Who's Who of experts in the field. Plan to spend some time searching his archives.

**Ketogenic Diet Resource** (www.Ketogenic-Diet-Resource.com) is a website that I've made several references to throughout my book. Ellen Davis has packed it full of vetted information and links to outside resources. Start by visiting her Cancer page.

**Low Carb USA** is relatively new to the scene, and it kicked off with an amazing event in San Diego in August 2016. Visit www.lowcarbusa.org to see what new events are planned.

**MaxLove** website and Facebook page (www.maxloveproject.org and https://www.facebook.com/maxloveproject). These are wonderful and supportive places for families with children who are facing life-threatening illnesses.

**Pablo Kelly** blogs about his brain cancer experience at www.facebook.com/pablosbrainjourney.

**Quest Nutrition's Keto Pet Sanctuary** (www.KetoPetSanctuary.com; blog.questnutrition.com/is-the-ketopet-sanctuary-curing-cancer; and www.facebook.com/KetoPet). This wonderful institution is treating dogs with cancer using ketogenic metabolic therapies. Watch an inspiring video presentation of their work at https://www.facebook.com/incrediblechap/posts/10109549918164309.

## Nutrition Resources

**Histamine Intolerance.** My friend and colleague Dr. Georgia Ede has an excellent post about this topic, including a brilliant slideshow, on her website: www.DiagnosisDiet.com/histamine-intolerance-science.

**Ideal Body Weight Calculator** (www.Calculator.net/ideal-weight-calculator.html). The *Ideal Weight Calculator* computes the ideal body weight as well as a healthy body weight range based on height, gender, and age. People have pursued an ideal weight formula for centuries, and hundreds of formulas and tables have been created. Although there is still no definite answer regarding the "best" weight for any individual, the results obtained by most formulas are very good. The *Ideal Weight Calculator* provides the results of all the popular formulas for comparison purposes.

**Oxalate Content of Foods** (https://regepi.bwh.harvard.edu/health/Oxalate/files/Oxalate
%20Content%20of%20Foods.xls)

**Spices Health Benefits** (www.webmd.com/food-recipes/features/spices-and-herbs
-health-benefits#1)

**Sugar Alcohols** (www.FoodInsight.org/articles/sugar-alcohols-fact-sheet)

**USDA Food Composition Database** (https://ndb.nal.usda.gov/ndb). All diet tracking apps
link to this vetted source of detailed nutrient information. Note that there are options to
search for both generic and brand-name products.

## Online Learning

**Biochemistry Topics** (www.aklectures.com/subject/biochemistry). Andrey Kopot does
an excellent job in walking you through the science of nutrient metabolism. I love his
presentations and hope that this link works forever.

**Blood Meters: Low Red Blood Cell (RBC) Counts.** Talk to your doctor or pharmacist
about blood meters designed to compensate for the effect that low red blood cell counts
have on glucose measurements. Here is a technical article describing the problem:
https://www.ncbi.nlm.nih.gov/pmc/articles/PMC3440048.

**Blood Testing Demonstration** (https://www.youtube.com/watch?v=rMMpeLLgdgY). A
quick demonstration of how to properly perform a finger prick test.

**Understanding Your Lab Tests** (https://LabTestsOnline.org). This is a good resource
designed to help patients learn more about the lab tests ordered by medical professionals.

**Yogic Breathing** (https://www.youtube.com/watch?v=9E09eO8BGDU). A straightforward
presentation of the science and practice. You have to breathe, so why not take 10 minutes
to work through this?

# Glossary

**Adjuvant/Adjunct therapy.** Usually, an intervention that is meant to enhance another therapy, especially when paired with a more conventional protocol.

**Antioxidant.** Used here to describe a substance that inhibits the action of free radicals.

**Apoptosis.** Also known as programmed cell death, this is the programmed self-destruction (suicide) of a cell when damage (e.g., mutated DNA) interferes with its optimal function. Evasion of apoptosis is one of the hallmarks of a cancer cell.

**Autophagy.** (Greek for "self-eating") A normal cellular mechanism in which dysfunctional or no longer needed parts of the cell are internally degraded and recycled.

**Clinical guideline.** A protocol (typically generated by teams of experts) that recommends how a patient should be treated for a given disease or condition.

**Clinical trial.** An investigation using humans to determine if a treatment is safe, effective, and therapeutic in managing a particular disease or condition. (Careful, here, as much pseudoscience claims to have evidence from clinical trials, but this can be misleading or patently false.)

**Confounding variable.** In a clinical trial, usually a condition that interferes with a clear and unbiased interpretation of the trial's results (e.g., not accounting for the past medical history of the individuals enrolled).

**Cytoplasm.** All the material (excluding the nucleus) contained within a cell's outer membrane.

**Evidence-based.** In medicine, a treatment or therapy based on both clinical experience and objective research obtained through clinical trials.

**Gluconeogenesis.** The making of new glucose in the liver using carbon molecules obtained from a variety of sources. This process typically occurs when the system perceives a shortage of glucose or when there is an abundance of one type of nutrient, such as amino acids or lactate.

**Glycolysis.** The enzymatic breakdown of glucose in the cytoplasm of the cell to produce either pyruvate (to enter the Krebs cycle) or lactate (fermentation within the cytoplasm).

**Heterogeneous.** A diverse or varied collection. In this instance the term is used to describe the wide variation in characteristics among cancer cells within a tumor.

**Hormesis.** The beneficial result to an organism from exposure to small doses of a cellular stressor (a toxin, a chemical, or even a change in temperature) that at large doses or higher levels would be harmful.

**Hypothesis.** In science, a theory that is then tested using reproducible methodology that yields results that can be statistically evaluated.

**Mitochondrion.** An organelle suspended within a cell's cytoplasm that is responsible for the majority of cellular energy production in complex organisms, including humans. Most cells contain a few mitochondria, while others, such as heart and muscle cells, contain thousands. Mitochondria also direct a number of cellular biochemical processes necessary for DNA repair and signaling to control activities such as cell replication and apoptosis.

**N-of-1 trial.** Term used to describe a trial involving only one participant. The study may be performed solely for oneself or for use as a case study.

**Organelle.** A structure within a cell with a particular function (e.g., nucleus, mitochondrion).

**Oxidation.** Oxidation generally refers to the addition of, or exposure to, oxygen. More specifically, it is a chemical reaction in which a substance loses electrons. The oxidation process can produce free radicals, which are damaging to cells or other molecules necessary for life.

**Oxidative phosphorylation.** The scientific term for respiration in organisms using oxygen and phosphate to form molecules of ATP, the "currency of energy" in humans and other animals.

**Peer review.** The formal evaluation of a study, trial, or research paper by others in that field of research. This evaluation is often required before an author's work can be published in a scientific journal.

**Preclinical data.** The raw data collected from a trial, often using animal models that can help determine whether to move to a level of inquiry that may include trials in humans. Promising preclinical data in animal models does not guarantee success in people, but may bolster interest in designing a study for humans.

**Prooxidant.** A compound or molecule that oxidizes other molecules, generally a particle with an electrical charge like oxygen that can damage cancer cells by altering them so that they die.

**Pseudoscience.** Beliefs promoted as having a basis in science even though they have not been tested using the scientific method (i.e., developing and testing a hypothesis). Often these beliefs are propagated by people with questionable motives and/or credentials.

**Reactive oxygen species (ROS).** Oxygen molecules with an extra negative charge. Depending on their quantity, these molecules can have either a positive effect—acting as signaling molecules—or a negative effect—causing damage and inflammation at the cellular level.

**Synergy.** In medicine, synergy refers to a positive interaction between treatments (such as two drugs used in combination) that produces an effect that is greater than that of each treatment used on its own.

# Notes

## Introduction

1. Kabat-Zinn J. *Wherever You Go, There You Are: Mindfulness Meditation in Everyday Life.* 10th ed. New York: Hyperion; 1994:189–190.
2. Schopick J. *Honest Medicine: Effective, Time-Tested, Inexpensive Treatments for Life-Threatening Diseases, Including Multiple Sclerosis, Epilepsy, Liver Disease, Lupus, Rheumatoid Arthritis, and Other Diseases.* Oak Park, IL: Innovative Health Pub; 2011.
3. Freeman JM, Vining EP, Kossoff EH, et al. A blinded, crossover study of the efficacy of the ketogenic diet. *Epilepsia.* 50(2), 322–325. doi:10.1111/j.1528-1167.2008.01740.x.
4. Cervenka MC, Henry BJ, Felton EA, et al. Establishing an adult epilepsy diet center: experience, efficacy and challenges. *Epilepsy Behav.* 2016;58:61–68. doi:10.1016/j.yebeh.2016.02.038.
5. Lambrechts DAJE, de Kinderen RJA, Vles JSH, et al. A randomized controlled trial of the ketogenic diet in refractory childhood epilepsy. *Acta Neurologica Scandinavica.* 2016;135(2):231–239. doi:10.1111/ane.12592.
6. Fine EJ, Segal-Isaacson CJ, Feinman RD, et al. Targeting insulin inhibition as a metabolic therapy in advanced cancer: a pilot safety and feasibility dietary trial in 10 patients. *Nutrition.* 2012;28(10):1028–1035. doi:10.1016/j.nut.2012.05.001.
7. Klement RJ, Kämmerer U. Is there a role for carbohydrate restriction in the treatment and prevention of cancer? *Nutr Metab (Lond).* 2011;8:75. doi:10.1201/b16308-18.

## Chapter 1: Cancer: Genetics or Metabolism?

1. Ledford H. End of cancer-genome project prompts rethink. *Nature.* 2015;517(7533):128–129. doi:10.1038/517128a.
2. Hanahan D, Weinberg RA. The hallmarks of cancer. *Cell.* 2000;100(1):57–70. doi:10.1016/s0092-8674(00)81683-9.
3. Hanahan D, Weinberg R. Hallmarks of cancer: the next generation. *Cell.* 2011;144(5):646–674. doi:10.1016/j.cell.2011.02.013.
4. Seyfried TN, Mukherjee P. Targeting energy metabolism in brain cancer: review and hypothesis. *Nutr Metab.* 2005;2:30. doi:10.1186/1743-7075-2-30.
5. Seyfried TN. Cancer as a mitochondrial metabolic disease. *Front Cell Dev Biol.* 2015;3:43. doi:10.3389/fcell.2015.00043.
6. Chang HT, Olson L, Schwartz KA. Ketolytic and glycolytic enzymatic expression profiles in malignant gliomas: implication for ketogenic diet therapy. *Nutr Metab.* 2013;10(1):47. doi:10.1186/1743-7075-10-47.
7. Lodish MB, Stratakis CA. Endocrine side effects of broad-acting kinase inhibitors. *Endocr Relat Cancer.* 2010;17(3):R233–R244. doi:10.1677/erc-10-0082.

8. Hudson CD, Hagemann T, Mather SJ, et al. Resistance to the tyrosine kinase inhibitor axitinib is associated with increased glucose metabolism in pancreatic adenocarcinoma. *Cell Death Dis.* 2014;5(4):e1160. doi:10.1038/cddis.2014.125.

9. Linneberg A, Madsen F, Skaaby T. Allergen-specific immunotherapy and risk of autoimmune disease. *Allergy Clin Immunol.* 2012;12(6):635–639. doi: 10.1097/ACI.0b013e3283588c8d.

10. Seyfried TN, Yu G, Maroon JC, et al. Press-pulse: a novel therapeutic strategy for the metabolic management of cancer. *Nutr Metab (Lond).* 2017;14(19). doi:10.1186/s12986-017-0178-2.

## Chapter 2: "Show Me the Evidence"

1. Nebeling LC, Miraldi F, Shurin SB, et al. Effects of a ketogenic diet on tumor metabolism and nutritional status in pediatric oncology patients: two case reports. *J Am Coll Nutr.* 1995;14(2):202–208. doi:10.1080/07315724.1995.10718495.

2. Zhou W, Mukherjee P, Kiebish MA, et al. The calorically restricted ketogenic diet, an effective alternative therapy for malignant brain cancer. *Nutr Metab.* 2007;4:5. doi:10.1186/1743-7075-4-5.

3. Poff AM, Ari C, Seyfried TN, et al. The ketogenic diet and hyperbaric oxygen therapy prolong survival in mice with systemic metastatic cancer. *PLoS ONE.* 2013:8(6):e65522. doi:10.1371/journal.pone.0065522.

4. Fine EJ, Segal-Isaacson CJ, Feinman RD, et al. Targeting insulin inhibition as a metabolic therapy in advanced cancer: a pilot safety and feasibility dietary trial in 10 patients. *Nutrition.* 2012;28(10):1028–1035. doi:10.1016/j.nut.2012.05.001.

5. Tan-Shalaby JL, Carrick J, Edinger K, et al. Modified Atkins diet in advanced malignancies—final results of a safety and feasibility trial within the Veterans Affairs Pittsburgh Healthcare System. *Nutr Metab.* 2016;13(1):52. doi:10.1186/s12986-016-0113-y.

## Chapter 3: "Show Me the Science"

1. Winter SF, Loebel F, Dietrich J. Role of ketogenic metabolic therapy in malignant glioma: a systematic review. *Crit Rev Oncol Hematol.* 2017;112:41–58. doi:10.1016/j.critrevonc.2017.02.016.

2. Nutrition for the Person with Cancer During Treatment: A Guide for Patients and Families. https://old.cancer.org/acs/groups/cid/documents/webcontent/002903-pdf.pdf. Published 2015. Updated January 9, 2017. Accessed January 10, 2017.

3. Derr RL, Ye X, Islas MU, et al. Association between hyperglycemia and survival in patients with newly diagnosed glioblastoma. *J Clin Oncol.* 2009;27(7):1082–1086. doi:10.1200/jco.2008.19.1098.

4. Chaichana KL, McGirt MJ, Woodworth GF, et al. Persistent outpatient hyperglycemia is independently associated with survival, recurrence and malignant degeneration following surgery for hemispheric low grade gliomas. *Neurol Research.* 2010;32(4):442–448. doi:10.1179/174313209x431101.

5. Cahill GF, Veech RL. Ketoacids? Good medicine? *Trans Am Clin Climatol Assoc.* 2003;114:149–163. https://www.ncbi.nlm.nih.gov/pubmed/12813917.

6. Noh HS, Hah Y-S, Nilufar R, et al. Acetoacetate protects neuronal cells from oxidative glutamate toxicity. *J Neurosci Research.* 2006;83(4):702–709. doi:10.1002/jnr.20736.

7. Rho JM. Substantia(ting) ketone body effects on neuronal excitability. *Epilepsy Curr.* 2007;7(5):142–144. doi:10.1111/j.1535-7511.2007.00206.x.

8. Volek JS, Freidenreich DJ, Saenz C, et al. Metabolic characteristics of keto-adapted ultra-endurance runners. *Metabolism.* 2016;65(3):100–110. doi:10.1016/j.metabol.2015.10.028.

9. Volek JS, Phinney SD, Kossoff E, et al. *The Art and Science of Low Carbohydrate Living: An Expert Guide to Making the Life-Saving Benefits of Carbohydrate Restriction Sustainable and Enjoyable.* Lexington, KY: Beyond Obesity; 2011:5.

## Chapter 4: Is the Ketogenic Diet Right for You?

1. Kossoff E, Turner Z, Doerrer S, et al. *The Ketogenic and Modified Atkins Diets: Treatments for Epilepsy and Other Disorders.* New York: Demos Medical Publishing, LLC; 2016:33.

2. Lu Z, Xie J, Wu G. Fasting selectively blocks development of acute lymphoblastic leukemia via leptin-receptor upregulation. *Nature Medicine.* 2017;23(1):79–90. doi:10.1038/nm.4252.

3. Xie J, Zhang C, Lu Z. Study shows fasting kills cancer cells of common childhood leukemia. Medical Press. http://medicalxpress.com/news/2016-12-fasting-cancer-cells-common-childhood.html. Published December 12, 2016. Accessed January 11, 2017.

4. How is shared decision-making different from informed consent? The American Cancer Society. http://www.cancer.org/treatment/findingandpayingfortreatment/understandingfinancialandlegalmatters/informedconsent/informed-consent-shared-decision-making. Updated July 28, 2014. Accessed January 11, 2017.

5. Merriam-Webster. Wellness. MedlinePlus. Accessed January 11, 2017. http://c.merriam-webster.com/medlineplus/wellness.

6. "About Wellness," National Wellness Institute, accessed July 23, 2017, http://www.nationalwellness.org/?page=AboutWellness. The Six Dimensions of Wellness were developed by Dr. Bill Hettler.

## Chapter 5: Understanding the Origins of the Ketogenic Diet

1. Newburgh LH, Marsh PL. The use of a high fat diet in the treatment of diabetes mellitus. *Arch Intern Med.* 1920;26(6):647. doi:10.1001/archinte.1920.00100060002001.

2. Banting W. Letter on Corpulence. 1864. http://www.thefitblog.net/ebooks/LetterOnCorpulence/LetteronCorpulence.pdf. [Web blog post]. (n.d.).

3. Groves B. William Banting father of the low-carbohydrate diet. The Weston A. Price Foundation. https://www.westonaprice.org/health-topics/know-your-fats/william-banting-father-of-the-low-carbohydrate-diet. Published April 30, 2003. Accessed March 14, 2017.

4. McClellan WS, DuBois EF. Clinical calorimetry: XLV, prolonged meat diets with a study of kidney functions and ketosis. *J Biol Chem.* 1930;87:651–668. http://www.jbc.org/content/87/3/651. Accessed January 11, 2017.

5. Atkins RC. *Dr. Atkins' Diet Revolution: The High Calorie Way to Stay Thin Forever.* New York: Bantam Books; 1973.

6. Kossoff EH, Dorward JL. The Modified Atkins Diet. *Epilepsia.* 2008;49(suppl 8):37–41. doi:10.1111/j.1528-1167.2008.01831.

7. Cervenka MC, Henry BJ, Felton EA, et al. Establishing an adult epilepsy diet center: experience, efficacy and challenges. *Epilepsy Behav.* 2016;58:61–68. doi:10.1016/j.yebeh.2016.02.038.
8. Schmidt R, Ropele S, Ebenbauer N, et al. P2-074: effects of memantine on brain volume, glucose metabolism and cognition in Alzheimer's disease patients: a neuroimaging study. *Alzheimers Dement.* 2008;4(4). doi:10.1016/j.jalz.2008.05.1147.
9. Bredesen DE. Reversal of cognitive decline: a novel therapeutic program. *Aging (Albany NY).* 2014;6(9):707–717, table 1.

## Chapter 6: Diet *Does* Matter!

1. Kossoff E, Turner Z, Doerrer S, et al. *The Ketogenic and Modified Atkins Diets: Treatments for Epilepsy and Other Disorders.* New York: Demos Medical Publishing, LLC; 2016.
2. NMR LipoProfile Blood Test. Walk-In Lab. http://www.walkinlab.com/heart-health-tests/nmrlipoprofilebloodtest.html. Accessed January 12, 2017.
3. Servan-Schreiber D. *Anticancer: a new way of life.* New York: Viking; 2009.
4. Bazzano LA, Hu T. Effects of low-carbohydrate and low-fat diets. *Ann Intern Med.* 2015;162(5):393. doi:10.7326/L15-5057-5.
5. Harvard University. Low fat, low carb, or Mediterranean: which diet is right for you? Harvard Health Publications. http://www.health.harvard.edu/staying-healthy/low-fat-low-carb-or-mediterranean-which-diet-is-right-for-you. Accessed January 12, 2017.

## Chapter 7: Fasting for Health

1. Faris MA, Kacimi S, AlKurd RA, et al. Intermittent fasting during Ramadan attenuates proinflammatory cytokines and immune cells in healthy subjects. *Nutr Res.* 2012;32(12):947–955. doi:10.1016/j.nutres.2012.06.021.
2. Mizushima N. Autophagy: process and function. *Gene Dev.* 2007;21(22):2861–2873. doi:10.1101/gad.1599207.
3. Jin S, White E. Role of autophagy in cancer: management of metabolic stress. *Autophagy.* 2007;3(1):28–31. doi:10.4161/auto.3269.
4. Institute of Medicine (US) Panel on Macronutrients. Chapter 12: Physical activity. In: *Dietary Reference Intakes: For Energy, Carbohydrate, Fiber, Fat, Fatty Acids, Cholesterol, Protein, and Amino Acids.* Washington, D.C.: National Academies Press; 2005:880–935.
5. Office of Dietary Supplements. Nutrient recommendations: dietary reference intakes (DRI). National Institutes of Health. https://ods.od.nih.gov/Health_Information/Dietary_Reference_Intakes.aspx. Accessed February 02, 2017.
6. Mukherjee P, El-Abbadi MM, Kasperzyk JL, et al. Dietary restriction reduces angiogenesis and growth in an orthotopic mouse brain tumour model. *Br J Cancer.* 2002;86(10):1615–1621. doi:10.1038/sj.bjc.6600298.
7. Hanahan D, Weinberg RA. The hallmarks of cancer. *Cell.* 2000;100(1):57–70. doi:10.1016/s0092-8674(00)81683-9.
8. González O, Tobia C, Ebersole J, et al. Caloric restriction and chronic inflammatory diseases. *Oral Dis.* 2012;18(1):16–31. doi:10.1111/j.1601-0825.2011.01830.x.
9. Seyfried TN, Kiebish M, Mukherjee P, et al. Targeting energy metabolism in brain cancer with calorically restricted ketogenic diets. *Epilepsia.* 2008;49(suppl 8):114–116. doi:10.1111/j.1528-1167.2008.01853.x.

10. Sinclair DA. Toward a unified theory of caloric restriction and longevity regulation. *Mech Ageing Dev.* 2005;126(9):987–1002. doi:10.1016/j.mad.2005.03.019.

11. Masoro EJ. History of caloric restriction, aging and longevity. In: Everitt AV, Rattan SIS, eds. *Calorie Restriction, Aging and Longevity.* Netherlands: Springer Netherlands; 2010:3–14. doi:10.1007/978-90-481-8556-6_1.

12. Zhou W, Mukherjee P, Kiebish MA, et al. The calorically restricted ketogenic diet, an effective alternative therapy for malignant brain cancer. *Nutr Metab.* 2007;4(1):5. doi:10.1186/1743-7075-4-5.

13. Lv M, Zhu X, Wang H, et al. Roles of caloric restriction, ketogenic diet and intermittent fasting during initiation, progression and metastasis of cancer in animal models: a systematic review and meta-analysis. *PLoS ONE.* 2014;9(12): e115147. doi:10.1371/journal.pone.0115147.

14. Longo VD, Panda S. Fasting, circadian rhythms, and time-restricted feeding in healthy lifespan. *Cell Metab.* 2016;23(6):1048–1059. doi:10.1016/j.cmet.2016.06.001.

15. Safdie FM, Dorff T, Quinn D, et al. Fasting and cancer treatment in humans: a case series report. *Aging.* 2009;1(12):988–1007. doi:10.18632/aging.100114.

16. Shukla SK, Gebregiworgis T, Purohit V, et al. Metabolic reprogramming induced by ketone bodies diminishes pancreatic cancer cachexia. *Cancer Metab.* 2014;2(1):18. doi:10.1186/2049-3002-2-18.

17. Nair KS, Welle SL, Halliday D, et al. Effect of beta-hydroxybutyrate on whole-body leucine kinetics and fractional mixed skeletal muscle protein synthesis in humans. *J Clin Invest.* 1988;82(1):198–205. doi:10.1172/JCI113570.

18. Tisdale MJ, Brennan RA, Fearon KC. Reduction of weight loss and tumour size in a cachexia model by a high fat diet. *Br J Cancer.* 1987;56(1):39–43. https://www.ncbi.nlm.nih.gov/ pmc/articles/PMC2001676.

19. Tisdale MJ, Brennan RA. A comparison of long-chain triglycerides and medium-chain triglycerides on weight loss and tumour size in a cachexia model. *Br J Cancer.* 1988;58(5):580–583. https://www.ncbi.nlm.nih.gov/pmc/articles/PMC2246820.

20. Beck SA, Tisdale MJ. Effect of insulin on weight loss and tumour growth in a cachexia model. *Br J Cancer.* 1989;59(5):677–681. https://www.ncbi.nlm.nih.gov/pmc/articles/PMC2247211.

21. Fearon K, Strasser F, Anker SD, et al. Definition and classification of cancer cachexia: an international consensus. *Lancet Oncol.* 2011;12(5):489–495. doi:10.1016/s1470-2045(10)70218-7.

22. Fearon K, Arends J, Baracos V. Understanding the mechanisms and treatment options in cancer cachexia. *Nat Rev Clin Oncol.* 2013;10(2):90–99. doi:10.1038/nrclinonc.2012.209.

23. Kim JS, Khamoui AV, Jo E, et al. β-hydroxy-β-methylbutyrate as a countermeasure for cancer cachexia: a cellular and molecular rationale. [Abstract]. *Anticancer Agents Med Chem.* 2013;13(8):1188–1196. https://www.ncbi.nlm.nih.gov/pubmed/23919746.

24. Mirza KA, Pereira SL, Voss AC, et al. Comparison of the anticatabolic effects of leucine and Ca-β-hydroxy-β-methylbutyrate in experimental models of cancer cachexia. [Abstract]. *Nutrition.* 2014;30(7–8):807–813. doi:10.1016/j.nut.2013.11.012.

25. Pedroso JAB, Nishimura LS, de Matos-Neto EM, et al. Leucine improves protein nutritional status and regulates hepatic lipid metabolism in calorie-restricted rats. *Cell Biochem Funct.* 2014;32(4):326–332. doi:10.1002/cbf.3017.

# Chapter 8: Get Started!

1. O'Connor A. How the sugar industry shifted blame to fat. *New York Times*. September 12, 2016. http://www.nytimes.com/2016/09/13/well/eat/how-the-sugar-industry-shifted-blame-to-fat.html. Accessed January 26, 2017.

2. Singerman D. The shady history of big sugar. *New York Times*. September 16, 2016. http://www.nytimes.com/2016/09/17/opinion/the-shady-history-of-big-sugar.html. Acessed January 26, 2017.

3. O'Connor A. Coke and Pepsi give millions to public health, then lobby against it. *New York Times*. October 10, 2016. http://www.nytimes.com/2016/10/10/well/eat/coke-and-pepsi-give-millions-to-public-health-then-lobby-against-it.html. Accessed January 26, 2017.

4. Daley CA, Abbott A, Doyle PS, et al. A review of fatty acid profiles and antioxidant content in grass-fed and grain-fed beef. *Nutr J*. 2010;9(1):10. doi:10.1186/1475-2891-9-10.

5. Suez J, Korem T, Zilberman-Schapira G, et al. Non-caloric artificial sweeteners and the microbiome: findings and challenges. *Gut Microbes*. 2015;6(2):149–155. doi:10.1080/19490976.2015.1017700.

6. Suez J, Korem T, Zeevi D, et al. Artificial sweeteners induce glucose intolerance by altering the gut microbiota. *Nature*. 2014;514(7521):181–186. doi:10.1038/nature13793.

7. Abhilash M, Alex M, Mathews VV, et al. Chronic effect of aspartame on ionic homeostasis and monoamine neurotransmitters in the rat brain. *Int J Toxicol*. 2014;33(4):332–341. doi:10.1177/1091581814537087.

8. Lau K, McLean WG, Williams DP, et al. Synergistic interactions between commonly used food additives in a developmental neurotoxicity test. *Toxicol Sci*. 2006;90(1):178–187. doi:10.1093/toxsci/kfj073.

9. Soffritti M, Belpoggi F, Esposti DD, et al. Aspartame induces lymphomas and leukaemias in rats. *Eur J Oncol*. 2005;10(2):107–116.

10. Soffritti M, Belpoggi F, Tibaldi E, et al. Life-span exposure to low doses of aspartame beginning during prenatal life increases cancer effects in rats. *Environ Health Perspect*. 2007;115(9):1293–1297. doi:10.1289/ehp.10271.

11. Cong W-N, Wang R, Cai H, et al. Long-term artificial sweetener acesulfame potassium treatment alters neurometabolic functions in C57BL/6J mice. *PLoS ONE*. 2013:8(8):e70257. doi:10.1371/journal.pone.0070257.

12. Soffritti M, Padovani M, Tibaldi E, et al. Sucralose administered in feed, beginning prenatally through lifespan, induces hematopoietic neoplasias in male swiss mice. *Int J Occup Environ Health*. 2016;22(1):7–17. doi:10.1080/10773525.2015.1106075.

13. Arrigoni E, Brouns F, Amadò R. Human gut microbiota does not ferment erythritol. *Br J Nutr*. 2005;94(05):643–646. https://www.ncbi.nlm.nih.gov/pubmed/16277764.

14. Robey IF, Nesbit LA. Investigating mechanisms of alkalinization for reducing primary breast tumor invasion. *BioMed Res Int*. 2013;2013:1–10. doi:10.1155/2013/485196.

15. Vitaglione P, Morisco F, Mazzone G, et al. Coffee reduces liver damage in a rat model of steatohepatitis: the underlying mechanisms and the role of polyphenols and melanoidins. *Hepatology*. 2010;52(5):1652–1661. doi:10.1002/hep.23902.

16. Lee WJ, Zhu BT. Inhibition of DNA methylation by caffeic acid and chlorogenic acid, two common catechol-containing coffee polyphenols. *Carcinogenesis*. 2006;27(2):269–277. doi:10.1093/carcin/bgi206.

## Chapter 9: Create Your Personal Plan

1. USDA. Dietary Reference Intakes: Macronutrients. (n.d.). National Agricultural Library. https://www.nal.usda.gov/sites/default/files/fnic_uploads//macronutrients.pdf. Accessed January 29, 2017.

## Chapter 11: Put Your Plan into Action

1. Seyfried TN, Mukherjee P. Targeting energy metabolism in brain cancer: review and hypothesis. *Nutr Metab.* 2005;2(1):30. doi:10.1186/1743-7075-2-30.
2. Deberardinis RJ, Chandel NS. Fundamentals of cancer metabolism. *Sci Adv.* 2016;2(5):e1600200. doi:10.1126/sciadv.1600200.
3. Diabetes.co.uk. How to test your blood glucose (sugar) levels. YouTube. https://www.youtube.com/watch?v=rMMpeLLgdgY. Published December 3, 2010. Accessed January 29, 2017.
4. Meidenbauer JJ, Mukherjee P, Seyfried TN. The glucose ketone index calculator: a simple tool to monitor therapeutic efficacy for metabolic management of brain cancer. *Nutr Metab.* 2015;12(1):12. doi:10.1186/s12986-015-0009-2.

## Chapter 12: Get to Know Your Macros

1. USDA. Welcome to the USDA Food Composition Databases. USDA Food Composition Database. https://ndb.nal.usda.gov/ndb. Accessed January 29, 2017.
2. Seyfried TN, Yu G, Maroon JC, et al. Press-pulse: a novel therapeutic strategy for the metabolic management of cancer. *Nutr Metab.* 2017;14:19. doi:10.1186/s12986-017-0178-2.
3. Li S, Zhou T, Li C, et al. High metastatic gastric and breast cancer cells consume oleic acid in an AMPK dependent manner. *PLoS ONE.* 2014;9(5):e097330. doi:10.1371/journal.pone.0097330.
4. Menendez JA, Vellon L, Colomer R, et al. Oleic acid, the main monounsaturated fatty acid of olive oil, suppresses Her-2/*neu* (*erbB*-2) expression and synergistically enhances the growth inhibitory effects of trastuzumab (Herceptin™) in breast cancer cells with Her-2/*neu* oncogene amplification. *Ann Oncol.* 2005;16(3):359–371. doi:10.1093/annonc/mdi090.
5. Weil A. Is chicory good for you? Weil Lifestyle. http://www.drweil.com/diet-nutrition/food-safety/is-chicory-good-for-you. Published December 14, 2016. Accessed January 29, 2017. http://www.drweil.com/diet-nutrition/food-safety/is-chicory-good-for-you.

## Chapter 14: Nutritional Supplements

1. NIH. Vitamin D. Office of Dietary Supplements. https://ods.od.nih.gov/factsheets/VitaminD-HealthProfessional. Accessed January 30, 2017. https://ods.od.nih.gov/factsheets/VitaminD-HealthProfessional.
2. Civitelli R, Villareal DT, Agnusdei D, et al. Dietary L-lysine and calcium metabolism in humans. *Nutrition.* 1992;8(6):400–405. https://www.ncbi.nlm.nih.gov/pubmed/1486246.
3. Poff AM, Ari C, Arnold P, et al. Ketone supplementation decreases tumor cell viability and prolongs survival of mice with metastatic cancer. *Int J Cancer.* 2014;135(7):1711–1720. doi:10.1002/ijc.28809.

4. Meidenbauer JJ, Mukherjee P, Seyfried TN. The glucose ketone index calculator: a simple tool to monitor therapeutic efficacy for metabolic management of brain cancer. *Nutr Metab.* 2015;12(1):12. doi:10.1186/s12986-015-0009-2.

5. Murray AJ, Knight NS, Cole MA, et al. Novel ketone diet enhances physical and cognitive performance. *FASEB J.* 2016;30(12):4021–4032. doi:10.1096/fj.201600773R.

6. Kirste S, Treier M, Wehrle SJ, et al. *Boswellia serrata* acts on cerebral edema in patients irradiated for brain tumors. *Cancer.* 2011;117(16):3788–3795. doi:10.1002/cncr.25945.

7. Flavin DF. A lipoxygenase inhibitor in breast cancer brain metastases. *J Neuro-Oncol.* 2007;82(1):91–93. doi:10.1007/s11060-006-9248-4.

8. Sanchez-Barcelo EJ, Mediavilla MD, Alonso-Gonzalez C, et al. Melatonin uses in oncology: breast cancer prevention and reduction of the side effects of chemotherapy and radiation. *Expert Opin Investig Drugs.* 2012;21(6):819–831. doi:10.1517/13543784.2012.681045.

9. Ferreira GM, Martinez M, Camargo ICC, et al. Melatonin attenuates Her-2, p38 MAPK, p-AKT, and mTOR levels in ovarian carcinoma of ethanol-preferring rats. *J Cancer.* 2014;5(9):728–735. doi:10.7150/jca.10196.

10. Lissoni P, Barni S, Ardizzoia A, et al. Randomized study with the pineal hormone melatonin versus supportive care alone in advanced non-small cell lung cancer resistant to a first-line chemotherapy containing cisplatin. *Oncology.* 1992;49(5):336–339. doi:10.1159/000227068.

11. Johnson JR, Burnell-Nugent M, Lossignol D, et al. Multicenter, double-blind, randomized, placebo-controlled, parallel-group study of the efficacy, safety, and tolerability of THC:CBD extract and THC extract in patients with intractable cancer-related pain. *J Pain Symptom Manage.* 2010;39(2):167–179. doi:10.1016/j.jpainsymman.2009.06.008.

12. Kesari S. Dexanabinol in patients with brain cancer. ClinicalTrials.gov. https://clinicaltrials.gov/ct2/show/NCT01654497?term=cannabinoids%2BAND%2Bcancer&cntry1=NA%3AUS&rank=9. Published July 16, 2012. Updated December 19, 2016. Accessed January 30, 2017.

13. NIH. Botanical dietary supplements: background information. Office of Dietary Supplements. https://ods.od.nih.gov/factsheets/BotanicalBackground-HealthProfessional. Updated June 24, 2011. Accessed January 30, 2017.

14. Search about Herbs. Memorial Sloan Kettering Cancer Center. https://www.mskcc.org/cancer-care/treatments/symptom-management/integrative-medicine/herbs/search?keys=Cromoglicic%2Bacid&letter=. Accessed January 30, 2017.

15. Vitamins & Supplements Center. WebMD. http://www.webmd.com/vitamins-supplements/default.aspx. Accessed January 30, 2017.

16. Cancer and acid-base balance. American Institute for Cancer Research. http://preventcancer.aicr.org/site/News2?id=13441. Published May 2008. Accessed January 30, 2017.

17. Whitson JM, Cooperberg MR, Stackhouse GB, et al. Urinary citrate levels do not correlate with urinary pH in patients with urinary stone formation. *Urology.* 2007;70(4):634–637. doi:10.1016/j.urology.2007.04.052.

18. Robey IF, Baggett BK, Kirkpatrick ND, et al. Bicarbonate increases tumor pH and inhibits spontaneous metastases. *Cancer Res.* 2009;69(6):2260–2268. doi:10.1158/0008-5472.can-07-5575.

19. Robey IF, Nesbit LA. Investigating mechanisms of alkalinization for reducing primary breast tumor invasion. *BioMed Res Int.* 2013;2013:1–10. doi:10.1155/2013/485196.

20. Finley JW, Kong A, Hintze KJ, et al. Antioxidants in foods: state of the science important to the food industry. *J Agric Food Chem*. 2011;59(13):6837–6846. doi: 10.1021/jf2013875.

## Chapter 15: Other Health Challenges and Keto

1. Mayo Clinic Staff. Constipation. Mayo Clinic. http://www.mayoclinic.org/diseases -conditions/constipation/basics/risk-factors/con-20032773. Published October 19, 2016. Accessed February 12, 2017.

2. Mercola. For best toilet health: squat or sit? Mercola.com. http://articles.mercola.com /sites/articles/archive/2012/12/03/toilet-squatting-position.aspx. Published December 3, 2012. Accessed February 12, 2017.

3. Abbott R, Ayres I, Hui E, et al. Effect of perineal self-acupressure on constipation: a randomized controlled trial. *J Gen Intern Med*. 2015;30(4):434–439. doi:10.1007 /s11606-014-3084-6.

4. Niv G, Grinberg T, Dickman R, et al. Perforation and mortality after cleansing enema for acute constipation are not rare but are preventable. *Int J Gen Med*, 2013;6:323–328. doi:10.2147/ijgm.s44417.

5. About Lab Tests Online. Lab Tests Online. https://labtestsonline.org. Accessed February 12, 2017.

6. Medicines that can cause pancreatitis—topic overview. Web MD. http://www.webmd .com/digestive-disorders/tc/medicines-that-can-cause-pancreatitis-topic-overview. Accessed February 12, 2017.

7. Onitilo AA, Kio E, Doi SAR. Tumor-related hyponatremia. *Clin Med Res*. 2007;5(4):228– 237. doi:10.3121/cmr.2007.762.

8. Gallstone disease. Johns Hopkins Medicine. http://www.hopkinsmedicine.org /gastroenterology_hepatology/_pdfs/pancreas_biliary_tract/gallstone_disease.pdf. Published 2013. Accessed February 12, 2017.

9. NIH. Gallstones. National Institute of Diabetes and Digestive and Kidney Diseases. https://www.niddk.nih.gov/health-information/digestive-diseases/gallstones. Published November 2013. Accessed February 12, 2017.

10. Youm Y-H, Nguyen KY, Grant RW, et al. The ketone metabolite β-hydroxybutyrate blocks NLRP3 inflammasome–mediated inflammatory disease. *Nat Med*. 2015;21:263– 269. doi:10.1038/nm.3804.

11. Goldberg EL, Asher JL, Molony RD, et al. "β-Hydroxybutyrate deactivates neutrophil NLRP3 inflammasome to relieve gout flares." *Cell Reports* 18, no. 9 (2017): 2077–087. doi:10.1016/j.celrep.2017.02.004.

12. Feinman RD, Pogozelski WK, Astrup A, et al. Dietary carbohydrate restriction as the first approach in diabetes management: critical review and evidence base. *Nutrition*. 2015;31(1):1–13. doi:10.1016/j.nut.2014.06.011.13.

13. Poplawski MM, Mastaitis JW, Isoda F, et al. Reversal of diabetic nephropathy by a ketogenic diet. *PLoS ONE*. 2011;6(4):e18604. doi:10.1371/journal.pone.0018604.

14. Mavropoulos JC, Yancy WS, Hepburn J, et al. The effects of a low-carbohydrate, ketogenic diet on the polycystic ovary syndrome: a pilot study. *Nutr Metab*. 2005;2:35. doi:10.1186/1743-7075-2-35.

15. Volek JS, Feinman RD. Carbohydrate restriction improves the features of Metabolic Syndrome. Metabolic Syndrome may be defined by the response to carbohydrate restriction. *Nutr Metab*. 2005;2:31. doi:10.1186/1743-7075-2-31.

16. Lheureux PE, Hantson P. Carnitine in the treatment of valproic acid-induced toxicity. *Clin Toxicol*. 2009;47(2):101–111. doi:10.1080/15563650902752376.

17. Cross Reactive Food. American Latex Allergy Association. http://latexallergyresources .org/cross-reactive-food. Accessed February 12, 2017.

## Chapter 16: Evaluate Your "Response to Treatment"

1. Volek JS, Freidenreich DJ, Saenz C, et al. Metabolic characteristics of keto-adapted ultra-endurance runners. *Metabolism*. 2016;65(3):100–110. doi:10.1016/j.metabol.2015.10.028.

2. Donga E, Dijk MV, Dijk JG, et al. A single night of partial sleep deprivation induces insulin resistance in multiple metabolic pathways in healthy subjects. *Endocrinology*. 2010;151(5):2399. doi:10.1210/endo.151.5.9998.

3. Irwin M, Mascovich A, Gillin JC, et al. Partial sleep deprivation reduces natural killer cell activity in humans. *Psychosomatic Medicine*. 1994;56(6):493–498. doi:10.1097/00006842 -199411000-00004.

4. Meidenbauer JJ, Mukherjee P, Seyfried TN. The glucose ketone index calculator: a simple tool to monitor therapeutic efficacy for metabolic management of brain cancer. *Nutr Metab*. 2015;12(1):12. doi:10.1186/s12986-015-0009-2.

5. Gong Z, Aragaki AK, Chlebowski RT, et al. Diabetes, metformin and incidence of and death from invasive cancer in postmenopausal women: results from the women's health initiative. *Int J Cancer*. 2016;138(8):1915–1927. doi:10.1002/ijc.29944.

6. Poff AM, Ari C, Arnold P, et al. Ketone supplementation decreases tumor cell viability and prolongs survival of mice with metastatic cancer. *Int J Cancer*. 2014;135(7):1711–1720. doi:10.1002/ijc.28809.

## Chapter 17: Your Anticancer Life

1. Kiecolt-Glaser JK, Bennett JM, Andridge R, et al. Yoga's impact on inflammation, mood, and fatigue in breast cancer survivors: a randomized controlled trial. *J Clin Oncol*. 2014;32(10):1040–1049. doi:10.1200/jco.2013.51.8860.

2. Zupec-Kania B. *Modified Ketogenic Diet Therapy*. The Charlie Foundation for Ketogenic Diet Therapies; 2013.

# Index

Note: Page numbers in italics refer to photographs and figures; page numbers followed by *t* refer to tables.

vitamin B family, 240–41, 244
vitamin C
    antioxidant supplement concerns during
      cancer treatment, 265
    intravenous therapy precautions for
      supplements, 110
    overview, 241, 243
vitamin D, 242, 244, 279, 301
vitamin E, 243, 265
vitamin K₂, 243, 244
vitamins
    choosing supplements, 240–44
    overview, 239–240
    *See also specific vitamins*
Volek, Jeff
    keto-adaptation research, 52
    ketone supplement research, 297
    low carbohydrate living books, 73, 139,
      148, 300, 336
    magnesium supplement choice, 248
    metabolic adaptation research, 296
    nutritional ketosis definition, 255
vomiting, suggestions for, 318, 329

Wahls, Terry, 84, 283, 336
Wahls Paleo Plus plan, 84, 283, 336
*The Wahls Protocol* (Wahls), 283, 336
Walsh, Raffi Kalamian, *v*
    breath practice, 314
    diagnosis, ix
    diet ratio calculations, 147
    gift of life, 323–24
    gingerbread house, 47
    gratitude practice, 312
    gum-chewing, 138
    imaging study errors, 307
    ketogenic diet for, xi, 79, 122, 317
    progression of illness, xii–xvi
    soccer injury, 300
    switch to new oncologist, 56–57
Warburg, Otto, xiii, 3, 4, 5
Warburg effect, xiv, 3–5, 32
war on cancer, xxii, 1
wasting. *See* cachexia

water
    alkalizers and ionizers, 266–67
    importance of, 143, 215–16
water-only fasts, 91, 163
weakness
    potential causes of, 282
    as side effect of diet, 182
WebMD, 263
websites and blogs, 342
weighing foods, 160, 173, 212
weight. *See* body weight
weight loss
    cachexia vs., 103–5
    with carbohydrate restriction, 63
    from chemotherapy and radiation, 97–98
    concerns of healthcare providers, 72
    concerns with ketogenic diet, 51
    considerations in personalizing the diet,
      156–160
    low-carb diet vs. ketogenic diet, 145
    rate of, 158–59
    troubleshooting, 327
Weinberg, Robert, 2–3
wellness, defining, 54–55
Westman, Eric, 148, 278, 336
*Wheat Belly* (Davis), 117
whey, insulin release from, 131
whipped cream canisters, 174
Wilder, Russell, 61
Wilford, Justin, 48
Winters, Nasha, 77, 130, 263, 335
Women's Health Initiative, 308
Woodyatt, Rollin, 61

XCT oil, 101
    *See also* MCT oils
xylitol, 138, 139

"yeah, but" thinking, 44, 45
yoga, benefits of, 312
Yong, Ed, 259

zinc supplements, 249
Zupec-Kania, Beth, 146–47, 287, 337

# About the Author

**Miriam Kalamian** is a nutrition consultant, educator, and author specializing in the implementation of ketogenic therapies. She earned her master of education (EdM) from Smith College and her master of human nutrition (MS) from Eastern Michigan University. She is board certified in nutrition (CNS) by the Board for Certification of Nutrition Specialists.

Inspired by the work of Thomas N. Seyfried, PhD, Miriam draws on a decade of experience to provide comprehensive guidelines that specifically address the many diet and lifestyle challenges associated with a cancer diagnosis.

Miriam is a leading voice in the keto movement. Her passion for helping others implement this diet comes directly from her personal experience. Her son Raffi was diagnosed with a brain tumor in December 2004. Standard of care therapies failed to stop the relentless progression of his disease, and it became painfully clear that she needed to switch gears quickly. That is what originally led her to Dr. Thomas Seyfried's research supporting the use of the ketogenic diet for cancer.

Beyond cancer, Miriam integrates nutritional strategies with metabolic therapies and lifestyle modifications to develop personalized treatments that address a broad spectrum of conditions that are currently considered intractable, including age-related, neurodegenerative, and bariatric diseases.

Miriam lives with her husband in Montana.

## About the Foreword Author

**Thomas N. Seyfried** received his PhD in genetics and biochemistry from the University of Illinois at Urbana-Champaign in 1976. He was a postdoctoral fellow in the Department of Neurology at the Yale School of Medicine, and then served on the faculty as an assistant professor in neurology. Awards and honors have come from such diverse organizations as the American Oil Chemists' Society, National Institutes of Health, American Society for Neurochemistry, and the Ketogenic Diet Special Interest Group of the American Epilepsy Society. Dr. Seyfried previously served as chair on the Scientific Advisory Committee for the National Tay-Sachs and Allied Diseases Association and presently serves on several editorial boards, including those for *Nutrition & Metabolism, Neurochemical Research, The Journal of Lipid Research*, and *ASN Neuro*. He is the author of *Cancer as a Metabolic Disease: On the Origin, Management, and Prevention of Cancer* (Wiley Press, 2012). Dr. Seyfried's research focuses on gene–environment interactions related to complex diseases, such as epilepsy, autism, brain cancer, and neurodegenerative (the GM1 and GM2 gangliosidoses) diseases.